MASS TRAUMA AND VIOLENCE

SOCIAL WORK PRACTICE WITH CHILDREN AND FAMILIES

Nancy Boyd Webb, *Series Editor*

Mass Trauma and Violence: Helping Families and Children Cope
Nancy Boyd Webb, *Editor*

Culturally Competent Practice with Immigrant and Refugee Children and Families
Rowena Fong, *Editor*

Social Work Practice with Children, Second Edition
Nancy Boyd Webb

Complex Adoption and Assisted Reproductive Technology: A Developmental Approach to Clinical Practice
Vivian B. Shapiro, Janet R. Shapiro, and Isabel H. Paret

Child Development: A Practitioner's Guide
Douglas Davies

Group Work with Adolescents: Principles and Practice
Andrew Malekoff

MASS TRAUMA AND VIOLENCE

Helping Families and Children Cope

Edited by
Nancy Boyd Webb

Foreword by Victor M. Fornari

THE GUILFORD PRESS
New York   London

© 2004 The Guilford Press
A Division of Guilford Publications, Inc.
72 Spring Street, New York, NY 10012
www.guilford.com

Printed in the United States of America

This book is printed on acid-free paper.

Last digit is print number: 9 8 7 6 5 4 3 2 1

Library of Congress Cataloging-in-Publication Data

Mass trauma and violence : helping families and children cope / edited by Nancy
Boyd Webb.
    p. cm.–(Social work practice with children and families)
Includes bibliographical references and index.
  ISBN 1-57230-976-8 (hardcover : alk. paper)
  1. Posttraumatic stress disorder. 2. Posttraumatic stress disorder in children.
3. Victims of violence–Treatment. 4. Victims of terrorism–Treatment.
5. Disasters–Psychological aspects. I. Webb, Nancy Boyd, 1932– II. Series.
  RC552.P67M363 2004
  616.85′21–dc22

                                                              2003022300

To the families and friends of those who died
as a result of acts of terrorism:
The memory of your loved ones
will always be in our hearts.

About the Editor

Nancy Boyd Webb, DSW, BCD, RPT-S, is a leading authority on play therapy with children who have experienced loss and traumatic bereavement. Her bestselling books, which are considered essential references for clinical courses and agencies that work with children, include *Helping Bereaved Children, Second Edition: A Handbook for Practitioners* (Guilford Press), *Play Therapy with Children in Crisis, Second Edition: Individual, Group, and Family Treatment* (Guilford Press), *Culturally Diverse Parent–Child and Family Relationships* (Columbia University Press), and *Social Work Practice with Children, Second Edition* (Guilford Press). In addition, she has published widely in professional journals and produced a video, *Techniques of Play Therapy: A Clinical Demonstration*, which won a bronze medal at the New York Film Festival's International Non-Broadcast Media Competition. Dr. Webb is the editor of The Guilford Press book series Social Work Practice with Children and Families. She is a board member of the New York Association for Play Therapy and on the editorial advisory board for the journal *Trauma and Loss: Research Interventions*.

A board-certified diplomate in clinical social work and a registered play therapy supervisor, Dr. Webb presents frequently at play therapy, social work, and bereavement conferences in the United States and abroad. She has been a professor on the faculty of the Fordham University School of Social Service since 1979, and in October 1997 was named University Distinguished Professor of Social Work. In 1985, she founded Fordham's Post-Master's Certificate Program in Child and Adolescent Therapy to meet the need in the New York metropolitan area for training in play therapy. In April 2000, Dr. Webb appeared as a panelist in a satellite teleconference *Living with Grief: Children, Adolescents, and Loss*, sponsored by the Hospice Foundation of America. Hosted by Cokie Roberts, the conference was beamed to more than 2,100 sites. Dr. Webb was appointed to the endowed James R. Dumpson Chair in Child Welfare Studies at Fordham in 2002, and the same year was honored as Social Work Educator of the Year by the New York State Social Work Education Association.

In addition to teaching, writing, and consulting, Dr. Webb maintains a clinical practice and supervises and consults with schools and agencies. She lectures and conducts workshops throughout the United States, Canada, Australia, Europe, Hong Kong, and Taiwan on play therapy, trauma, and bereavement.

Contributors

Charlotte Burrough, MSW, The Kids' Place, Edmond, Oklahoma

Lois Carey, MSW, BCD, RPT-S, private practice, Upper Grandview, New York

Teddy Chen, MSSW, PhD, Charles B. Wang Community Health Center, New York, New York

Stephen Coulter, MSW, MSocSc, Family Trauma Centre, Belfast, Northern Ireland, United Kingdom

Maddy Cunningham, DSW, Graduate School of Social Service, Fordham University, New York, New York

Lin Fang, MSW, CSW, Charles B. Wang Community Health Center, New York, New York

Robin F. Goodman, PhD, ATR-BC, Department of Psychiatry, New York University School of Medicine, New York, New York

Thomas Hardaway, MD, Departments of Behavioral Medicine and Psychiatry, Brooke Army Medical Center, San Antonio, Texas

Beth Hartley, LCSW, The Den for Grieving Kids, Family Centers, Inc., Greenwich, Connecticut

Haya Itzhaky, PhD, School of Social Work, Bar-Ilan University, Ramat Gan, Israel

David Koch, PhD, Graduate School of Social Service, Fordham University, New York, New York

Joanne V. Loewy, DA, Louis and Lucille Armstrong Music Therapy Program, Department of Social Work and Home Care Services, Beth Israel Medical Center, New York, New York

Idalia Mapp, PhD, Graduate School of Social Service, Fordham University, Tarrytown, New York

Matt McDermott, MA, MSocSc, MSW, CQSW, CPT-P, Department of Child and Family Psychiatry, Mater Misericordiae Hospital, Dublin, Republic of Ireland

Danny Mize, MA, MRE, The Kids' Place, Edmond, Oklahoma

Kathleen Nader, DSW, Two Suns, Cedar Park, Texas

Isobel Reilly, BSS, DipSW, MSocSc, Family Trauma Centre and School of Social Work, Queens University, Belfast, Northern Ireland, United Kingdom

Kristen Stewart, MA, MT-BC, Louis and Lucille Armstrong Music Therapy Program, Department of Social Work and Home Care Services, Beth Israel Medical Center, New York, New York

Nancy Boyd Webb, DSW, BCD, RPT-S, Graduate School of Social Service, Fordham University, Tarrytown, New York

Mary Beth Williams, PhD, LCSW, CTS, Trauma Recovery Education and Counseling Center, Warrenton, Virginia

Tova Yedidia, PhD, School of Social Work, Bar-Ilan University, Ramat Gan, Israel

Foreword

Stressful life events and loss are both unpredictable and a normal part of life. Severe trauma and violent occurrences are prevalent throughout the world and profoundly affect people of all ages. This important text reminds us that grief can be considered the cost of commitment (Parkes, 1972) and that when death occurs as secondary to traumatic events, the grief process becomes complicated. Traumatic occurrences demonstrate the fragility of human life and the enormous medical, financial, and emotional needs of victims and their families.

This book presents the aftermath of mass trauma and violence in different parts of the world and the different therapeutic helping interventions that practitioners have created to help the children, youth, and families who were affected by these chaotic events. When large groups of people experience trauma together, helping efforts often occur in settings such as schools or other community settings where the possible stigma of receiving mental health services is reduced. However, some individuals do not admit their need for help and they cope instead by minimizing or denying the significance of the traumatic event on them. Even in New York, Pennsylvania, and Washington, DC, following the events of September 11, 2001, some people tended to play down their own responses. Determined to view themselves as strong and not easily influenced by tragedy, these people put on a mask of resolve to carry on with their lives as if nothing had happened.

My belief is that everyone is affected by such events, and I wish to emphasize the inevitable influence of mass trauma on everyone, whether or not he or she is physically injured or loses a loved one. I will illustrate this point through the following case example:

Laura is a young woman who consulted me for the first time 2 months after 9/11. In obtaining Laura's history, I learned that she had grown up on Long Island and is now enrolled in college there. However, when I asked her about how the events of 9/11 had affected her, she said,

"Not at all." Further questioning revealed that her father was a New York City firefighter whose best friend had relieved him from work that day so that her parents could celebrate their 25th anniversary. Laura stated that after her father witnessed the first plane hit the tower, he decided to spend the remainder of the day in the city working. He learned later that his friend had died. He actually lost a number of colleagues. Laura is aware that her father's behavior has subsequently changed; he is drinking more and having trouble sleeping. However, Laura continued to state that the changes in her father had not affected her at all. She described the family's belief that this is "No big deal!"

Traumatic events affect all of us in some way. Sometimes the way we protect ourselves is by denying the ways in which we are affected. Even people who are very influenced by a trauma may not be aware of just how powerful the consequences are. They may genuinely believe that they weren't affected and that they are fine. One self-protective mechanism is to believe that bad things happen to others and not to us. So, 9/11 and other bad events can happen to other people, but "I am fine," we insist.

Helping traumatized and bereaved victims of mass trauma navigate the complex journey to adaptation with dignity, optimism, and inner peace is no small task. *Mass Trauma and Violence* is destined to become a sought-after guide in an area where road maps are lacking. Nancy Boyd Webb is a courageous pioneer who provides us with a valuable reference on how to respond, from a public health perspective, to what has become our *new reality*.

VICTOR M. FORNARI, MD
*North Shore University Hospital
and New York University School of Medicine*

REFERENCE

Parkes, C. M. (1972). *Bereavement: Studies of grief in adult life.* New York: International Universities Press.

Preface

This book developed as a direct outgrowth of the September 11, 2001, terrorist attacks on New York and Washington, after which mental health practitioners and professional organizations struggled to put together guidelines to help parents, teachers, and agencies deal with large-scale destruction and numerous traumatic deaths. There had never been acts of terrorism of this scope in the United States before, and the entire country experienced various degrees of disbelief, fear, panic, anger, and sadness associated with the terrible events of that day. Since then, the country has experienced ongoing stress from anthrax attacks, snipers, and a full-scale war—all mass traumas that create anxiety, fear, and grief in children and families.

The professional literature is sparse on topics related to helping children following terrorism and other mass trauma situations. There are more books about children and disasters than about children and traumatic stress and terrorism. However, the stress induced by single-incident events, such as natural disasters (caused by "acts of God") and technological disasters (caused by accidents), are quite different from the traumatic stress caused by deliberate actions that can be repeated. The circumstances of war and terrorism create an ongoing climate of fear of recurrence among survivors who become acutely aware of their own increased vulnerability.

This book highlights the impact of traumatic stress on children and families and presents a framework for helping based on the literature on stress and coping, trauma, bereavement, attachment, and risk and resilience. Contributors present detailed clinical examples to demonstrate methods that have been found helpful in allaying children's anxieties, including:

- Short-term school-based debriefing soon after the crisis events
- Bereavement groups for children who suffered losses of family members, relatives, friends, and neighbors
- Individual play therapy for children whose intense and ongoing responses continue to disrupt their lives
- Psychoeducational approaches for teachers, parents, and communities
- Cognitive-behavioral methods

The book illustrates the use of a range of creative methods such as art, story, music, and sandtray in individual and group therapy and in family treatment. In recognition that other countries have been coping with the ongoing stresses of terrorism for decades, the book includes a section on living with traumatic memories and continuous fears, with chapters about the situations in Israel and in Northern Ireland. A chapter on the special circumstances of children in military families conveys the multiple pressures and anxieties for children whose parents are deployed to dangerous assignments or war. The book also addresses distinctive cultural responses to terrorism and resistance to accepting mental health services, as demonstrated in work with Chinese immigrant families in New York following the events of 9/11.

The conceptual framework for the book is developmental–transactional theory within the context of stress, coping, traumatic bereavement, attachment, and risk and resiliency. Assessment of the impact of any traumatic event must include an appreciation of the multiple factors that influence the meaning of any crisis for an individual. The introductory section of the book presents both an overview of terrorism and its impact as well as the theoretical basis for helping victims and a synopsis of different helping methods.

Our nation continues to be "on alert" about possible future terrorist attacks in retaliation for the United States' initiative in Iraq. This constitutes a relatively new area for mental health practitioners, who may be unfamiliar with methods to help children and families cope in a climate of ongoing national stress.

In addition, the incidence of posttraumatic stress disorder (PTSD) in schoolchildren in grades 4–12 in New York City is reported as 10.5% since 9/11 (Goodnough, 2002). The need for treatment and monitoring of children showing traumatic stress responses (PTSD, depression, and anxiety) is evident and will continue. The professional community will watch and learn from New York's and Washington's experiences, in the same way that wise practitioners welcome information about helping approaches that have proved effective in other countries. A quote from Maya Angelou's comments at the inauguration of President Clinton on

January 20, 1993, aptly offers a hopeful philosophy for confronting trauma:

> History, despite its wrenching pain, cannot be unlived, but, if faced with courage, need not be lived again.

The contributors to this volume demonstrate methods for helping traumatized children and families harness their courage and move on with their lives.

REFERENCES

Angelou, M. (1993). *On the pulse of morning.* New York: Random House.

Goodnough, A. (2002, May 2). Post-9/11 pain found to linger in young minds. *New York Times*, p. A1.

Acknowledgments

Nothing can quite match the excitement of completing an edited book in which a group of 21 mental health professionals from different areas of the United States and the world have collaborated to express and share their combined wisdom for the benefit of readers they will never see, who will adapt the clinical methods presented here to assist traumatized children and adults. I am always impressed by the generosity of practitioner-scholars whose writings contribute to the knowledge base of the profession, even as their work assists those in direct practice who are eager and grateful to learn new helping approaches.

I am also pleased that I was able to convince my publisher that this book was needed, and that it would fill a gap in the literature about helping people following mass trauma situations. Whereas some people initially believed that the impact of September 11, 2001, would fade and that a book focused primarily on the events of 9/11 would soon become dated, I knew that there was a dearth of literature about mass trauma, and I doubted that we had seen the last of terrorism (although I inwardly hoped to be proven wrong!).

Clearly, the situation of living in the shadow of possible trauma creates an undercurrent of anxiety that leads to feelings of vulnerability. The authors from Israel and from Northern Ireland (Chapters 13 and 14) have presented the special challenges associated with living in an atmosphere of danger, as does the author who discusses children in military families (Chapter 12). Thankfully, at this writing, the United States has not experienced other large-scale terrorist attacks since 9/11, but the country has gone to war, and the terror alert has not been removed.

This book was written over the course of a year—due in part to the authors' willingness to meet deadlines, and in part to the diligence of my assistants at Fordham's Graduate School of Social Service, who efficiently tackled various assignments (from conducting library and Internet searches, to creating tables, to contacting authors about necessary contract information). I wish to acknowledge and thank the following individuals, in alphabetical order: Beth Carroll, Alison Hamonds, Marla Mendillo, and Nivea Pelicier. I also appreciate the professionalism of the staff members of The Guilford Press, who provided expert copyediting, excellent promotion and publicity, and consistent assistance with the myriad tasks related to publishing a book.

My husband, Kempton, once again endured my long hours at the computer and the necessary transport of books and other materials to our different residences in Vermont and Florida, where I do most of my writing. He believes in the importance of my work, and provides support in every possible way.

As we move into the new century, we face new challenges. Educators and practitioners must prepare themselves, their students, and fellow staff members to provide clinical services in climates of uncertainty and fear. This book was written in the hope that this goal can be achieved—that people can learn to live well despite anxiety, to survive traumatic events, and to carry on productively with their lives.

Contents

MASS TRAUMA AND VIOLENCE

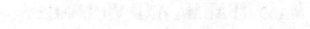

PART I

Theoretical Framework for Assessment and Treatment

CHAPTER 1

The Impact of Traumatic Stress and Loss on Children and Families

NANCY BOYD WEBB

Experiences of stress and loss occur inevitably and unpredictably over the normal course of human life, from infancy to old age. Even the birth process itself requires both the mother and the infant to endure physical and emotional strain and pain. And this is just the beginning, since both mother and baby must adjust and cope with the infant's inherent helplessness and dependency. No one can survive in this world alone, and the proximity-seeking behavior of young children, based on their biologically based survival instinct, results in the formation of protective attachment relationships (Bowlby, 1969, 1973, 1980). Attachment (whether to parents or to other caretakers) is universal across cultures (Bowlby, 1969; LeVine & Miller, 1990). It serves the four functions of (1) providing a sense of security, (2) regulating affect and arousal, (3) promoting the expression of feelings and communication, and (4) serving as a base for exploration (Davies, 1999). When an attachment relationship is disrupted by separation or death, the child's development may be compromised, depending on various circumstances (as will be discussed in this and the next chapter). Thus attachment can be a source of both positive and sad feelings. Parkes (1972) has referred to grief as the cost of commitment. When a death occurs in *traumatic* circumstances, the grief process becomes more complicated and more difficult to resolve. This is the topic of this book.

The book was conceived in the months following the terrorist attacks of September 11, 2001—when thousands of children and adults in New York City, in Washington, D.C., and elsewhere experienced the traumatic deaths of loved ones at the World Trade Center, at the Pentagon, and aboard Flight 93 in rural Pennsylvania. This sudden confrontation with large-scale, intentional violence literally pulled the rug out from under the U.S. national persona of invulnerability, as a total of over 3,000 individuals were eventually declared dead or "missing and presumed dead." Thousands of these individuals' family members and friends mourned their personal losses; in addition, all Americans suffered a sense of loss of safety regarding the future. Mental health professionals struggled to help, using makeshift guidelines about how to assist grieving communities in a tragedy of unprecedented magnitude. All U.S. residents, and indeed all residents of Western countries, felt degrees of anxiety, grief, and fear.

This book focuses on the concept of "mass trauma"—that is, on the impact of traumatic events that occur to many people at the same time. As a foundation for the presentation of various helping interventions later in the book, this introductory section provides a theoretical framework for assessment and treatment. The present chapter focuses on the impact of mass trauma that is deliberately precipitated, as in terrorism and war. These circumstances engender specific responses, such as group outpourings of disbelief and outrage—in addition to anxiety and traumatic grief responses, which often are experienced by victims of any mass trauma. Chapter 2 focuses on the assessment of individuals who have experienced a trauma, including the typical trajectories of responses over time; Chapter 3 provides an overview of child and adolescent treatment issues. The current chapter deals with the specific circumstances of the trauma itself and how these may contribute to particular responses, such as a search for causality and meaning, and the desire for revenge. Other components of the traumatic event that may influence reactions are also considered, such as whether it qualifies as Type I or Type II (Terr, 1991) and whether it occurs in conjunction with other and/or ongoing traumas. The concepts of "traumatic grief," "complicated grief," "stress," "traumatic stress," and "coping" are presented as these pertain to situations of mass trauma.

MASS TRAUMA

Definition

The term "mass trauma" refers to trauma that occurs as a result of a frightening, potentially life-threatening event that is experienced by a large number of people simultaneously. According to Criterion A for posttraumatic stress disorder (PTSD) in the most recent revision of the

Diagnostic and Statistical Manual of Mental Disorders (DSM-IV-TR), the trauma-inducing event is characterized by one or both of the following:

(1) the person experienced, witnessed, or was confronted with an event or events that involved actual or threatened death, or serious injury, or a threat to the physical integrity of self or others

(2) the person's response involved intense fear, helplessness, or horror. **Note:** In children, this may be expressed instead by disorganized or agitated behavior

(American Psychiatric Association, 2000, p. 467)

Again, to qualify as a "mass" trauma, the event must affect numerous people. Examples of situations that can result in trauma to masses of people include the following:

- Natural disasters (earthquakes, fires, hurricanes, floods, tornadoes, mudslides, dam collapses)
- Transportation disasters (plane, train, bus, ship/ferryboat, accidents)
- Technology-related disasters (industrial/chemical/nuclear accidents/explosions)
- Spacecraft disasters
- Shootings, kidnappings, hostage, internment situations
- War and civil/political/community violence
- Terrorism

An extensive literature exists related to interventions following natural, transportation, and technology-related disasters, thereby providing guidance for helping families and communities when terrible events occur as a result of "acts of God" or human mistakes (Barnard & Morland, 1999; Chemtob, Tomas, Law, & Cremniter, 1997; Fornari, 1999; Gordon, Farberow, & Maida, 1999; La Greca, Silverman, Vernberg, & Roberts, 2002; Saylor, 1993; Wilson & Raphael, 1993; Zakour, 1996; Zinner & Williams, 1999). Less is known about the special challenges of helping when mass trauma occurs as a result of acts deliberately caused by one person or group. This book focuses on the aftermath of situations in which humans have created or intentionally precipitated a mass trauma. As will be discussed more fully below, the range of responses among people in the community often includes intense reactions of rage and confusion, combined with a loss of belief in the essential goodness of humankind. These reactions, combined with other responses to acute stress and loss, present special challenges for treatment.

Distinctive Factors in Various Mass Trauma Situations

Although clinicians tend to view trauma primarily from the perspective of the suffering individual, it is possible to refer to traumatized families (Figley, 1988), schools (Stevenson, 2002), communities (Zinner & Williams, 1999), and nations (Apfel & Simon, 1996). Unlike the private experience of a teen who is traumatized in a rape or mugging, mass traumas—which, by definition, are shared—offer the possibility of comparing stories and receiving support from others who experienced the same or similar frightening events. Although responses to trauma ultimately occur on an individual basis, the reactions of others can be influential nonetheless. And, as noted by many researchers, children are particularly sensitive to the emotional climate around them; they may exhibit calm or panic, depending on the reactions of the behavior of influential adults, such as parents and teachers (Arroyo & Eth, 1996; McFarlane, 1987).

The particular circumstances of different traumatic situations vary, as do the nature of affected persons' responses. In Chapter 2, I present my full tripartite conceptualization of the interactive components of mass trauma, which include (1) the nature of the traumatic event, (2) factors affecting individual responses, and (3) factors in the support system. This chapter focuses on the first group of factors (the nature of the traumatic event). Many components of any mass trauma situation can be evaluated to determine the nature of its potential impact, as depicted in Table 1.1.

TABLE 1.1. Components of Mass Trauma Events

Single versus recurring traumatic event:
  Type I (acute) or Type II (chronic or ongoing) trauma

Proximity to the traumatic event:
  On site, on the periphery, or through the media

Extent of exposure to violence/injury/pain:
  Witnessed and/or experienced

Nature of losses/deaths/destruction:
  Personal, community, and/or symbolic loss
  Danger, loss, and/or responsibility traumas
  Loved one "missing"/no physical evidence
  Death determined by retrieval of body or fragment
  Loss of status/employment/family income
  Loss of a predictable future

Attribution of causality:
  Random/"act of God" or deliberate/human-made

Note. Some of these concepts have been discussed in earlier volumes on children in various kinds of crises (e.g., Webb, 1991, 1999, 2002). Here they pertain particularly to mass trauma events.

Single versus Recurring Traumatic Event: Type I (Acute)
or Type II (Chronic or Ongoing) Trauma

Terr (1991) first presented the concepts of "Type I" and "Type II" trauma. Type I trauma occurs following *one* sudden shock, such as a rape; by contrast, Type II trauma is "precipitated by a *series* of external blows" (p. 19, emphasis added), such as ongoing incest. Although the present book does not focus on traumatic abuse events occurring to an individual, I believe that the concepts of Type I (acute) and Type II (chronic or ongoing) trauma also apply to situations of mass trauma, which may occur as either a single event (e.g., the shootings at Columbine High School in 1999) or as ongoing traumatic events (e.g., war and repeated terrorist bombings). Terr (1991) emphasized that Type I traumas follow from *unanticipated* single events, whereas in Type II events the individual lives with a sense of fear, dread, and rage related to the expectation of repetition of the trauma. Both types of trauma generate extreme fright and responses that, if untreated, can lead to serious disorders in both childhood and adulthood. Furthermore, because of the unpredictable likelihood of repeated traumas throughout life, persons who survive a Type I trauma remain vulnerable to subsequent traumas and may react powerfully when these occur, even when there is no ostensible connection between the traumatic events.

Proximity to the Traumatic Event: On-Site, on the Periphery,
or through the Media

Research by Pynoos and Nader (1989) documented that children who were closer to a shooting on a playground showed more symptoms of PTSD than children who were on the periphery or not on the playground when the attack occurred. The severest responses, including fear of a recurrence, occurred in children who were closest to the shooting; this was true both soon after the event and 14 months later (Pynoos & Nader, 1989). These findings, which seem intuitively valid, confirm the importance of proximity to a traumatic event as potentially significant in the subsequent development of symptoms. Therefore, Chemtob et al. (1997) asserted that preventive interventions (e.g., debriefing) should be offered to people closest to the scene of a trauma, such as the 1993 World Trade Center bombing.

   However, proximity can be viewed as emotional, as well as geographic. For example, many employees who worked in the World Trade Center at the times of both the 1993 and 2001 events lived some distance from the site (even out of state) and commuted to work by car or public transportation. Their families certainly qualified as being in high-risk "proximity," even though they lived on the periphery. Other people also living far away may have been profoundly affected through the detailed and repeated media coverage that literally brought the traumatic events into the living rooms of the observers. This could qualify as "vicarious traumatization" (McCann & Pearlman, 1990), since it consisted of the secondary exposure to traumatic events through verbal and visual depictions of scenes of horror. Most research on the effects of television programs on behavior focuses on the interrelationship between watching violent scenes and children's aggressive behavior (Murray, 1997; Joy, Kimball, & Zabrack, 1986; Williams, 1986). However, the viewing of violence in entertainment programs is quite different from watching graphic news reports that depict *actual* traumatic events. The distinction between cartoon-enacted violence and a real-life scene of firefighters digging in debris for dead bodies may be quite apparent even to young children. A preliminary study of PTSD and grief among the children of Kuwait following the 1990–1991 Gulf War found that viewing media images of real violence was associated with increased symptoms (Nader, Pynoos, Fairbanks, Al-Ajeel, & As-Asfour, 1993). More research is needed to understand the complex factors determining who develops symptoms of PTSD and who does not following media exposure to mass trauma events.

Extent of Exposure to Violence/Injury/Pain: Witnessed and/or Experienced

As noted above, we live in a violent world in which children and their parents may watch fictional murders and other crimes in movies or television shows, or actual violent events on television news. Nonetheless, watching a violent episode in the safety of one's living room is very different from, say, witnessing actual drug-related murders on street corners in one's own neighborhood. Pynoos and Eth (1985, p. 19) believe that "children who [personally] witness extreme acts of violence represent a population at significant risk of developing anxiety, depressive, phobic, conduct, and posttraumatic stress disorders." The child witness who, in addition to *observing* violence, also suffers personal injury may develop numerous posttraumatic symptoms, in addition to losing trust in adults as protectors and developing diminished, demoralized ideas about people, life, and the future (Terr, 1991).

Nature of Losses/Deaths/Destruction

Posttraumatic loss takes many forms. From one perspective, it can involve the death of a family member, the mass destruction of a community, and/or the symbolic loss of a sense of security about the future and of the ability to trust other people. Indeed, situations of mass trauma are particularly likely to involve personal, community, and symbolic loss all at once.

Another way of looking at the nature of losses and deaths following many different types of traumatic events has been proposed by Weisaeth and Eitinger (1993). These authors suggest that the significance of such events can be viewed in terms of the following three categories of traumas:

1. "Danger traumas" (caused by threats to one's own life).
2. "Loss traumas" (such as deaths of beloved persons, sometimes witnessed by the survivors).
3. "Responsibility traumas" (attacks on the psychological self, resulting in reduced belief in one's ability to deal effectively with danger).

These categories often overlap, but nonetheless are helpful in considering the general nature of expected responses. Specifically, these would include reactions of anxiety and fear following danger traumas, grief and mourning following loss traumas, and guilt related to responsibility traumas.

A further variable influencing the nature of losses, deaths, and destruction following a traumatic event in general and a mass trauma in particular is the extent to which the remains of those who perished in the event are recoverable. A fact needing to be faced by many families and friends at first, and by some on a long-term basis or forever, is that no physical evidence at all may be obtainable. Other survivors will have to live with the reality that the death of their loved ones has been established only through the retrieval of isolated body parts or even a single fragment. In either case, the psychological effects can be serious (see the case of Bobby, presented later in this chapter).

A factor often compounding the misery of those who survive a traumatic event (either one they have experienced themselves or one in which they have lost a family member) is that personal status, employment, and/or family income are jeopardized as well. If an individual's own injuries are too serious to permit a return to work at his or her previous level (or at all), if their workplace is destroyed, or if a family's principal breadwinner is killed, both the financial and the psychological effects of this can be devastating. Moreover, as many families discovered after the events of "9/11," it can take months or even years for various benefits to be approved and allocated when the circumstances of an event are highly unusual.

Finally, the loss of a predictable future can be among the most profound losses following a situation of mass trauma. This factor is discussed more fully below in connection with the attribution of causality.

Attribution of Causality: Random/"Acts of God" or Deliberate/Human-Made

With some exceptions, children's morality leans toward the polarities of good–bad and right–wrong; they do not show much flexibility in their moral judgments until the early teen years (Kohlberg, 1981; Piaget, 1932/ 1965). These rigid beliefs contribute to strong impulses to identify and punish wrongdoers and to seek revenge on persons who have caused deaths and destruction. Of course, adults as well as children may exhibit wishes for revenge. When numerous deaths have occurred as a result of deliberate actions, all people struggle to answer the question "Why?" For example, a child asked (in regard to the 9/11 attacks), "Why did they do it, when we taught them to fly?" For adults, their internal conflicts often included questioning on a deeper scale: "How could they use their religious beliefs to justify these mass killings?" Reiker and Carmen (1986, p. 362) point out that "confrontations with violence challenge one's most basic assumptions about the self as invulnerable and intrinsically worthy and about the world as orderly and just." In all the terrorist attacks of 9/11, the assumptions of American citizens that their country was invulnerable and worthy were challenged by a group of people who totally disapprove of the U.S. way of life. In addition to disbelief about the reason for this attack, some people may have felt underlying feelings of dismay that a small group of men could cause such extensive destruction to two of the largest and most powerful cities in the world. van der Kolk (1996, p. 15) states that "trauma is usually accompanied by intense feelings of humiliation . . . [related to the] capacity to be able to count on [protect] oneself." In this case, Americans learned that their country was neither invincible nor omniscient, and this attribution of meaning based on the facts of the situation led many people to a loss of faith.

This discussion of causality in connection with the 9/11 attacks on the United States illustrates mass trauma situations when a *deliberate* human act or acts produced the traumatic event. Similar dynamics and attributions of meaning would apply to situations involving shootings, mass kidnappings, hostage takings, internments, war, and civil/political/community violence. Once again, all of these situations involve deliberate actions by an individual or group intended to intimidate, control, or otherwise do harm to another group of people. These forms of mass trauma are very different from those traumatic events in which death and destruction occurs because of forces of nature or because of accidents. Although natural disasters, and disasters connected to transportation or technology, can also cause massive injuries and pain (including acute losses and deaths), the damage in these circumstances is unintentional, inadvertent, and essentially fortuitous, without the complicating factor of the attribution of evil purposes. All forms of trauma can cause survivors to conclude that the world is not and may never be the same because of what happened, but this conclusion can be particularly compelling after a deliberately inflicted trauma. For some, it leads to a profound sense of alienation that, without treatment, can persist and negatively affect the individuals' future recovery (Shalev & Ursano, 2003).

TRAUMATIC GRIEF

Trauma

The word "trauma" comes from the Greek, meaning "wound." In Terr's (1990) landmark book about the kidnapping of 29 children on a school bus in Chowchilla, California, she defines trauma as occurring "when a sudden, unexpected, overwhelmingly intense blow or series of blows assaults the person from the outside" (p. 8). Other writers have emphasized the stress involved with memories of the experience that shatter the person's sense of invulnerability to harm (Figley, 1985; van der Kolk, 1996). The personal meaning of the traumatic experience evolves over time, according to van der Kolk (1996), and may include feelings of irretrievable loss, anger, betrayal, and helplessness. Thus it is evident that loss is always part of trauma, whether in the symbolic form of a loss of a sense of safety and security or in the form of a specific loss, such as that of a familiar neighborhood or one's home.

Grief and Mourning

The terms "grief" and "mourning" apply to "the sequence of subjective states that follow loss" (Bowlby, 1960, p. 11). The simplest definition of grief is that it is a reaction to loss (Corr, Nabe, & Corr, 2000). Usually grief and mourning refer to responses after a *death*, but there is growing acceptance that other types of losses can result in emotional reactions similar to those associated with death. For example, a loss of employment that brings with it a change of status, reduced income, and separation from a familiar work environment and former colleagues can precipitate feelings of anger, sorrow, and despair, culminating in a depressed state similar to that of a bereaved person.

The Distinction between "Grief" and "Traumatic Grief"

According to Jacobs (1999), "traumatic grief" creates responses of intrusive, distressing preoccupation with the deceased person in the form of yearning, longing, and searching. Although these emotions are typical in all mourning situations, one difference in traumatic grief is in the intensity and duration of these responses, which can appear to dominate the bereaved person's life. When these strong separation reactions are teamed with revenge fantasies, the individual (whether child, adolescent, or adult) may become preoccupied, have difficulty concentrating in school or work, and demonstrate other behavioral problems as well.

Another distinctive aspect of traumatic grief is that when a loss occurs in a *traumatic* situation, the usual grief responses of yearning are mixed with frightening memories of the traumatic event. Thus the feelings of sadness and longing for the person who died combine with anxiety and fear associated with the trauma, and actually may disrupt or derail the usual grief process (Eth & Pynoos, 1985; Nader, 1997). Nader notes that the intrusiveness and intensity of traumatic memories can interfere with the normal bereavement process of remembering the dead person. The horror of the traumatic event blocks recall of pretrauma memories about the person. Therefore, traumatic grief requires special treatment involving cognitive and emotional reprocessing of the traumatic memories in order to permit mourning to proceed. Further discussion and examples of treatment of traumatic grief appear in Chapters 4, 7, 8, 9, 10, 13, and 14.

The Case of Bobby, Age 7[1]

Background

Bobby, age 7, was a second grader who lived in the New York City suburbs, about 30 miles from the World Trade Center. He was absent from school for 2 days after 9/11, and when he returned he told his teacher that his father was in one of the buildings that was hit by an airplane. After calling Bobby's home to verify this, the teacher announced to the class that she had some sad news. She then said that Bobby's father was missing because of the World Trade Center attack. She suggested that the children should be "extra nice" to Bobby, because he now didn't have a father at home. Tim raised his hand and said that he would "loan" Bobby his own father, "until they find all the pieces and put him back together again." Bobby looked devastated, and the teacher said that although Tim was trying to be helpful, nobody else could take the place of your *own* father.

That afternoon when he went home from school, Bobby asked his mother if his father's body was in pieces. His mother, horrified and unsure what to say, said that she didn't know for sure and that they still were trying to find the people who were "lost." She also told Bobby that the next day they would go into the city to give some "samples" to help the rescuers find his daddy. When they went to the center that had been set

---

[1]This is a composite case, with elements drawn from cases in clinical practice and from the literature.

up for family members, Bobby's mother took his father's toothbrush and gave it to a nurse there, who also took a swab from Bobby's cheek. Bobby asked the nurse whether this would help bring his father back.

About a month later, while Bobby was in school, the medical examiner's office telephoned his mother and told her that a part of her husband's body had been found. It was his finger, which still had his college class ring on it, and which had been positively identified through DNA tests. The caller wanted to know whether Bobby's mother wanted the examiner's office to keep the finger or whether she wanted to claim it; he explained that if she took it, she would need to sign a statement about whether or not she wanted to be notified if additional body parts were identified in the future. Bobby's mother, who had been bracing herself for a call of this nature, said that she wanted to have a memorial service; that the finger had convinced her that her husband was really dead; and that she would not need to claim any future evidence. The service was held the following weekend and was attended by family, friends, and many of Bobby's classmates.

Development of Symptoms

Soon after the service Bobby began to have bad dreams; he would wake up crying and run to his mother's bed. The mother was also beginning to have great difficulty sleeping, because she missed her husband terribly and was very preoccupied about whether or not he had suffered. In addition, she was worried about finances and the responsibilities of raising Bobby and his older sister alone. At night, Bobby and his mother would cry together. Bobby began to resist going to school; he said he had stomachaches in the morning, and would beg to stay home. Though he did not tell his mother this, he was afraid that the other children knew that his father was "in parts," and this embarrassed and bothered him. He also worried about his mother, and didn't know what to say to her when she cried.

Assessment

Many of Bobby's reactions would be considered within the range of normal grief responses after a situation of sudden traumatic death. The boy's sleep disturbance, and his desire to cling to his surviving parent following the other parent's death, are typical reactions following parental death; such reactions usually subside in time. His school avoidance, however, was more problematic, and could have led to additional problems if not treated in a timely manner. Bobby's mother and the school personnel did not know his reason for wanting to stay home, and might have attributed it to his understandable concern about his mother's seemingly fragile mental state.

Comment and Suggested Intervention

In this particular situation, both the mother and Bobby were inhibited in their mourning by the thought of the father's/husband's dismemberment. This was a horrible reality to deal with, and both would have benefited from help in expressing their feelings about the *traumatic* aspects of this death, before they would be able to recall other memories. My own suggestion would be to help the mother and child, in separate sessions, describe what they thought actually happened to the father's/husband's body, permitting whatever feelings of horror and fear each might be imagining in their internal views of his "death scene." Bobby could be asked to draw a picture of what he thought his father's body looked like after he died. They each needed to express whatever feelings they had in connection with the death, and to mourn and cry about it. These separate sessions would be followed immediately by a joint session in which both mother and child would be encouraged to draw a picture of the way they *wished* to remember their father/husband, and to reminisce about these positive memories. They also would be urged to look at family photographs together, to assist them in replacing their traumatic images with positive recollections.

MULTIPLE AND ONGOING TRAUMAS: COMPLICATED GRIEF

Persons who have past experience with trauma, and persons who are living in dangerous situations in which trauma is likely to recur, may be more likely to develop PTSD after exposure to a new trauma (Academic Highlights, 2001). However, early distressing experiences do not *always* create a sensitivity to later trauma, since past experiences of mastery can sometimes "help steel the child (or adult) against later traumatization from stressful circumstances" (Fletcher, 1996, p. 263). Individuals' strengths (resilience) and weaknesses (vulnerabilities) vary greatly and lead to particular responses in particular situations. Some authors suggest that the meaning that people give to their experiences affects the way they cope; that is, coping style derives from a personal assessment of "how much one is harmed, threatened, and challenged by an experience" (McFarlane & Yehuda, 1996, p. 175). For example, Anne Frank's statement to the effect that, after all, she still believed in the goodness of people illustrates a teenager's ability to retain a positive view of the world (her personal meaning), despite the very dangerous circumstances in which she was hiding with her family (Frank, 1952/1993). Similarly, John F. Kennedy was able to keep his stressful, traumatic memories related to his war experiences from interfering with his later work functioning (as reported in the Grant study, cited by McFarlane & Yehuda, 1996). We must conclude that traumatic experiences may or may not result in disabling traumatic grief. As Arroyo and Eth (1996, p. 54) state, "It is impossible to predict exactly who will develop psychic trauma." My tripartite assessment of the interactive components of the assessment of children and family's responses to traumatic stress and loss (see Chapter 2) identifies factors intrinsic to the individual person, to the traumatic event, and to the recovery environment that can influence and mediate specific responses.

"Complicated grief" refers to situations involving multiple losses and sudden, traumatic death (Goldman, 1996). Typical responses involve denying, repressing, and avoiding aspects of the loss, while at the same time holding on to memories of the lost loved one (Rando, 1993). Common sense suggests that repeated experiences of loss and death will require an increased ability to cope with the associated pain and anguish. Some psychological responses that may be employed include avoidance (including dissociation), which serves to protect the individual from recalling details of what happened, and hypervigilance, which keeps the person alert for possible additional traumatic events. Obviously, a child living in a war zone must pay attention to sounds and signs of imminent attack, but in order to concentrate on his or her homework and be able to fall asleep at night, the child may need to deliberately push away thoughts about the dangerous situation.

The Case of Mary, Age 7[2]

Background

Mary, a 7-year-old girl, was one of the children who were trapped in the elevator with her kindergarten class during a class trip to the World Trade Center at the time of the February 1993 bombing. During this crisis, the children were stuck in the dark elevator for several hours with their teacher and several adult chaperones, who engaged them in singing songs and reciting the rosary while they waited to be rescued. It was only after their rescue that news about the bombing became known. When the children returned to school the following Monday, a crisis team was in the classroom to engage the children in posttraumatic play related to the bombing. The team checked in again later that week, but school personnel tended to discount the impact of the experience on the children, and the class soon resumed its usual activities. Some parents later reported that their children continued to experience sleep disruptions, and that some were afraid to go on elevators.

A little more than 2 years after the 1993 World Trade Center bombing, Mary happened to be in Oklahoma City in April 1995, visiting rela-

---

[2]This example was reported in *The New York Times*; see Martin (1997). See also Webb (1999).

tives. She arrived 1 day before the attack on the Murrah Federal Building that killed 168 people, including 19 children. After this attack, Mary became convinced that she had somehow caused both bombings, according to her mother. Two years later, when a reporter spoke with Mary's mother, she said that the girl (then 9 years old) would become very upset and cry if anyone referred to any kind of bombing.

Comment

This child clearly needed counseling following the first bombing to help her understand how it happened, and also to deal with her anxiety about a possible recurrence of a similar trauma. Even if reassurance about future safety had been emphasized, Mary's reactions following the second bombing can be understood in terms of developmental considerations (see Chapter 2): Because of their immature reasoning powers, young children can come to believe that they cause bad things to happen. Whereas *anyone*, child or adult, might react intensely in circumstances like this of a repeated trauma, we would need more information about Mary's precrisis adjustment and about her family in order to understand why she continued to experience traumatic symptoms and was not able to put her past traumas behind her.

STRESS AND TRAUMATIC STRESS

Stress

A certain amount of stress is part of life and can even add an element of excitement to otherwise routine activities. However, when events become too exciting/stressful, a person can become overstimulated and uncomfortable. As I wrote in *Play Therapy with Children in Crisis* (Webb, 1999, p. 3),

> Although stress in itself is not harmful (Selye, 1978), it may precipitate a crisis if the anxiety accompanying it exceeds the individual's ability to adapt. . . . People have different levels of stress tolerance as well as different modes of responding to stress. The formation of psychological defenses and symptoms typically occurs as a result of attempts to "fight" the anxiety or flee from it (the "fight or flight" responses; Selye, 1978). Young children are particularly vulnerable to stress because of their youth, immature defenses, and lack of life experience. They often require assistance to obtain relief from their anxiety and to learn new coping methods.

This view of stress is based on a principle of balance or homeostasis. That is, stress is seen as a physical or emotional response that taxes an individual's personal resources; if it exceeds these, it can endanger his or her well-being (Lazarus & Folkman, 1984; Resick, 2001). Another view of stress, called the "conservation-of-resources" theory (Hobfoll, 1989), proposes that psychological stress is a reaction to actual or threatened losses of a person's resources. These resources include four categories of assets, according to Resick (2001, p. 58, citing Hobfoll): "objects (car, belongings), conditions (good marriage, seniority), personal characteristics (self-esteem, skills), and energies (knowledge, money, time). Stress responses occur when these resources are threatened or lost."

Traumatic Stress

Although traumatic events are not everyday occurrences, many people do experience at least one or more traumatic events in their lifetime, according to Resick (2001). A review of the literature on the prevalence of trauma found that in different studies, between 21% and 39% of adults reported having experienced at least one traumatic event, such as criminal victimization (rape, assaults, robberies, homicides), natural disasters, war, or technological accidents.

According to several population surveys (Kessler, Sonnega, Bromet, Hughes, & Nelson, 1995; Norris, 1992; Stein, Walker, Hazen, & Forde, 1997) the likelihood of experiencing a natural disaster is about 8–11% in a lifetime, whereas other hazards were found to have forced evacuations from home for about 15% of the population. Clearly, a substantial number of people do experience traumatic events of various types over the normal course of their lives, and these may make them more vulnerable in future mass trauma situations.

Whether one subscribes to the homeostatic or the conservation-of-resources model of stress, it is evident that traumatic events in general and situations of mass trauma in particular certainly create extreme stress for the individuals involved. For example, war creates profound traumatic stress for multitudes of people. Resick (2001) comments that because of the massive social upheaval caused by war, it is impossible to estimate its traumatic effects with any precision. However, we know that the range of people traumatized by war includes combat soldiers, their families, citizens of warring countries, and other parts of the international community (which often become involved in some phase of the conflict or peace efforts). The Red Cross estimated that as of 1993, 40 million persons had been killed in wars since World War II, and millions of refugees had had to leave their countries and seek asylum (International Federation of Red Cross and Red Crescent Societies, 1996). Chapters 12, 13, and 14 discuss some of the critical challenges in helping people who are experiencing traumatic stress, traumatic grief, and ongoing anxiety due to war-related circumstances.

Coping

"Coping," or the manner in which an individual deals with stress, is discussed at greater length in Chapter 2 as a factor affecting individual responses to mass trauma. As noted in that chapter, coping styles may involve either approach to or avoidance of a stressor; coping efforts may be either effective or ineffective; and different types of coping responses may be appropriate at different phases of a traumatic event and its aftermath. However, it is worth noting here that properly applied coping efforts can be very effective even in helping people deal with such massive stressors as those created by war. The examples of Anne Frank and John F. Kennedy have been mentioned earlier in this chapter; the case vignette that follows gives another example.

The Case of Zlata, Age 11[3]

Background

Zlata, an 11-year-old girl, was living with her parents in Sarajevo (then a city in Yugoloslavia, now the capital of Bosnia and Herzegovina) and keeping a diary when war broke out in April 1992. She described the war's impact on herself and her family through her diary until the family finally escaped to Paris in December 1993. Over the course of this year and a half, Zlata experienced daily shelling, noise, destruction, and killings. The deaths included that of her best friend in the park across the street from her house. Her school was closed for long periods of time; she was not allowed to go out and play because it was too dangerous; the windows of her home were shattered; and her family spent many nights in their own or a neighbor's cellar because they were afraid that their home might be bombed.

Coping

Zlata dealt with this constant danger and stress in several ways that helped her. The diary, especially, helped her get some "distance" from what she was witnessing through recording the events. She admitted at times that her stomach was in knots, and that she had trouble concentrating on reading and schoolwork. She also admitted that she got angry and wanted to scream; she asked (in her personal search for meaning) what she had done to "deserve" being in a war.

However, Zlata took pleasure in feeding and playing with her cat, in planning birthday celebrations for relatives, and in trying to keep up with various family members and friends throughout the city. She also referred

---

[3]This is summarized from Filipovic (1994).

to some conscious methods for dealing with her anxiety, such as putting her fingers in her ears to keep out the sounds of shooting and shellings.

Like Anne Frank, Zlata tried through her diary to find meaning in what she was experiencing. Although she said at one point that she didn't like to write about the war because it made her remember it, the diary helped her get through and process her thoughts and feelings. It would be interesting to know how she is coping now as a young woman in her 20s, and whether and to what extent her wartime memories remain a part of her current life.

CONCLUDING COMMENTS

Traumatic events, by definition, make a terrifying impact on those who experience them. Some traumas are so intense that their force continues to reverberate through time and place, making it impossible for people to escape their horrible memories. Nonetheless, it is the *meaning* of the event, not the trauma itself, that gives it power—and the attribution of meaning is very personal and unique. This explains why a group of people (e.g., soldiers in the Vietnam War) can experience the same traumatic event and some will suffer PTSD over the course of their lifetime, while others manage to put the experience in the recesses of their memories and to direct their thoughts and energies toward living in the present.

Proneness to the development of PTSD may increase, depending on the following factors (Weisaeth & Eitinger, 1993, p. 74):

- High-risk *situations* (particularly severe trauma)
- High-risk *persons* (vulnerability in exposed persons)
- High-risk *reactions* (early responses that predict later illness)

This chapter has discussed the nature of the traumatic event (the situation) as contributing to different stress responses, including traumatic and complicated grief. Chapter 2 focuses on the assessment of factors pertaining to the individual; it also considers the role of possible mediating factors in the culture, the family, and other aspects of the environment.

REFERENCES

Academic Highlights. (2001). Trauma and stress. Diagnosis and treatment. *Journal of Clinical Psychiatry, 62*(11), 906–915.

American Psychiatric Association. (2000). *Diagnostic and statistical manual of mental disorders* (4th ed., text rev.). Washington, DC: Author.

Apfel, R. J., & Simon, B. (Eds.). (1996). *Minefields in their hearts: The mental health of children in war and communal violence.* New Haven, CT: Yale University Press.

Arroyo, W., & Eth, S. (1996). Post-traumatic stress disorder and other stress reactions. In R. J. Apfel & B. Simon (Eds.), *Minefields in their hearts. The mental health of children in war and communal violence* (pp. 52–74). New Haven, CT: Yale University Press.

Barnard, P., & Morland, I. (1999). When children are involved in disasters. In P. Barnard, I. Morland, & J. Nagy (Eds.), *Children, bereavement, and trauma: Nurturing resilience* (pp. 21–30). London: Jessica Kingsley.

Bowlby, J. (1960). Grief and mourning in infancy. *Psychoanalytic Study of the Child, 15*, 3–39.

Bowlby, J. (1969). *Attachment and loss: Vol. 1. Attachment.* London: Hogarth Press.

Bowlby, J. (1973). *Attachment and loss: Vol. 2. Separation: Anxiety and anger.* London: Hogarth Press.

Bowlby, J. (1980). *Attachment and loss: Vol. 3. Loss.* London: Hogarth Press.

Chemtob, C. M., Tomas, S., Law, W., & Cremniter, D. (1997). Post disaster psychosocial intervention: A field study of the impact of debriefing on psychological distress. *American Journal of Psychiatry, 154*(3), 415–417.

Corr, C. A., Nabe, C. M., & Corr, D. M. (2000). *Death and dying, life and living* (3rd ed.). Belmont, CA: Wadsworth.

Davies, D. (1999). *Child development: A practitioner's guide.* New York: Guilford Press.

Eth, S., & Pynoos, R. (1985). Interaction of trauma and grief in childhood. In S. Eth & R. Pynoos (Eds.), *Post-traumatic stress disorder in children* (pp. 169–186). Washington, DC: American Psychiatric Press.

Figley, C. R. (Ed.). (1985). *Trauma and its wake: Vol. 1. The study and treatment of post-traumatic stress disorder.* New York: Brunner/Mazel.

Figley, C. R. (1988). Post-traumatic family therapy. In F. M. Ochberg (Ed.), *Post-traumatic therapy and victims of violence* (pp. 83–109). New York: Brunner/Mazel.

Filipovic, Z. (1994). *Zlata's diary: A child's life in Sarajevo.* New York: Penguin.

Fletcher, K. E. (1996). Childhood posttraumatic stress disorder. In E. J. Mash, & R. A. Barkley (Eds.), *Child psychopathology* (pp. 242–276). New York: Guilford Press.

Fornari, V. (1999). The aftermath of a plane crash—helping a survivor cope with deaths of mother and sibling: Case of Mary, age 8, and follow-up at age 17. In N. B. Webb (Ed.), *Play therapy with children in crisis* (2nd ed): *Individual, group, and family treatment* (pp. 407–429). New York: Guilford Press.

Frank, A. (1993). *The diary of a young girl.* New York: Bantam. (Original work published 1952)

Goldman, L. (1996). *Breaking the silence: A guide to help children with complicated grief.* Washington, DC: Accelerated Development.

Gordon, N. S., Farberow, N. L., & Maida, C. A. (1999). *Children and disasters.* New York: Brunner/Mazel.

Hobfoll, S. (1989). Conservation of resources: A new attempt at conceptualizing stress. *American Psychologist, 44*, 513–524.

International Federation of Red Cross and Red Crescent Societies. (1996). *World disasters report, 1996.* Oxford: Oxford University Press.

Jacobs, S. C. (1999). *Traumatic grief: Diagnosis, treatment, and prevention.* New York: Brunner/Mazel.

Joy, L. A., Kimball, M., & Zabrack, M. L. (1986). Television exposure and children's aggressive behavior. In T. M. Williams (Ed.), *The impact of television: A natural experiment in three communities* (pp. 303–360). Orlando, FL: Academic Press.

Kessler, R., Sonnega, A., Bromet, E., Hughes, M., & Nelson, C. (1995). Posttraumatic stress disorder in the National Comorbidity Survey. *Archives of General Psychiatry, 52,* 1048–1060.

Kohlberg, L. (1981). *Philosophy of moral development.* New York: Harper & Row.

La Greca, A. M., Silverman, W. K., Vernberg, E. M., & Roberts, M. C. (Eds.). (2002). *Helping children cope with disasters and terrorism.* Washington, DC: American Psychological Association.

Lazarus, R. S., & Folkman, S. (1984). *Stress, appraisal, and coping.* New York: Springer.

LeVine, R. A., & Miller, P. M. (1990). Commentary. *Human Development, 33,* 73–80.

Martin, D. (1997, November 16). Bomb attack's terrifying hold. *The New York Times,* p. 43.

McCann, L. I., & Pearlman, L. (1990). Vicarious traumatization: A framework for understanding the psychological effects of working with victims. *Journal of Traumatic Stress, 3*(1), 131–149.

McFarlane, A. C. (1987). Family functioning and overprotection following a natural disaster: The longitudinal effects of post-traumatic morbidity. *Australian and New Zealand Journal of Psychiatry, 21,* 210–218.

McFarlane, A. C., & Yehuda, R. (1996). Resilience, vulnerability and the course of posttraumatic reactions. In B. A. van der Kolk, A. C. McFarlane, & L. Weisaeth (Eds.), *Traumatic stress: The effects of overwhelming experience on mind, body, and society* (pp. 155–181). New York: Guilford Press.

Murray, J. P. (1997). Media violence and youth. In J. Osofsky (Ed.), *Children in a violent society* (pp. 72–96). New York: Guilford Press.

Nader, K. O. (1997). Childhood traumatic loss: The interaction of trauma and grief. In C. R. Figley, B. E. Bride, & N. Mazza (Eds.), *Death and trauma: The traumatology of grieving* (pp. 17–41). Washington, DC: Taylor & Francis.

Nader, K., Pynoos, R., Fairbanks, L., Al-Ajeel, M., & Al-Asfour, A. (1993). A preliminary study of PTSD and the children of Kuwait following the Gulf crisis. *British Journal of Clinical Psychology, 32,* 407–416.

Norris, J. (1992). Epidemiology of trauma: Frequency and impact of different potentially traumatic events on different demographic groups. *Journal of Consulting and Clinical Psychology, 60,* 409–418.

Parkes, C. M. (1972). *Bereavement: Studies of grief in adult life.* New York: International Universities Press.

Piaget, J. (1965). *The moral judgment of the child.* New York: Free Press. (Original work published 1932)

Pynoos, R. S., & Eth, S. (1985). Children traumatized by witnessing acts of personal violence: Homicide, rape, or suicide behavior. In S. Eth & R. S. Pynoos (Eds.), *Post-traumatic stress disorder in children* (pp. 19–43). Washington, DC: American Psychiatric Press.

Pynoos, R. S., & Nader, K. (1989). Children's memory and proximity to violence. *Journal of the American Academy of Child and Adolescent Psychiatry, 28,* 236–241.

Rando, T. (1993). *Treatment of complicated mourning.* Champaign, IL: Research Press.

Reiker, P. P., & Carmen, E. H. (1986). The victim-to-patient process: The disconfirmation and transformation of abuse. *American Journal of Orthopsychiatry, 56,* 360–370.

Resick, P. A. (2001). *Stress and trauma.* Philadelphia: Psychology Press.

Saylor, C. F. (1993). *Children and disasters.* New York: Plenum Press.

Selye, H. (1978). *The stress of life* (rev. ed.). New York: McGraw-Hill.

Shalev, A. Y., & Ursano, R. J. (2003). Mapping the multidimensional picture of acute responses to stress. In R. Orner & U. Schnyder (Eds.), *Reconstructing early interventions after trauma: Innovations in the care of survivors* (pp. 118–129). New York: Oxford University Press.

Stein, M., Walker, J., Hazen, A., & Forde, D. (1997). Full and partial posttraumatic stress disorder: Findings from a community survey. *American Journal of Psychiatry, 154,* 1114–1119.

Stevenson, R. G. (2002). Sudden death in schools. In N. B. Webb (Ed.), *Helping bereaved children: A handbook for practitioners* (2nd ed., pp. 194–213). New York: Guilford Press.

Terr, L. C. (1990). *Too scared to cry: Psychic trauma in childhood.* New York: Harper & Row.

Terr, L. C. (1991). Childhood traumas: An outline and overview. *American Journal of Psychiatry, 148*(1), 10–20.

van der Kolk, B. A. (1996). The black hole of trauma. In B. A. van der Kolk, A. C. McFarlane, & L. Weisaeth (Eds.), *Traumatic stress. The effects of overwhelming experience on mind, body, and society* (pp. 3–23). New York: Guilford Press.

Webb, N. B. (Ed.). (1991). *Play therapy with children in crisis.* New York: Guilford Press.

Webb, N. B. (Ed.). (1999). *Play therapy with children in crisis* (2nd ed.): *Individual, group, and family treatment.* New York: Guilford Press.

Webb, N. B. (Ed.). (2002). *Helping bereaved children: A handbook for practitioners* (2nd ed.). New York: Guilford Press.

Weisaeth, L., & Eitinger, L. (1993). Posttraumatic stress phenomena: Common themes across wars, disasters, and traumatic events. In J. P. Wilson & B. Raphael (Eds.), *International handbook of traumatic stress syndromes* (pp. 69–77). New York: Plenum Press.

Williams, T. M. (Ed.). (1986). *The impact of television: A natural experiment in three communities.* Orlando, FL: Academic Press.

Wilson, J. P., & Raphael, B. (1993). (Eds.). *International handbook of traumatic stress syndromes.* New York: Plenum Press.

Zakour, M. J. (1996). Disaster research in social work. In C. L. Streeter & S. A. Murty (Eds.), *Research on social work and disasters* (pp. 7–25). New York: Haworth Press.

Zinner, E. S., & Williams, M. B. (Eds.). (1999). *When a community weeps: Case studies in group survivorship.* Philadelphia: Brunner/Mazel.

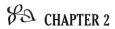

CHAPTER 2

A Developmental–Transactional Framework for Assessment of Children and Families Following a Mass Trauma

NANCY BOYD WEBB

Traumatic events have different effects on the people exposed to them. Just as everyone has distinctive fingerprints, everyone's history and personality are unique, and these determine what meanings we attach to traumatic events. These attributions, in turn, activate a wide range of responses to these events—terror and horror for some people, anger and sadness for others. Because so many different factors blend together to create one's personal meaning associated with a traumatic event, it is impossible to predict any person's specific reactions (Arroyo & Eth, 1996). However, we do know that a number of factors can influence an individual's responses, such as his or her past experiences with trauma and loss, age, general level of adjustment, coping style, and qualities of resilience. These individual factors interact with particular elements of the traumatic event, and with the type of support and cultural factors in the family and community, to produce different personal responses.

For over 10 years now, I have been developing different versions of a tripartite assessment model to illustrate the interactive components of bereavement and other life crises (Webb, 1991, 1993, 1996, 1999, 2002, 2003). This chapter presents the adaptation of my tripartite model for as-

23

sessment of an individual child or family member following a mass trauma.

APPLYING THE TRIPARTITE ASSESSMENT MODEL TO THE CHILD'S AND FAMILY'S RESPONSES IN SITUATIONS OF MASS TRAUMA

Whereas it may seem foolhardy to try to make sense of the confusing jumble of factors contributing to different responses to a traumatic event, numerous theorists, including myself, have attempted to do so (Arroyo & Eth, 1996; Shalev, 1996; McFarlane & Yehuda, 1996; Fletcher, 1996; Silverman & La Greca, 2002). Table 2.1 specifies factors reported by other authors that resonate with my own tripartite assessment model.

As noted in Chapter 1, my model of assessment specifies three different sets of variables (hence the term "tripartite") as determining an individual's specific responses to a mass trauma situation: (1) factors related to the nature of the traumatic event, (2) factors affecting individual responses, and (3) factors in the support system.

Figure 2.1 depicts the specific components in each category. These components, especially those in the second and third categories, are discussed in detail below.

TABLE 2.1. Factors Contributing to Different Responses to a Traumatic Event

Author (Year)	Contributing factors	Category[a]
Arroyo & Eth (1996)	Anxiety of parents (may encourage children's clinging)	S
Fletcher (1996)	Developmental factors: Coping style	I
	Degree of distress caused by traumatic event	E
	Social characteristics	S
	Nature of response to past stress	I
McFarlane & Yehuda (1996)	Vulnerability and resilience factors	I
	Personal meaning of trauma	I
Shalev (1996)	Magnitude of the stressor	E
	Pretrauma vulnerability	I
	Preparation for a stressful event	S
Silverman & La Greca (2002)	Preexisting characteristics	I
	Psychological resources	I
	Aspects of traumatic exposure	E
	The postdisaster recovery environment	S
Nader (2001)	Developmental influences: Age	I
	Influence of parental attachment style	S
	Impact of previous traumatic experiences	E

[a]S, the social environment; I, factors in the individual; E, factors related to the traumatic event.

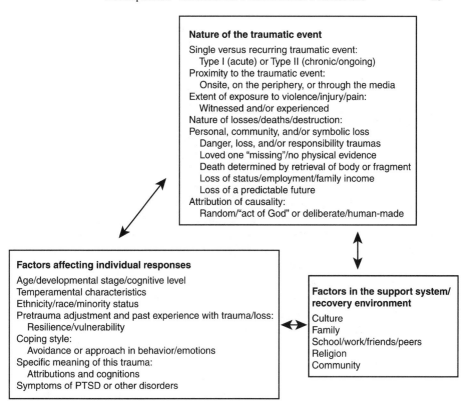

FIGURE 2.1. Interactive components of the assessment of a child's or family member's responses to traumatic stress and loss: Webb.

Nature of the Traumatic Event

Chapter 1 has reviewed and discussed the various factors associated with the traumatic event that may create stress for an individual child or family member. By definition, mass trauma leads to extensive numbers of deaths and/or widespread destruction of property. Because an entire community is often affected, its resources for rescue and recovery may be strained or exhausted. This can add another layer of distress for surviving family members and friends; they may be aware, for example, that a medical staff is engaged in triaging the most serious casualties and postponing care for those whose injuries, while serious, are not considered life-threatening. When everyone is suffering in the aftermath of a trauma, no one seems to have sufficient emotional resources to provide support.

Another characteristic of mass trauma situations, as compared with other types of traumas, is the possible traumatization of helpers themselves—whose effectiveness may be reduced by their physical and emotional exhaustion in dealing with large numbers of victims, as well as their preoccupation with their personal losses. Moreover (as happened following the Oklahoma City bombing and the attacks of September 11, 2001), well-meaning mental health professionals from other communities who are eager to volunteer their services may stream into the disaster area and create a situation of "too many helpers" (Webb, 1999). This was portrayed in a cartoon depicting two vultures consuming a carcass in a desert with a cloud of other birds on the distant horizon, as one vulture says to the other, "Here come the grief counselors!" Obviously, the altruistic desire to help others in situations of mass trauma requires sensitive organizational response. In Oklahoma City, a procedure was implemented to protect the survivors from the potentially stressful involvement of numerous clinicians and researchers trying to help and/or study them (Krug, Nixon, & Vincent, 1996).

The large numbers of people involved in situations of mass trauma can create positive as well as negative effects among the survivors. For example, more than a year after "9/11," many widows continued to meet in both formal and informal support groups; the fact that they suffered similar losses provided a bond and facilitated mutual aid. Other people, by contrast, found themselves unemployed and without fellow workers or resources, because the buildings in which they worked were destroyed in the attacks. Losses are great for *all* survivors of mass traumatic events, but the particular nature of responses to these losses depends on a combination of individual factors and factors in the support system and the recovery environment, as discussed in the remainder of this section.

Factors Affecting Individual Responses

Age/Developmental Stage/Cognitive Level

Children's age affects their ability to understand, and this understanding ultimately contributes to the meaning associated with traumatic events. For example, a 4-year-old who saw the plane hitting one of the twin towers of the World Trade Center on 9/11 asked his mother why the airplane flew into the building, without any realization that people had died as a result. Similarly, many young children who witnessed people jumping from the windows of the towers wondered whether they were going to land on trampolines! In contrast, a 10-year-old girl wrote to a preteen chat room about her fears that terrorists might crash into a building and cause her own death or that of someone she knew (Merrick, 2001), and a 16-year-old honor student commented to his father that there was no point in studying any more, since everyone was going to die soon in a war or by anthrax poisoning. People of all ages struggle to find meaning in unusual events;

the younger children cited above simply did not comprehend the reality of danger and of death, whereas the two older youth clearly did.

There is a developmental progression in children's ability to comprehend the reality of death (Webb, 2002; Nagy, 1948), with most experts agreeing that children do not have a mature conception of death until about age 7 or 8 (Speece & Brent, 1996). This may not be firmly in place, however, until their ability to think abstractly is consistently evident. Therefore, a child's response to death will be influenced by whether he or she thinks it is temporary and reversible (beliefs typical of the preschool child), or whether the child knows that death is final and irreversible and that it is beyond the dead person's ability to return (knowledge typical of the school-age youngster). The nature of the child's grief reaction relates to his or her understanding. Death inevitably creates a separation experience, whether or not the reason for it is understood. The preschooler who loses a parent or other caretaker in a traumatic event cannot fathom the absence of the attachment figure, and his or her responses may reflect Bowlby's (1960, 1973, 1980) stages of protest, anger, and eventual detachment. An older child, who realizes that the death was beyond the control of the person who died, may struggle to comprehend the reason for it; the child may think that something he or she might have done could have caused it, or wonder whether he or she could have prevented it. In circumstances when the death was the result of a deliberate act, the child may fantasize about getting revenge on the perceived perpetrator.

Age and developmental level clearly affect cognitive understanding and appraisal of danger. Since "trauma," by definition, requires the occurrence of an event in which a person witnessed or was confronted with a situation that involved actual or threatened death or serious injury to self or others, young children who do not comprehend the danger and who do not understand the finality of death are less likely to experience intense stress or fear. This was illustrated in a study of children following the nuclear disaster at Three Mile Island, when few children exhibited posttraumatic stress disorder (PTSD) symptoms because they did not perceive that any lives were in danger (Wroble & Baum, 2002). However, children do notice and can become anxious when they witness terrified reactions among the adults around them. The association between the symptoms of parents and their children has been documented in a number of studies (Breton, Valla, & Lambert, 1993; Laor, Wolmer, Mayes, et al., 1996; Sullivan, Saylor, & Foster, 1991) and is discussed more fully later in this chapter. The responses of adolescents and adults to a traumatic event are more likely to depend on their temperament, their general coping style, and their own past history of trauma and loss (see below).

One possible qualification of the preceding is that when deaths occur as a result of a mass trauma situation, a great deal of attention may be given to the event and to the families of the victims. Because of repeated exposure, young children may come to realize the finality of a death far sooner than they would in nontraumatic circumstances. According to Baker (1997, p. 140), "Children commonly experience four primary emotional reactions to death: fear, anger, sadness, and guilt. Especially powerful are feelings of fear and anxiety. The world has suddenly become to them a very unsafe place in which beloved people can disappear forever." All these things are especially likely in cases of mass trauma.

Temperamental Characteristics

Because temperament may modulate a person's responses to stress, it should be considered in the assessment of a particular individual's reactions (Wertlieb, Weigel, Springer, & Feldstein, 1987). For example, a child who has been sensitive and high-strung all his or her life may respond with anxious behaviors following a mass trauma. Thomas and Chess outlined nine different dimensions of temperament, which they subsequently grouped into three specific profiles of child behavior (Thomas & Chess, 1981; Chess & Thomas, 1986). These three general clusters of temperamental style, identified from parental reports, are referred to as "the difficult child," "the easy child," and "the slow-to-warm or shy child."

Studies of children exposed to extreme stressors report that temperament plays an important role in a child's response (Wertlieb et al., 1987; Werner & Smith, 1982). For example, anxious children were more vulnerable to developing PTSD after Hurricane Andrew, even when their exposure to the disaster was relatively limited (La Greca, Silverman, Vernberg, & Prinstein, 1996). Similarly, young people who scored with high levels of depression and stress symptoms before an earthquake in California had higher levels of these symptoms after the disaster (Silverman & La Greca, 2002). Temperamental characteristics are evident early in childhood and tend to endure. Children who were ranked as "stress-resistant" after exposure to four or more stressors in their lives were more likely to have been considered by their parents as easygoing rather than difficult as infants (Marsten et al., 1988; Werner & Smith, 1982). Although temperament can be modified somewhat by environmental responses, in general a person's overall temperamental style tends to remain stable throughout life.

Ethnicity/Race/Minority Status

Another fact that affects an individual's response to stress is his or her ethnicity. Findings from community studies report that minority children and youth exhibit higher levels of PTSD symptoms and have lower recovery rates following exposure to natural disasters (La Greca et al., 1996; La Greca, Silverman, & Wasserstein, 1998; Lonigan, Shannon, Taylor, Finch, & Sallee, 1994). We can speculate that this might be related to higher levels of predisaster exposure to trauma, due to community violence in the poorer urban neighborhoods where minority populations reside (Silverman & La Greca, 2002). This possibility seems to have been corroborated in a study of more than 8,000 school children in New York City 6 months following the 9/11 attacks. About 10.5% of children in 4th through 12th grades were found to have symptoms of PTSD or other disorders, such as agoraphobia and depression; Hispanic students were disproportionately affected, followed by non-Hispanic blacks, who were affected more than either non-Hispanic whites or Asians (Goodnough, 2002). A reporter from *The New York Times* interviewed the principal of one of the schools that participated in the study. This principal said, "We have kids in trauma all the time. Some come to school hurt. Some have housing problems. Some don't sleep. Our kids were fragile *before*" (quoted in Purnick, 2002, p. B1, italics added). A therapist at the New York University Study Center also confirmed the role of preexisting stressors such as family and community violence, which compounded the traumatic impact of 9/11 for the children in this study (Purnick, 2002).

Pretrauma Adjustment and Past Experience with Trauma/Loss: The Foundation for Resilience or Increased Vulnerability?

An individual's general adjustment in school/work and in family life serves as a baseline against which the stress of a traumatic event rebounds. Logic suggests that a person who was coping adequately with the everyday stresses of life will respond with more agility and effectiveness in a traumatic situation than someone who was struggling and barely managing to get through the daily hassles of work or school. However, a person who has experienced previous traumas may or may not have difficulty coping with future stresses. There is a lack of agreement about this. On the one hand, Fletcher (1996) points out that it is the *outcome* of past stressful experiences, rather than the exposure itself, that results in increased strength and resilience or in increased vulnerability to future stress. He maintains that persons who have successfully mastered past stressful challenges may face future traumatic circumstances with a positive attitude, due to their increased sense of self-efficacy.

On the other hand, Brady (2001) states that a history of a previous trauma may be associated with vulnerability to the development of PTSD after a subsequent traumatic event. Some vulnerability factors stem from the biological effects of early traumatic experiences that interfere with an individual's ability to reduce or modulate his or her physiological distress in later stressful encounters. For example, in the year after the Columbine High School shootings, school counselors and students became aware of "trauma triggers" (e.g., fire alarms, loud noises, and certain areas of the school), which stimulated automatic fear responses in those who had witnessed the shootings (Arman, 2000). The implication is that the tendency toward heightened physiological arousal is automatic following trauma. van der Kolk (1996) conveys this concept compellingly in a chapter titled "The Body Keeps the Score." This biological vulnerability means that persons who have been exposed to early trauma—even after they have recovered—may have a unique biological profile that makes it more difficult for them to recover following subsequent traumas (Yehuda, 2001).

These different views among the experts suggest that the matter of previous exposure is complex and needs to be evaluated together with other facets of a person's life. Thus an assessment of a child or family member includes weighing the impact of traumatic events, in addition to the history of the person's past and current losses, with special attention given to experiences of multiple and/or traumatic losses.

Coping Style: Degree of Avoidance or Approach in Behavior and Emotions

"Coping" refers to the manner in which people deal with stress. Folkman (1991, p. 5) defined it as "the changing thoughts and acts that the individual uses to manage the external and/or internal demands of a specific person–environment transaction that is appraised as stressful." Ayalon (1983) refers to coping as a formula for survival. However, Resick (2001) reminds us that despite its positive connotation, coping may have either effective or ineffective outcomes, depending on whether negative consequences result. This supports Fletcher's (1996) views, as mentioned previously.

Coping styles can be classified as primarily avoidance or approach strategies, involving both behavior (action) and emotions (affects). For example, following a school shooting incident, some students who were witnesses may eagerly give evidence to try to catch the sniper; others may prefer to go home and avoid any discussion of their traumatic experience. Similarly, some students will readily express their feelings of fear, anger, and sadness, while others will suppress and hide their emotions. Following a natural disaster, children and adolescents who used negative coping strategies such as blaming others showed higher levels of PTSD symptoms than did youth who used problem-solving and other adaptive coping skills (La Greca et al., 1996; Vernberg, La Greca, Silverman, & Prinstein, 1996; Berman, Kurtines, Silverman, & Serafini, 1996). Of course, patterns of coping are intrinsically related to a youngster's developmental level (Compas & Epping, 1993; Saylor & Deroma, 2002), and his or her temperament.

According to Resick (2001), research has consistently shown that withdrawal and avoidance responses are associated with greater posttrauma distress and failure to recover. However, different coping responses may be appropriate at different phases of a traumatic situation. For example, resignation and stoic acceptance might be appropriate responses in some war or hostage conditions, whereas action resulting in escape might be effective in other such situations. "In order to succeed one's coping must match the circumstances of the event and the survivor's resources" (Shalev & Ursano, 2003, p. 126). Effective coping results in the following four outcomes, according to Pearlin and Schooler (1978):

- Relief of distress
- Sense of personal worth
- Ability to enjoy rewarding interpersonal contacts
- Sustained task performance

These results may be only partially achieved, however. Furthermore, Ayalon (1983) warns against drawing up a blueprint for how people *should* cope with situations of extreme stress, because complicating factors such as personal appraisals and attributions about the situation may control various coping efforts.

Specific Meaning of This Trauma: Attributions and Cognitions

It is human nature to try to understand the reasons why events happen. As discussed earlier in this chapter, even young children search for explanations of an upsetting experience in their attempts to resolve their confusion (Arroyo & Eth, 1996). When they lack correct information they create their own meaning, as in the fairy tale about "Chicken Little," who thought the sky was falling and who actually convinced some of her animal friends of this as well. A child's age ultimately determines his or her ability to understand the full significance of a traumatic event, and this in turn affects the nature of the child's subsequent coping (Compas & Epping, 1993; Saylor & Deroma, 2002).

The intense fear associated with traumatic events often leads to feelings of helplessness and hopelessness about being unable to do anything to stop or reduce the unfolding sequence of harm and horror. For example, traumatic events such as terrorist attacks can cause people to question their beliefs that the world is safe, secure, and predictable; that other people can be trusted; and that they themselves and/or responsible adults are in charge and can cope successfully. Terr (1991) has described changed attitudes about people and life among traumatized children who came to realize the vulnerability of all humans, especially themselves, and who lived with the expectation that more traumas would follow. Apprehension about the future can also take the form of a sense of a foreshortened future, as identified by Terr (1983) in her study of the kidnapped children of Chowchilla.

Beliefs that are most likely to be disrupted after a traumatic event are those regarding safety, trust, power/control, esteem, and intimacy

(McCann, Sakheim, & Abrahamson, 1988). According to Resick (2001), the more someone attributes blame to him- or herself and feels guilt related to the trauma, the greater the stress and the symptoms are likely to be. We know that children typically blame themselves when bad things happen, so this increases their risk of symptom development following a trauma.

Another factor that influences a child's reaction is the nature of his or her caregiver's responses. The younger the child is, the more he or she depends on the parent(s) or other caregiver as the source of security and safety. The attachment object provides comfort, love, and dependability. When this adult becomes frightened, hurt, or bereaved in a mass crisis situation, the child then becomes bereft of his or her source of security. Lifton and Olson (1976) refer to the shattering of the shield of invincibility, with damage to the foundation of basic trust on which future development rests (Erikson, 1950). More discussion of how family responses influence children's reactions appears later in the chapter.

Symptoms of PTSD or Other Disorders

Chapter 1 has presented the definition of a "traumatic event" given in the *Diagnostic and Statistical Manual of Mental Disorders*, fourth edition, text revision (DSM-IV-TR; American Psychiatric Association, 2000). Situations of terrorist bombings, war, and community violence clearly qualify as traumatic events, according to this definition; the potentially dangerous circumstances of military families, in contrast, create ongoing stress and chronic anxiety about the future *possibility* of death and trauma. This chapter emphasizes that the responses of children and their families to stressful and/or traumatic situations vary according to (1) the circumstances of the event, (2) the unique backgrounds of each individual, and (3) the level and type of support in their social environments. Although all exposed persons do not develop symptoms of PTSD (or other psychiatric disorders), and those who do may recover spontaneously after a period of time (McFarlane & Yehuda, 1996; Shalev, 1996; Brady, 2001), practitioners need to be aware of some of the typical difficulties that can develop.

Fletcher (1996) has prepared a table of incidence rates of PTSD symptoms, and other associated symptoms and diagnoses, among children and adults following exposure to traumatic events. Here, I draw on this and other reports in the literature to discuss the diagnoses of acute stress disorder (ASD) and PTSD, together with other diagnoses that may develop following situations of mass trauma and ongoing anxiety. It is important to recognize that symptoms from several different diagnostic clusters may exist together (this coexistence is referred to as "psychiatric comorbidity"), and that children may have some symptoms, but not enough to qualify fully for a particular diagnosis (Drake, Bush, & van Gorp, 2001; Gurwitch, Sullivan, & Long, 1998). Among adults, epidemiological studies have shown a high rate of comorbidity between PTSD and depression, substance abuse or dependence, and anxiety disorders (Brady et al., 2000).

The diagnosis of PTSD first appeared in the DSM-III (American Psychiatric Association, 1980) based on the study and treatment of combat veterans. As such, the diagnosis focused on adult experience and ignored the distinct and special symptoms of children (Shelby, 1997). The DSM-III-R (American Psychiatric Association, 1987) included some child corollaries of the adult PTSD symptoms, but still failed to include many of children's typical responses to stress, such as increased dependency, decreased bladder and bowel control, and loss of confidence in parents' ability to protect them (Shelby, 1997). Later versions of the DSM (American Psychiatric Association, 1994, 2000) have included more criteria related to children, but many child therapists continue to believe that children's specific responses to traumatic events are inadequately represented in the DSM, possibly because of children's limited verbal abilities and/or their unwillingness to revisit or reveal their frightening memories (Shelby, 1997; Scheeringa, Zeanah, Drell, & Larrieu, 1995; McFarlane, Policansky, & Irwin, 1987). Use of parents' or teachers' reports to assess children's symptoms has been found to be unreliable, since adults tend to minimize children's responses (McFarlane et al., 1987).

A diagnosis of PTSD requires the presence of specific symptoms in three distinct areas following the experience of the frightening traumatic event, as specified above. These areas are as follows:

- Reexperiencing (one or more symptoms)
- Avoidance and numbing (three or more symptoms)
- Hyperarousal (two or more symptoms)

Fletcher (1996) maintains that the diagnostic symptoms of PTSD apply to traumatized children of all ages, and he acknowledges variations related to age and developmental level. For example, he mentions that younger children are more likely to be overwhelmed in stressful circumstances than are older children and adults; he also notes that preschoolers typically exhibit regressed behavior in response to trauma, whereas regression is less frequent in older children. It is important to specify the timing of the assessment, because responses may change over time, and initial responses may later subside (Shalev, 1996). McFarlane and Yehuda (1996) state:

> The typical pattern for even the most catastrophic experiences is resolution of symptoms and not the development of PTSD. Only a minority of

the victims will go on to develop PTSD, and with the passage of time the symptoms will resolve in approximately two thirds of these. (p. 156)

Some authors have identified three stages of response to trauma (McFarlane & Yehuda, 1996; Gurwitch et al., 1998). These include the acute stress response (the immediate posttrauma phase); the early, short-term phase (1 week to 3 months after the trauma); and the long-term adaptation phase (over 3 months after the trauma). Other theorists conceptualize four stages following trauma: the impact phase, the immediate postimpact rescue phase, the early recovery phase, and the "return-to-life phase" (Shalev & Ursano, 2003). Whichever conceptualization is used, the point is that symptoms change over time. Early responses can be viewed as survival-driven and adaptive to the perception of harm to the self or others, whereas later (during the rescue phase, in Shalev & Ursano's [2003] scheme) the individual begins to cope with his or her drastically changed reality. The recovery stage overlaps with this phase and consists of survivors' efforts to try to understand the meaning of what happened, at the same time they are trying emotionally to distance themselves from the traumatic event (Shalev & Ursano, 2003).

These proposals regarding *stages* of responses to traumatic events have important implications for treatment, as will be discussed in Chapter 3. In the early phases following a traumatic event, the assessment looks at the degree to which the symptoms are tolerated by the survivor and the degree to which they interfere with normal functioning (Shalev & Ursano, 2003). Since we know that many symptoms will subside, early interventions often focus on what has been referred to as "psychological first aid" (Pynoos & Nader, 1988; Nader, 1997).

The fear associated with traumatic events produces intense stress and anxiety in survivors, who often are coping simultaneously with multiple losses and complicated grief. Both grief and PTSD reactions can involve symptoms of intrusion and avoidance (Jacobs, 1999; Simpson, 1997), thereby making diagnosis challenging. In addition, some deaths may have strong traumatic features in addition to the loss repercussions. When trauma and grief overlap, treatment requires special attention to the trauma in order to permit mourning to proceed (Nader, 1997; Eth & Pynoos, 1985). Again, this will be discussed further in Chapter 3.

Because the diagnosis of PTSD requires that symptoms must be present for at least 4 weeks, the diagnosis of ASD was added to the DSM-IV (American Psychiatric Association, 1994) to acknowledge and classify persons who exhibit symptoms similar to PTSD *prior to* the 1-month time requirement. ASD actually includes most of the same criteria as PTSD, with the addition of symptoms of dissociation. Studies have found that the presence of full or partial ASD was associated with increased risk of developing PTSD, especially among persons who dissociated during the traumatic event (Shalev, Peri, Canetti, & Schreiber, 1996). However, many persons develop PTSD without first exhibiting signs of ASD. Although dissociative disorders are rarely diagnosed in children, studies have found high rates of dissociative symptoms among sexually and physically abused children (Wolfe & Birt, 1997). I am not aware of studies of children's dissociative responses in situations of mass trauma, although logic suggests that children would employ such methods as fantasy and intense daydreaming to shut out their anxiety and fright connected with war and terrorism, just as many do to cope with incest and other forms of abuse.

In addition to the symptoms associated with ASD and PTSD, various other symptoms and reactions are common in children following traumatic events. These include anxiety and fear, depression, regressive behavior, somatic complaints, and other problem behaviors (Gurwitch et al., 1998). Anxiety reactions take the form of separation anxiety and specific fears, especially in situations that generate reminders of the actual traumatic event, as previously mentioned with regard to survivors of the Columbine shooting (Arman, 2000). The physical separations that often occur in the aftermath of traumas can be particularly frightening to children and create anxiety reactions. In addition, depression often accompanies chronic PTSD among children and adolescents (Goenjian et al., 1995), as it does with approximately half the adult men and women who have PTSD (Kessler, Sonnega, Bromet, Hughes, & Nelson, 1995). The assessment of the individual who has survived a mass trauma situation is complex and has many components. A review of some assessment issues and selected methods follows a discussion of the mediating factors in the recovery environment.

Factors in the Support System and Recovery Environment

A mass trauma occurs to numerous people simultaneously, with multiple and concurrent repercussions in the recovery environment. These include consequences to the physical surroundings (e.g., destruction of buildings and disruption of transport and communications networks), as well as to the social network (e.g., the impact on and responses of medical and religious facilities and personnel). Many circumstances can help or hinder a person's efforts to obtain aid and to regain a precrisis state of functioning. This section focuses on factors in the *social* environment, since the circumstances of the physical environment have been discussed to some extent in Chapter 1 as components of the traumatic event. The overlapping and interacting factors in the support system and the recovery environment include the following:

- Culture
- Family

- School/work/friends/peers
- Religion
- Community

Culture

The concept of "culture" encompasses the beliefs, morals, values, customs, world view, behaviors, and communication styles that are socially transmitted and held in common by a group, and to which the group's members are expected to conform (Banks, 1991; Webb, 2001). Cultural issues permeate all aspects of life; for the purposes of this discussion, they include the different meanings attributed to traumatic experiences by various cultures, and their distinctive preferences for seeking help when symptoms and/or needs become acknowledged.

Cultural beliefs are shaped by specific religious practices and are expressed within a family context. For example[1], when a Chinese adolescent who attended a high school close to the World Trade Center began to have nightmares and difficulty concentrating in school during the months that followed the 9/11 attacks, he did not say anything to his parents because they were preoccupied with their own concerns. Several months later, the school counselor notified the parents about their son's poor grades, and they informed the boy that his failure was "shaming" the family. The boy knew that something was wrong with him, and told his parents that he thought he should talk to the counselor about his nightmares and poor concentration. His mother responded that she would prefer to have him consult his uncle or the family minister, rather than have this "weakness" recorded on his school documents. His father said that he should just pay more attention to his studies, and when the boy spoke to the minister, he suggested that the boy should pray to God to heal him. This brief vignette illustrates the impact of cultural beliefs and the interplay of culture, religion, and family expectations in how symptoms are acknowledged (or not) and how acceptable sources for obtaining relief are defined.

Resistance to mental heath services is typical among many cultures, which equate such counseling with an admission of "mental illness" (Joyner & Swensen, 1993; Wu, 2001; Shibusawa, 2001). Chapter 11 of this book discusses the use of community outreach and education to deal with cultural resistance to mental health services in the Chinese community of New York City. A strategy to counteract the stigma and shame that affected persons and their families might otherwise encounter in cultures that view psychological problems as disgraceful consists of emphasizing the normality of traumatic responses (Nader, Dubrow, & Stamm, 1999).

---

[1]This example is a composite drawn from my consultation experience.

This takes the form of educating family members and the community about typical and expected symptoms, such as sleep disturbances and loss of concentration after traumatic exposure. Each culture defines normality and pathology in its own terms, and these beliefs may be quite different from those of a mental health practitioner from a different cultural background. Kinzie (2001) points out that culture determines both the nature of the problems presented by a client and the manner in which a clinician understands and classifies them. For instance, the term *nervios* is used by some Hispanic groups to refer to symptoms of distress, anxiety, demoralization, and somatic problems (Dutton, 1998). This condition might be inaccurately diagnosed as pathology by a clinician unfamiliar with its frequent occurrence and cultural acceptance among Hispanics. Similar cultural knowledge must inform practice with Southeast Asian groups such as the Hmong, who have no words in their language for mental-health-related stress, and who instead express their anxieties through somatic and bodily complaints (Fong, 2004). All people experience stress, but its acceptable manifestations in human behavior pass through fine cultural filters.

The DSM for the first time in 2000 contained information about culturally manifested symptoms that otherwise might be unknown and misdiagnosed by clinicians with mainstream European American values. It is increasingly important for such practitioners to maintain a stance of openness and "cultural curiosity" about different cultures and their beliefs, as the United States progresses toward becoming a society in which the former "minorities" constitute the majority (Ozawa, 1997).

Family

The family is the preferred source of support for most people when they are experiencing stress. During experiences of mass trauma in particular, people make great efforts to assemble with their loved ones and to find out whether all their extended family members are safe. Attachment reactions stimulate proximity-seeking behavior at times of perceived danger. If long separations from family members occur at such times, anxiety mounts, and desperate searching may ensue. Children between the ages of 6 months and 4 years are particularly vulnerable to distress when separated from their parents, since they do not yet have firm object constancy and the ability to cognitively maintain their attachment relationships (Bingham & Harmon, 1996). Whereas separation anxiety decreases as children age, awareness of the danger associated with traumatic events increases (Fletcher, 1996). This sense of increased vulnerability makes children especially responsive to their parents' stress (Pfefferbaum, 1997). A child's reaction to trauma is often closely related to the reactions of the child's parents or other important adults, especially the mother (Fletcher,

1996). Anna Freud's reports of children exposed to trauma in World War II (Freud & Burlingham, 1943) found that children in the care of their own mothers or familiar substitutes were not psychologically devastated by their wartime experiences, because the caretakers maintained day-to-day routines and projected high morale (Garbarino, Kostelny, & Dubrow, 1991). In other words, calm mothers or other attachment figures influenced their children to be calm, even during the stress of wartime. Conversely, interventions with mothers who are anxious may ultimately help their children.

A practitioner working with a family after a mass trauma may attempt to construct a genogram in order to help the family identify the members of the extended family who need to be notified and who might be able to provide shelter or other forms of support. Such a genogram contains information about the names of, geographic locations of, frequency of contact with, and the quality of the relationships among various family members. Although this tool can serve as a valuable resource, some families in conditions of acute stress may be unable or unwilling to give personal information to an unknown clinician who is trying to help following a mass trauma. Cultural factors may also preclude the sharing of personal family data. Practitioners in traumatic situations often must modify and adapt their assessment procedures to fit the circumstances of the recovery environment. Sometimes, for example, they will need to rely on limited information initially, until a relationship of trust has been established that increases family members' willingness to share their history.

When a traumatic event has involved the death of a family member, special attention needs to be paid to the role and function of the person who died and to the family's history of past losses (Webb, 2002). Religious beliefs also must be ascertained and respected, especially in regard to expected procedures following death. The extent to which children are included or excluded in religious memorials, funerals, and burials varies among different cultures and religions, as does the open expression of emotions.

School/Work/Friends/Peers

A return to the regular routine of school or work helps people assume some control over their lives as they begin to put the traumatic event in the past, although distressing memories may still surface frequently and unpredictably. Although children often feel isolated and embarrassed when the death of a family member makes them feel "different" (Webb, 2002), in situations of *mass* trauma other children are similarly bereaved, and the shared experience can provide the opportunity for mutual support. Debriefing groups in schools, as discussed in Chapter 6, can assist young people with their necessary postrecovery tasks of trying to understand and cope with their terrible experience. A classroom exercise involving a draw-a-picture, tell-a-story intervention provides an opportunity to address issues of loss in a group format (Nader & Pynoos, 1991). Sometimes when many people have died in a mass trauma at a workplace or school, memorial services may be organized by the employer or school administration to provide an opportunity for tributes and shared mourning.

Religion

Religious beliefs permeate cultural and family practices related to death and to the search for meaning about the mysteries of life and death. Outreach counselors working with the survivors of Hurricane Hugo learned that many people in the ethnically divergent south Florida community at that time believed that the disaster was "God's will," and that God had sent the storm to "teach them a lesson" (Joyner & Swenson, 1993). The unknown causes of natural disasters contrast sharply with the situations of bombings and wars that occur as a result of deliberate actions. For example, many people were confused by the mixing of religious and political motives in the terrorist acts of 9/11, which caused peaceful Muslim Americans to express their great disapproval of the fatal suicide attacks in the name of Allah. This example emphasizes the caveat against making generalizations about any single cultural or religious group. Individuals often look for religious interpretations as part of their search for meaning following mass trauma events. When traumatic situations occur as a result of deliberate human-made actions, such as war, shootings, or terrorism, this can create serious questions about how or why a deity could allow such suffering. Buddhists may find their answer in "karma" (destiny), whereas some Christian faiths teach acceptance of life's "mysteries" and forgiveness of human wrongdoing. From a psychological/mental health viewpoint, individuals recovering from human-caused mass traumas have to make major accommodations to deal with their justified anger related to their extensive losses and the associated complicated mourning.

As noted above, religious practices have a major role in prescribing how people mourn their dead and the specific rituals for this purpose. The structure of rituals and expectations for mourning, funerals, and disposal of the dead body helps focus and facilitate the grief process.

Community

Situations of mass trauma, by definition, affect a large number of people who are going through a mourning process together. Anger is a part of normal grief, and an even greater part of traumatic grief. Indeed, it can be viewed as justified after a human-made, potentially avoidable tragedy. Effective community leaders try to channel this anger into recovery efforts, and to convey determination to carry on despite multiple losses. However, anxiety about possible recurrence of future traumatic events may immobilize individuals temporarily, until they become gradually reassured about their present safety.

When there have been many deaths in a mass trauma situation, often the community mourns together, and this global response can be very supportive and provide a sense of validation to the survivors. These collective demonstrations of grief may actually contribute to group recovery (Zinner & Williams, 1999).

The extent to which a mass trauma constitutes a crisis for an entire community—but also an opportunity—is captured in the following quote:

> It may stagnate a community's future development or propel a community into new areas of growth. The crisis may be one of attachment and identity as it disrupts stability and structure. The first task of healing after a crisis is to acknowledge what has happened to the fullest extent possible. The second task is to try to restore community equilibrium. This latter task has many parts in meeting its goal, including experiencing group loss and finding meaning. (Williams, Zinner, & Ellis, 1999, p. 8)

Over time, Oklahoma City, New York City, and Washington, D.C. have reestablished their equilibrium following the terrorist attacks in those cities. Memorials have been built or are being planned; tributes have been made during anniversaries; and healing seems to be progressing. Single-event traumas (that may or may not require treatment) can be put in the past, even though their memory lingers. In contrast, situations of ongoing anxiety—such as military deployment, circumstances of continuing political violence, and fears of a possible biological or chemical attack—do not permit closure and relief. At the time of this writing, the United States is on alert, and threats of war suggest the probability of ongoing stress, certain death, and mass destruction throughout the world. Responses of anxiety, stress, and depression will certainly affect countless numbers of children and families, both in the United States and abroad. Mental health practitioners must be prepared to carry out assessments and interventions in the most efficient and compassionate manner possible to help the hundreds who will require assistance.

ASSESSMENTS OF CHILDREN AND FAMILIES AFTER MASS TRAUMA: ISSUES AND SELECTED METHODS

An often-quoted statement is that the initial stress response to trauma constitutes "a normal response to an abnormal event" (Shalev, 1996, p. 77). As already discussed, the early symptoms of PTSD/ASD subside in many survivors. However, we do not know how many who initially present with symptoms of ASD will develop later symptoms of full-blown PTSD. Therefore, the matter of timing is of special importance in assessments of people who have been exposed to traumatic events. Those who are symptomatic in the early weeks following the trauma should be advised to return for an assessment for PTSD at a later time; in contrast, those who do not have any symptoms in the first few weeks after a trauma should be advised that these may develop later.

Over the past 10 years, a number of assessment tools in the forms of rating scales have been developed for the purpose of diagnosing PTSD and other conditions related to traumatic exposure. Barrios and Hartmann (1997) claim that there are more than 160 instruments for the assessment of children's fears and anxieties (PTSD falls into the category of an anxiety disorder). Some of these instruments are specific to particular types of trauma, such as sexual abuse; others have been developed primarily for research purposes related to documenting the incidence of particular diagnoses among specific populations following trauma. Depending on its purpose, a psychological assessment can include the use of questionnaires, checklists, structured interviews, and projective measures. It is beyond the scope of this chapter to provide a review of all these methods, and readers who want more information should consult Barrios and Hartmann (1997), Drake et al. (2001), Saylor and Deroma (2002), Finch and Daugherty (1993), and the data base of the National Center for PTSD (http://www.ncptsd.org). This section provides a brief overview of some issues involved in conducting assessments, and then describes and lists some selected assessment instruments that are practical for use following mass trauma.

Special considerations apply to the task of assessment of children and should influence the particular method selected. Among these are (1) the length and extensiveness of the assessment; (2) the format of the assessment (individual, group, family); (3) the child's ability and willingness to answer questions or respond to requests to describe his or her traumatic experience; and (4) the source(s) of information about the traumatic experience (child, parent, teacher).

With regard to the extensiveness of the evaluation, common sense suggests that children and families who have recently experienced a mass trauma should not be expected to tolerate an extensive evaluation procedure (Saylor & Deroma, 2002). Therefore, brief methods and group screening procedures that can be conducted in a natural setting, such as the school, are especially recommended (Pynoos & Eth, 1986; Nader & Pynoos, 1991, 1993). Once group screenings have occurred, children whose responses are problematic can be identified and offered more extensive assessments. Although parents and teachers are often asked for their input about children's posttrauma reactions, studies have found that they tend to underestimate PTSD symptomatology for children (McNally, 1998; Saylor, Belter, & Stokes, 1997). This argues for more utilization of methods that utilize children's *own* reports, in addition to obtaining input from other sources. However, children have limited verbal abilities and tend to avoid reminders of the trauma; this argues for *indirect* methods of child assessment through the use of play, art, and storytelling (Pynoos & Eth, 1986; Nader & Pynoos, 1991, 1993; Roje, 1996; Webb, 2003).

Pynoos and Eth's (1986) child interview is designed to be used in an initial meeting with a recently traumatized child who has witnessed a violent act. This single-session structured interview begins with a relationship-building phase in which the child is invited to draw and tell a story. This is followed by a second stage in which the clinician guides the child to reconstruct the traumatic experience, using an assortment of play materials. The third and final stage emphasizes recapitulation and closure. This 90-minute one-to-one interview was helpful to several hundred children, many of whom spontaneously expressed their relief in being able to explore the traumatic episode with an unaffected adult. The fact that these children were not reluctant to deal with their traumatic experience may relate to the special attention given by the clinician to establishing a "safe holding environment" for the child during the trauma reconstruction.

A different version of this structured drawing and storytelling method was reported by Nader (1997), who used it in a group format with children in schools following different types of traumatic events, including a tornado. The group drawing and storytelling exercise was viewed as a way to help children talk about some of the frightening things they had witnessed and to support each other through the group process. This classroom exercise directly preceded individual assessment screening via the use of the Childhood Post-Traumatic Stress Reaction Index.

Specific assessment instruments that have been used and that are recommended for screening of PTSD include the following:

- Childhood Post-Traumatic Stress Reaction Index (Frederick, Pynoos, & Nader, 1992)
- Traumatic Events Screening Inventory (Ribbe, 1996)
- Children's PTSD Inventory (Saigh et al., 2000)
- Trauma Symptom Checklist for Children (Briere, 1996)
- Clinician Administered PTSD Scale for Children and Adolescents for DSM-IV (Nader, Kriegler, Blake, & Pynoos, 1994; Nader et al., 1998)

Practice wisdom cautions that "a test result is not a diagnosis" (Drake et al., 2001, p. 15), and experts maintain that although a multidimensional approach to assessment is valid, the face-to-face interview is the gold standard for the accurate diagnosis of PTSD (Cohen, 1998). However, expediency suggests that we should try to identify persons who are showing symptoms following mass traumas through initial group screenings; we should then proceed to individual interviews, conducting further assessment through selected instruments (including information from parents and significant others, when feasible). In the case of children, a developmental history and a history of past losses add important information to the evaluation process (Webb, 2003). Interviews with children must respect their age and ability to engage and comprehend the traumatic event to which they have been exposed. Play and art materials can assist not only in developing the relationship, but also in providing a "child-friendly" method to permit a child to communicate his or her fears and anxieties symbolically through play (Webb, 2002).

Children and families exposed to mass traumas are fearful and fragile. The challenge for mental health professionals is to learn their unique stories through methods that will ease, not add to, their anxiety. An effective assessment should help an affected person begin to feel relief that someone understands his or her experience and will use that understanding to arrange help.

REFERENCES

American Psychiatric Association. (1980). *Diagnostic and statistical manual of mental disorders* (3rd ed.). Washington, DC: Author.

American Psychiatric Association. (1987). *Diagnostic and statistical manual of mental disorders* (3rd ed., rev.). Washington, DC: Author.

American Psychiatric Association. (1994). *Diagnostic and statistical manual of mental disorders* (4th ed.). Washington, DC: Author.

American Psychiatric Association. (2000). *Diagnostic and statistical manual of mental disorders* (4th ed., text rev.). Washington, DC: Author.

Arman, J. F. (2000). In the wake of tragedy at Columbine High School. *Professional School Counseling, 3*(3), 218–221.

Arroyo, W., & Eth, S. (1996). Post-traumatic stress disorder and other stress reactions. In R. J. Apfel & B. Simon (Eds.), *Minefields in their hearts: The mental health of children in war and communal violence* (pp. 52–74). New Haven, CT: Yale University Press.

Ayalon, O. (1983). Coping with terrorism: The Israeli case. In D. Meichenbaum & M. E. Jaremko (Eds.), *Stress reduction and prevention* (pp. 293–339). New York: Plenum Press.

Banks, J. (1991). *Teaching strategies for ethnic studies* (5th ed.). Boston: Allyn & Bacon.

Baker, J. E. (1997). Minimizing the impact of parental grief on children: Parent and family interventions. In C. R. Figley, B. E. Bride, & N. Mazza (Eds.),

Death and trauma: The traumatology of grieving (pp. 139–158). Washington, DC: Taylor & Francis.

Barrios, B.A., & Hartmann, D. P. (1997). Fears and anxieties. In E. J. Mash & L. G. Terdal (Eds.), *Assessment of childhood disorders* (3rd ed., pp 230–327). New York: Guilford Press.

Berman, S. L., Kurtines, W. M., Silverman, W. K., & Serafini, L. T. (1996). The impact of exposure to crime and violence on urban youth. *American Journal of Orthopsychiatry, 66*, 329–336.

Bingham, R. D., & Harmon, R. J. (1996). Traumatic stress in infancy and early childhood. Expression of distress and developmental issues. In C. R. Pfeffer (Ed.), *Severe stress and mental disturbance in children* (pp. 499–532). Washington, DC: American Psychiatric Press.

Bowlby, J. (1960). Grief and mourning in infancy. *Psychoanalytic Study of the Child, 15*, 3–39.

Bowlby, J. (1973). *Attachment and loss: Vol. 2. Separation: Anxiety and anger.* London: Hogarth Press.

Bowlby, J. (1980). *Attachment and loss: Vol. 3. Loss.* London: Hogarth Press.

Brady, K. T. (2001). Presentation and epidemiology of PTSD. *Journal of Clinical Psychiatry, 62*(11), 907–909.

Brady, K. T., Killeen, T. K., Brewerton, T., et al. (2000). Comorbidity of psychiatric disorders and posttraumatic stress disorder. *Journal of Clinical Psychiatry, 61*(Suppl.), 22–32.

Breton, J. J., Valla, J. P., & Lambert, J. (1993). Industrial disaster and mental health of children and their parents. *Journal of the American Academy of Child and Adolescent Psychiatry, 32*, 438–445.

Briere, J. (1996). *Trauma Symptom Checklist for Children (TSCC).* Odessa, FL: Psychological Assessment Resources.

Chess, S., & Thomas, A. (1986). *Temperament in clinical practice.* New York: Guilford Press.

Cohen, J. A. (1998). American Academy of Child and Adolescent Psychiatry Work Group on Quality Issues: Practice parameters for the assessment and treatment of children and adolescents with posttraumatic stress disorder. *Journal of the American Academy of Child and Adolescent Psychiatry, 37*(Suppl.) 4S–26S.

Compas, B. E., & Epping, J. E. (1993). Stress and coping in children and families. In C. F. Saylor (Ed.), *Children and disasters* (pp. 11–28). New York: Plenum Press.

Drake, E. B., Bush, S. E., & van Gorp, W. G. (2001). Evaluation and assessment of PTSD in children and adolescents. In S. Eth (Ed.), *PTSD in children and adolescents* (pp. 1–31). Washington, DC: American Psychiatric Association.

Dutton, M. A. (1998). Cultural issues in trauma treatment. *Centering. Newsletter of the Center: Posttraumatic Disorders Program, 3*(2), 1–3.

Erikson, E. (1950). *Childhood and society.* New York: Norton.

Eth, S., & Pynoos, R. (1985). Interaction of trauma and grief in childhood. In S. Eth & R. Pynoos (Eds.), *Posttraumatic stress disorder in children* (pp. 169–186). Washington, DC: American Psychiatric Press.

Finch, A. J., Jr., & Daugherty, T. K. (1993). Issues in the assessment of posttraumatic stress disorder in children. In C. F. Saylor (Ed.), *Children and disasters* (pp. 45–66). New York: Plenum Press.

Fletcher, K. E. (1996). Childhood posttraumatic stress disorder. In E. J. Mash & R. A. Barkley (Eds.), *Child psychopathology* (pp. 242–276). New York: Guilford Press.

Folkman, S. (1991). Coping across the life span: Theoretical issues. In M. Cummings, A. Greene, & K. N. Karrakar (Eds.), *Life span developmental psychology: Perspectives on stress and coping* (pp. 3–19). Hillsdale, NJ: Erlbaum.

Fong, R. (Ed.). (2004). *Culturally competent practice with immigrant and refugee children and families.* New York: Guilford Press.

Frederick, C., Pynoos, R., & Nader, K. (1992). Childhood Post-Traumatic Stress Reaction Index (CPTS-RI). A copyrighted semistructured interview for children with traumatic exposure. Available from Frederick or Pynoos at the University of California, Los Angeles or from Nader (Knader@twosuns.org).

Freud, A., & Burlingham, D. (1943). *War and children.* New York: Ernest Willard.

Garbarino, J., Kostelny, K., & Dubrow, N. (1991). What children can tell us about living in danger. *American Psychologist, 46*(4), 376–383.

Goenjian, A. K., Pynoos, R. S., Steinberg, A. M., Najarian, L. M., Asarnow, J. R., Karayan, I., Ghurabi, M., & Fairbanks, L. A. (1995). Psychiatric comorbidity in children after the 1988 earthquake in Armenia. *Journal of the American Academy of Child and Adolescent Psychiatry, 34*, 1174–1184.

Goodnough, A. (2002, May 2). Post 9/11 pain found to linger in young minds. *The New York Times*, p. 1.

Gurwitch, R. H., Sullivan, M. A., & Long, P. J. (1998). The impact of trauma and disaster on young children. *Child and Adolescent Psychiatric Clinics of North America, 7*(1), 19–32.

Jacobs, S. C. (1999). *Traumatic grief: Diagnosis, treatment, and prevention.* New York: Brunner/Mazel.

Joyner, C. D., & Swensen, C. C. (1993). Community-level intervention after disasters. In C. F. Saylor (Ed.), *Children and disasters* (pp. 211–231). New York: Plenum Press.

Kessler, R. C., Sonnega, A., Bromet, E., Hughes, M., & Nelson, C. (1995). Posttraumatic stress disorder in the National Comorbidity Study. *Archives of General Psychiatry, 52*, 1048–1060.

Kinzie, J. D. (2001). Cross-cultural treatment of PTSD. In J. P. Wilson, M. J. Friedman, & J. D. Lindy (Eds.), *Treating psychological trauma and PTSD* (pp. 255–277). New York: Guilford Press.

Krug, R. S., Nixon, S. J., & Vincent, R. (1996). Psychological response to the Oklahoma City bombing. *Journal of Clinical Psychology, 52*(1), 103–105.

La Greca, A. M., Silverman, W. K., Vernberg, E. M., & Prinstein, M. J. (1996). Symptoms of posttraumatic stress in children after Hurricane Andrew: A prospective study. *Journal of Consulting and Clinical Psychology, 64*, 712–723.

La Greca, A. M., Silverman, W. K., & Wasserstein, S. B. (1998). Children's predisaster functioning as a predictor of posttraumatic stress following Hurricane Andrew. *Journal of Consulting and Clinical Psychology, 66*, 883–892.

Laor, N., Wolmer, L., Mayes, L. C., et al. (1996). Israeli preschoolers under Scud missile attacks: A developmental perspective on risk-modifying factors. *Archives of General Psychiatry, 53*, 416–423.

Lifton, R., & Olson, E. (1976). The human meaning of total disaster. *Psychiatry, 39*, 1–18.

Lonigan, C. J., Shannon, M. P., Taylor, C. M., Finch, A. J., & Sallee, F. R. (1994). Children exposed to disasters! II. Risk factors for the development of post-traumatic symptomatology. *Journal of the American Academy of Child Psychiatry, 33*, 94–105.

Marsten, A. S., Garmezy, N., Tellegen, A., Pellegrini, D. S., Larkin, K., & Larsen, A. (1988). Competence and stress in school children: The moderating effects of individual and family qualities. *Journal of Child Psychology and Psychiatry, 29*, 745–764.

McCann, I. L., Sakheim, D. K., & Abrahamson, D. J. (1988). Trauma and victimization: A model of psychological adaptation. *Counseling Psychologist, 16*, 531–594.

McFarlane, A. C., Policansky, S. K., & Irwin, C. (1987). A longitudinal study of children following a natural disaster. *Psychological Medicine, 17*, 727–738.

McFarlane, A. C., & Yehuda, R. (1996). Resilience, vulnerability, and the course of posttraumatic reactions. In B. A. van der Kolk, A. C. McFarlane, & L. Weisaeth (Eds.), *Traumatic stress: The effects of overwhelming experience on mind, body, and society,* (pp. 155–181). New York: Guilford Press.

McNally, R. J. (1998). Measures of children's reactions to stressful life events. In T. W. Miller (Ed.), *Children of traumas: Stressful life events and their effect on children* (pp. 29–42). Madison, CT: International Universities Press.

Merrick, A. (2001, October 18). Youths turn to Web magazines to unload fears. *The Wall Street Journal*, p. B1.

Nader, K. O. (1997). Treating traumatic grief in systems. In C. R. Figley, B. E. Bride, & N. Mazza (Eds.), *Death and trauma: The traumatology of grieving* (pp. 159–192). Washington, DC: Taylor & Francis.

Nader, K. (2001). Treatment methods for childhood trauma. In J. P. Wilson, M. Friedman, & J. Lindy (Eds.), *Treating psychological trauma and PTSD* (pp. 278–334). New York: Guilford Press.

Nader, K., Dubrow, N., & Stamm, B. H. (Eds.). (1999). *Honoring differences: Cultural issues in the treatment of trauma and loss.* Philadelphia: Brunner/Mazel.

Nader, K., Kriegler, J., Blake, D., & Pynoos, R. (1994). *Clinician-administered PTSD scale for children and adolescents (CAPS-C): A semi-structured interview for children with traumatic exposure.* White River Junction, VT: National Center for PTSD.

Nader, K. O., Newman, E., Weathers, F. W., et al. (1998). *Clinician Administered PTSD Scale for Children and Adolescents for DSM-IV (CAPS-CA).* Lebanon, NH: Hitchcock Foundation.

Nader, K., & Pynoos, R. (1991). Play and drawing as tools for interviewing traumatized children. In C. Schaefer, K. Gitlin, & A. Sandgrund (Eds.), *Play diagnosis and assessment* (pp. 275–389). New York: Wiley.

Nader, K., & Pynoos, R. S. (1993). School disaster: Planning and initial interventions. *Journal of Social Behavior and Personality, 8*, 299–320.

Nagy, M. (1948). The child's theories concerning death. *Journal of Genetic Psychology, 73*, 3–7.

Ozawa, M. (1997). Demographic changes and their implications. In M. Reisch & E. Gambrill (Eds.), *Social work in the twenty-first century* (pp. 8–27). Thousand Oaks, CA: Pine Forge Press.

Pearlin, L. I., & Schooler, C. (1978). The structure of coping. *Journal of Health and Social Behavior, 22*, 337–356.

Pfefferbaum, B. (1997). Posttraumatic stress disorder in children: A review of the past 10 years. *Journal of the American Academy of Child and Adolescent Psychiatry, 36*(11), 1503–1509.

Purnick, J. (2002, May 20). Portraits of trauma, beyond 9/11. *The New York Times,* p. B1.

Pynoos, R. S., & Eth, S. (1986). Witness to violence: The child interview. *Journal of the American Academy of Child Psychiatry, 25,* 306–319.

Pynoos, R. S., & Nader, K. (1988). Psychological first aid and treatment approach to children exposed to community violence: Research implications. *Journal of Traumatic Stress, 1*(4), 445–473.

Resick, P. A. (2001). *Stress and trauma.* Philadelphia: Psychology Press.

Ribbe, D. (1996). Psychometric review of Traumatic Event Screening Instrument for Children (TESI-C). In B. H. Stamm (Ed.), *Measurement of stress, trauma, and adaptation* (pp. 386–387). Lutherville, MD: Sidran Press.

Roje, J. (1996). LA '94 earthquake in the eyes of children: Art therapy with elementary school children who were victims of disaster. *Art Therapy, 12,* 1263–1284.

Saigh, P. A., Yaskik, A. E., Oberfield, R. A., Green, B. L., Halamandaris, P. V., & Rubenstein, H. (2000). The Children's PTSD Inventory: Development and reliability. *Journal of Traumatic Stress, 13*(3), 369–380.

Saylor, C. F., Belter, R., & Stokes, S. J. (1997). Children and families coping with disaster. In S. A. Wolchik & I. N. Sandler (Eds.), *Handbook of children's coping* (pp. 361–383). New York: Plenum Press.

Saylor, C. F., & Deroma, V. (2002). Assessment of children and adolescents exposed to disaster. In A. M. La Greca, W. K. Silverman, E. M. Vernberg, & M. C. Roberts (Eds.), *Helping children cope with disasters and terrorism* (pp. 35–53). Washington, DC: American Psychological Association.

Scheeringa, M. S., Zeanah, C. H., Drell, M. J., & Larrieu, J. A. (1995). Two approaches to the diagnosis of posttraumatic stress disorder in infancy and early childhood. *Journal of the American Academy of Child and Adolescent Psychiatry, 34,* 191–200.

Shalev, A. Y. (1996). Stress versus traumatic stress. From acute homeostatic reactions to chronic psychopathology. In B. A. van der Kolk, A. C. McFarlane, & L. Weisaeth (Eds.), *Traumatic stress: The effects of overwhelming experience on mind, body, and society* (pp. 77–101). New York: Guilford Press.

Shalev, A. Y., Peri, T., Canetti, L., & Schreiber, S. (1996). Predictors of PTSD in injured trauma survivors: A prospective study. *American Journal of Psychiatry, 153,* 219–225.

Shalev, A. Y., & Ursano, R. J. (2003). Mapping the multidimensional picture of acute responses to stress. In R. Orner & U. Schnyder (Eds.), *Reconstructing early interventions after trauma: Innovations in the care of survivors* (pp. 118–129). New York: Oxford University Press.

Shelby, J. S. (1997). Rubble, disruption, and tears: Helping young survivors of natural disaster. In H. Kaduson & C. Schaefer (Eds.), *The playing cure* (pp. 143–169). Northvale, NJ: Aronson.

Shibusawa, T. (2001). Parenting in Japanese-American families. In N. B. Webb (Ed.), *Culturally diverse parent–child and family relationships: A guide for social workers and other practitioners,* (pp. 283–303). New York: Columbia University Press.

Silverman, W. K., & La Greca, A. M. (2002). Children experiencing disasters: Definitions, reactions, and predictors of outcomes. In A. M. La Greca, W. K. Silverman, E. M. Vernberg, & M. C. Roberts (Eds.), *Helping children cope with disasters and terrorism* (pp. 11–33). Washington, DC: American Psychological Association.

Simpson, M. A. (1997). Traumatic bereavements and death-related PTSD. In C. R. Figley, B. E. Bride, & N. Mazza (Eds.), *Death and trauma: The traumatology of grieving* (pp. 3–16). Washington, DC: Taylor & Francis.

Speece, M. W., & Brent, S. B. (1996). The development of children's understanding of death. In C. A. Corr & D. M. Corr (Eds.), *Handbook of childhood death and bereavement* (pp. 29–49). New York: Springer.

Sullivan, M. A., Saylor, C. F., Foster, K. Y. (1991). Post-hurricane adjustment of preschoolers and their families. *Advances in Behavior Research and Therapy, 13,* 163–171.

Terr, L. C. (1983). Chowchilla revisited: The effects of psychic trauma four years after a school bus kidnapping. *American Journal of Psychiatry, 140,* 1543–1550.

Terr, L. C. (1991). Childhood traumas: An outline and overview. *American Journal of Psychiatry, 148,* 10–20.

Thomas, A., & Chess, S. (1981). The role of temperament in the contributions of individuals to their development. In R. M. Lerner & N. A. Busch-Rossnagel (Eds.), *Individuals as producers of their development* (pp. 231–254). New York: Academic Press.

van der Kolk, B. A. (1996). The body keeps the score: Approaches to the psychobiology of posttraumatic stress disorder. In B. A. van der Kolk, A. C. McFarlane, & L. Weisaeth (Eds.), *Traumatic stress: The effects of overwhelming experience on mind, body, and society* (pp. 214–241). New York: Guilford Press.

Vernberg, E. M., La Greca, A. M., Silverman, W. K., & Prinstein, M. J. (1996). Predictors of children's post-disaster functioning following Hurricane Andrew. *Journal of Abnormal Psychology, 105,* 237–248.

Webb, N. B. (Ed.). (1991). *Play therapy with children in crisis: A casebook for practitioners.* New York: Guilford Press.

Webb, N. B. (Ed.). (1993). *Helping bereaved children: A handbook for practitioners.* New York: Guilford Press.

Webb, N. B. (1996). *Social work practice with children.* New York: Guilford Press.

Webb, N. B. (Ed.). (1999). *Play therapy with children in crisis* (2nd ed.). *Individual, group, and family treatment.* New York: Guilford Press.

Webb, N. B. (Ed.). (2001). *Culturally diverse parent–child and family relationships: A guide for social workers and other practitioners.* New York: Columbia University Press.

Webb, N. B. (Ed.). (2002). *Helping bereaved children: A handbook for practitioners* (2nd ed.). New York: Guilford Press.

Webb, N. B. (2003). *Social work practice with children* (2nd ed.). New York: Guilford Press.

Werner, E. E., & Smith, R. S. (1982). *Vulnerable but invincible: A longitudinal study of resilient children and youth.* New York: McGraw-Hill.

Wertlieb, D., Weigel, C., Springer, T., & Feldstein, M. (1987). Temperament as a moderator of children's stressful experiences. *American Journal of Orthopsychiatry, 57*(2), 234–245.

Williams, M. B., Zinner, E. S., & Ellis, R. R. (1999). The connection between grief and trauma: An overview. In E. S. Zinner & M. B. Williams (Eds.), *When a community weeps: Case studies in group survivorship* (pp. 3–17). Philadelphia: Brunner/Mazel.

Wolfe, V. V., & Birt, J. A. (1997). Child sexual abuse. In E. J. Mash & L. G. Terdal (Eds.), *Assessment of childhood disorders* (3rd ed., pp. 569–623). New York: Guilford Press.

Wroble, M. C., & Baum, A. (2002). Toxic waste spills and nuclear accidents. In A. M. La Greca, W. K. Silverman, E. M. Vernberg, & M. C. Roberts (Eds.), *Helping children cope with disasters and terrorism* (pp. 207–221). Washington, DC: American Psychological Association.

Wu, S. J. (2001). Parenting in Chinese-American families. In N. B. Webb (Ed.), *Culturally diverse parent–child and family relationships: A guide for social workers and other practitioners* (pp. 235–260). New York: Columbia University Press.

Yehuda, R. (2001). Pathophysiology of PTSD. *Journal of Clinical Psychiatry, 62*(11), 909–910.

Zinner, E. S., & Williams, M. B. (1999). Summary and incorporation: A reference frame for community recovery and restitution. In E. S. Zinner & M. B. Williams (Eds.), *When a community weeps: Case studies in group survivorship* (pp. 237–254). Philadelphia: Brunner/Mazel.

CHAPTER 3

Treating Traumatized Children and Adolescents

Treatment Issues, Modalities, Timing, and Methods

KATHLEEN NADER

In the last quarter of a century, a number of treatment methods have been developed and adapted to address the traumatic reactions of children and their families (Nader, 2001, 2002). Many clinicians have discovered the importance of including multiple methods, modalities, and settings for effective treatment, especially after mass traumas. Traumatic reactions and treatment issues vary in response to the nature of the traumatic experience; the individual characteristics of each child; and characteristics of the family, culture, and other elements of the support system (Fletcher, 2003; Nader, 2003; Webb, 2002; see also Chapter 2, this volume). Clinical and field studies suggest that failure to resolve some individual symptoms, moderate to severe traumatic reactions, and associated reactions may result in long-term consequences that interfere with the child's ability to engage over time in productive behaviors and to function adequately—socially, academically, professionally, and personally (La Greca, Silverman, Vernberg, & Roberts, 2002; Nader, 2003; Silverman, Reinherz, & Giaconia, 1996; Wilson & Raphael, 1993). Moreover, exposure to ongoing threat, multiple traumas, or some individual traumatic experiences may result in specific changes that dramatically affect the course of a child's life, such as changes to neurobiological and other brain functions, moral code, and personality (De Bellis, Baum, et al., 1999; De Bellis,

Keshavan, et al., 1999; Garbarino, Kostelny, & Dubrow, 1991; Nader, 2001). This chapter first examines various issues related to the treatment of child and adolescent trauma. It then discusses the modalities, timing, and methods used in treatment following mass traumatic events.

INFLUENCES ON TRAUMATIC REACTIONS

As discussed in Chapters 1 and 2, aspects of the event, the child, and the support system influence children's traumatic reactions. The nature of the traumatic experience—the type of event and manner in which it unfolds; its intensity, duration, and phase; the degree of threat or loss; the meaning to the child of the event and its individual episodic moments; and its link to other issues in the child's life—affects the issues to be addressed in treatment, as well as the interventions chosen to address aspects of the child's response. As diagrammed in Chapter 2, this volume, on tripartite assessment, characteristics of the child or adolescent that affect the manner and course of treatment include, for example, age at onset of the trauma, current age, pubertal stage, personality, temperament, attachment style, cognitive and coping skills, and history. In addition, the family's history and style (e.g., early and subsequent experience, socioeconomic status, and family lifestyle) help to shape traumatic reactions, responses to treatment, and recovery (Fletcher, 2003; Nader, 2003), as do other aspects of the recovery environment (culture, religion, school/work/friends/peers, and the community at large).

TREATMENT ISSUES FOLLOWING MASS TRAUMAS

Family/Community Factors

Parent, peer, and family reactions to the traumatic event and a youth's symptoms may affect the intensity and course of the youth's response. Lack of support from parents or schools has been linked to elevated and long-lasting trauma symptoms (Ruchkin, Eisemann, & Hagglof, 1998; Rossman, Bingham, & Emde, 1997; Udwin, Boyle, Yule, Bolton, & O'Ryan, 2000). Treating the adults in children's lives, and enlisting the aid of families, schools, and peers, are important to children's recovery (Scheeringa & Zeanah, 2001). Threats to caregivers, parents' own traumatic reactions and symptoms, increased anxiety, perceived rejecting or guilt- and anxiety-inducing behaviors, and parents' own history of psychiatric disorder have all been associated with children's increased symptoms (Deblinger & Heflin, 1996; Scheeringa & Zeanah, 2001; La Greca et al., 2002). A caregiver's own trauma or response to a young child's trauma may interfere with the ability to give appropriate care (Scheeringa & Zeanah, 2001). The trauma of one or both (i.e., a young child or a caregiver) may adversely affect the child's relationship style. When parents have denied or suppressed awareness of their children's symptoms, children have had more intense reactions (Burke, Borus, Burns, Millstein, & Beasley, 1982). Mothers' and fathers' widely disparate reactions, increased parental conflict, and increased family chaos have been associated with children's adverse reactions or difficulty in recovering (Pelcovitz et al., 1998; Scheeringa & Zeanah, 2001). Therefore, interventions aimed at enlisting support, assisting adults, and helping families are all part of a comprehensive intervention.

Attachment Factors (Style/Relationship Behavior)

Because traumas may affect attachment styles and attachment styles may affect reactions to traumas, some treatment methods for childhood trauma include or begin with treatments of the attachment relationship between parent (or other primary caregiver) and child (James, 1994; Copping, Warling, Benner, & Woodside, 2001). Relationships are not only encoded in memory, but also help to shape the very brain circuits that enable memories, relationships and self-regulatory processes (Siegel, 2003). Childhood traumas have affected child and adult attachment styles, psychological development, and interactional styles with peers and adults (Lyons-Ruth & Jacobvitz, 1999; Roche, Runtz, & Hunter, 1999). These changes sometimes reflect, for example, posttrauma increases in impulsiveness, fears, aggressive reactivity, irritability, or reactivity to reminders.

As discussed at the beginning of Chapter 1, early attachment styles become "working models" for significant social ties or interactions throughout life (Bowlby, 1973; Bretherton, 1993). Parental attachment styles may affect children's memory capacities, traumatic recall, and responses to stressful or novel situations (Goodman & Quas, 1996; Howe, 1997). They may also affect a youth's interactions with and expectations of a treating clinician, peers, and authority figures. Aspects of ongoing traumas or single-incident traumatic events (e.g., disruption to attachment styles, impaired functioning, feeling overwhelmed, prolonged separation, fear, anxiety, and misinterpretation of behaviors) can lead to patterns of child or parent behavior that seriously interfere with the attachment relationship. A parent may not be able to recognize or respond adequately to a child's needs; the child may not be able to express needs adequately or respond to the adult (Field, Seligman, Scafidi, & Schanberg, 1996; James, 1994; Scheeringa & Zeanah, 2001). A parent's own trauma or response to a young child's trauma has sometimes resulted in inadequate, withdrawn, overprotective/smothering, endangering, or constrictive caretaking (James, 1994; Scheeringa & Zeanah, 2001).

Attachment insecurity has been associated with a variety of symptoms and disorders (Greenberg, 1999; West, Adam, Spreng, & Rose, 2001) and with increased posttraumatic symptoms (Muller, Sicoli, & Lemieux, 2000). Studies suggest that toddlers with insecure attachments have higher cortisol levels in response to stressful or novel situations than children with secure attachments (Gunnar, Brodersen, Krueger, & Rigatuso, 1996; Nachmias, Gunnar, Mangelsdorf, Parritz, & Buss, 1996). Animal studies suggest that cortisol reactivity can be inherited by offspring (Suomi & Levine, 1998). Moreover, trauma-generated disorganized/disoriented insecure attachment may result in an inability to generate a coherent strategy for coping with relational stress (Schore, 2002).

In addition to the normal attachment bonds between infants and parents are the bonds that occur under traumatic circumstances (e.g., to other victims or to perpetrators). Children may develop increased attachments to those with whom they endure a traumatic experience. "Hostage syndrome" is the increase of attachment to perpetrators during traumatic events. A child victim perceives outside help as unavailable; a dominant person alternates between terroristic and nurturing behaviors, thus strengthening the bonds; responses such as dissociation, numbing, or self-blame, among others, lead to a confusion of pain and love; the victim's need for attachment overcomes fears (James, 1994; Ochberg & Soskis, 1982). This kind of trauma bonding is based on terror—the sense that one's life is in danger and the assailant is in total control. Relief over survival may be experienced as gratitude toward the perpetrator.

Culture and Religion

Applying issues of culture to traumatic response and recovery is not a simple task. For example, determining the need for cultural rituals is not as simple as determining whether a person is one, two, or more generations removed from a homeland. Acculturation, nationalization, regionalization, peer influence, and personal and family history all contribute to the differences within cultures. In addition to the recognized ethnic (e.g., African American, Asian, Hispanic, Native American), national (e.g., American, Croatian, Japanese, Italian), and religious (e.g., Christian, Hindu, Jewish, Muslim) cultures are those that develop, for example, regionally (e.g., the Southern, Northern, Western United States) and experientially (e.g., groups that emerge in response to a common experience such as trauma, loss, or injury). Aspects of personality (e.g., temperament, style, introversion vs. extraversion), location (e.g., specific community, rural vs. inner-city), and circumstance become intertwined with culture and religion and affect a child's readiness to share aspects of self and experience, pacing in treatment, world view, tendency to want to focus on the positive or the negative in a situation, and other treatment issues (Nader, 2003).

Trauma Recall

Even young children can and do accurately recall, over considerable time, participatory and nonparticipatory (e.g., witnessing) single-incident or ongoing traumatic experiences (Howe, 1997; Lewis, 1995; Nader, 2001). There is evidence that between ages 2½ and 4, recall increases with age. Preschool children are able to recall considerable information about their traumatic experiences, whether or not they had initial intrusive thoughts (Howe, Courage, & Peterson, 1995). Between 18 months and 2 years of age, children begin to use symbolic play and language to represent experience (Piaget, 1952) and may demonstrate in their play their perceptual memories of traumatic experiences (Terr, 1985). As early as age 2, children can show what did and did not happen. It is easier for preschoolers to identify familiar people and details relevant to their lives than unfamiliar individuals and details (Murray & Son, 1998). Young children are more concrete than older persons in their thinking (Lewis, 1995). Literal interpretations, animistic thinking, faulty hypotheses, and inaccurate associations are common (Murray & Son, 1998). For example, things occurring in spacial and temporal proximity may be seen as causal. Generalizations are common (e.g., from "one man is bad" to "all men are bad"). Unlike their interpretations, statements may not be literal; for example, "I hate you" may mean "I dislike what you are doing" (Murray & Son, 1998). Preschool children move easily from one focus to another and are easily distracted. Although they may become frightened during traumatic play and stop playing, young children may be able to continue after being comforted or after distracting themselves temporarily (Nader, 2001).

School-age children can form mental pictures and describe sequences of events without performing them. They can readily depict, in thought, in words and in play, the intense images and wishes that may have occurred during or after a traumatic event (e.g., fantasized interventions or escapes). They are able to focus on more than one aspect of a situation simultaneously and are aware that some actions can be reversed by subsequent actions (Brodzinsky, Gormly, & Ambron, 1986). Following traumatic experiences, children have included distortions of time and space (Terr, 1985; Pynoos & Nader, 1989) or have attempted to fill in gaps in their memories by confabulating. When given prompts or cues, however, children remember quite well (Lewis, 1995; Johnson & Foley, 1984). For example, Pynoos and Nader (1989) found that children who incorporated their wishful thinking into their unassisted retelling of a traumatic event were able to report their experiences accurately when assisted to begin at a specific point and proceed through the details of the event. Faulty pre- and postevent information can result in distortions in recall (Siegel, 1996). It is important that clinicians avoid introducing these confusions. In studies of small samples of adults, individuals with higher scores on measures of creative imagination or dissociation were more likely to recover false or previously unavailable true events when asked to form a mental image of an event (International Society for Traumatic Stress Studies, 1998).

Location of Treatment

Especially after mass traumas, the availability and location of treatment become significant issues. Assessment of traumatic reactions and progress in treatment requires an examination of children's emotional expressions, behaviors, and interactions in a variety of settings. Because children behave and respond differently in different contexts (i.e., to different settings and amidst different individuals), comprehensive assessment of children includes collecting information from multiple sources and in multiple contexts. Direct observation of children at school or day care, with caregivers, and in clinical settings has assisted the ongoing assessment and treatment-planning process (Achenbach & Rescorla, 2001; Friedrich et al., 2001; Nader, 2003; Reynolds & Kamphaus, 1998). Moreover, some interventions are best suited for specific settings. The course of and recovery from traumatization has been affected, for example, by whether or not a child's school was supportive (Udwin et al., 2000).

After mass traumas, assessment and interventions can be most effectively pursued within the school environment (Nader & Muni, 2002; Williams, 1994; Yule, Udwin, & Bolton, 2002; see also Chapter 6, this volume). School is a familiar, safe setting for youth. Because students are already in the building and transportation is not a problem, appointment attendance is assured. School assessment permits the enlistment of support and feedback from peers, teachers, and staff. When the trauma has occurred at the school, on-site treatment allows each individual, when ready, to work through traumatic material in the location where it occurred (Nader & Muni, 2002). Whether or not the event has affected the whole school or the larger community, schools are an excellent location for specific interventions, such as reintegration of severely traumatized or injured children into the classroom, collaboration with teachers and staff to assist traumatized children, and group treatments. For example, psychoeducational groups (e.g., for parents, teachers, or children), parent support groups (e.g., for grieving parents or parents of injured children), peer support groups (e.g., for a traumatized child and emotionally healthy peers or the child and other traumatized children), grief groups (e.g., for grieving children, grieving children and peers, or grieving children and children who have already recovered from loss; Nader & Mello, 2001; Webb, 2002), and injured children's groups (e.g., for injured children or injured children and physically and emotionally healthy supportive peers) have all been conducted at school sites (Nader & Mello, 2001). After mass traumas, private rooms in schools have been allotted for individual and group treatment sessions.

MODALITIES

Treatment for childhood trauma almost always includes more than one type of intervention (e.g., individual, conjoint, group). Successes have been demonstrated for a number of individual treatment methods (Nader, 2001; Terr, 1989, 2001; Webb, 1991, 1999, 2003). Most clinicians using individual methods include adjunctive treatment methods as well. Group methods have been used effectively as adjunctive (Cohen & Mannarino, 1997; Nader & Mello, 2001; Silberg, 1998) or as primary (March, Amaya-Jackson, Foa, & Treadwell, 1999; Yule & Williams, 1990) treatment methods for trauma symptoms. Some methods address specific symptoms that hinder progress or functioning (e.g., arousal symptoms such as sleep disturbance, irritability, or reduced impulse control; difficulty coping with trauma symptoms; Field et al., 1996; Glodich, 1999; Krakow et al., 2000, 2001; March et al., 1999). General adaptations are made in treatment methods for different age groups, for different types of experiences (e.g., child abuse, shootings), and for different types of problems (e.g., dissociative disorders) (Cohen, 1999; Nader, 2001, 2002; Putnam, 1997; Silberg, 1998).

Individual Treatment Methods

Individual methods differ according to a clinician's training, philosophy, and style. Although the primary method may be, for example, play, behavioral, or cognitive-behavioral therapy, a number of clinicians include aspects of each in the overall treatment process (Nader, 2001, 2002; Parson, 1996; Terr, 2001; Webb, 2003). Most individual treatment methods for school-age children include retelling (at least once, and sometimes repeatedly) of the traumatic experience, as well as work toward changing behaviors and thoughts that interfere with functioning and desirable emotional states.

Case of Jason[1]

Jason was a 14-year-old boy with a good grade point average who played an offensive position on the football team. He lived with his mother and a series of "stepfathers" who left, often after Jason had developed an attachment to them. One day when he was eating a school lunch with his team-

---

[1]This case has been disguised and is a composite of more than one mass trauma event.

mates, three male classmates entered the high school with guns and explosive devices. They rushed into the cafeteria and started firing. Three students were killed, and others were injured by bullets, flying glass, and debris, or in the rush to exit the cafeteria. With a bullet wound in his arm, Jason ran with other students into a janitor's closet. For more than an hour the students hovered quietly, fearing discovery and annihilation. Jason spent the time reliving the images of the bullets hitting his friends and the bone, flesh, and blood flying across the table; the sounds of gunfire, bullets hitting, and blood splattering; and the smells of blood and burning sulfur mixed with the smells of his lunch. Other students must have been having the same memories, because two of them threw up—new images and smells to add to the memories. Jason examined the blood on his shirt and tried to figure out how much was his and how much was a friend's. When he realized that some of his friend's flesh was stuck to his shirt, he struggled against regurgitating. He slipped into sleep a few times.

Jason's arm did not hurt until emergency room staff began to examine him. He remained in the hospital for 2 weeks, where he began his physical therapy—the bullet had cracked a bone. Jason had posttraumatic stress and additional symptoms. He experienced feelings of panic when he heard popping or splattering sounds, and had repeated memory flashes and nightmares about his friends being torn apart by the impact of bullets. He responded with nausea to smells that resembled those from his experience. Jason did not want to return to school. He was irritable and seemed to alternate between feelings of helplessness and rage.

After some physical recovery, Jason started school-based individual trauma treatment. In therapy sessions he recreated episodic experiences, using replicas of his peers, the cafeteria, the school, and the closet. Play/reenactment, cognitive reprocessing, abreactive reprocessing, and exposure techniques were utilized (see "Methods," below). Recognizing Jason's timing and readiness, specific perceptions, desires for intervention or retaliation, aspects of interactions and relationships, bereavement, previous experiences, and other meaningful aspects of the event became the prominent focus in different treatment sessions. Jason was unable to grieve until he had addressed aspects of his traumatic response. After a year of treatment, Jason seemed to regress; he began to play with elementary-school-age toys. This continued until he had completed some developmental tasks into which he incorporated traumatic imagery. He then returned to symbolically and directly working through aspects of trauma and grief.

Parent and Family Treatment

Ample evidence suggests that including parents in the treatment process (e.g., parent meetings, conjoint sessions, psychoeducation, family sessions) may aid children's recovery (Deblinger, Lippmann, & Steer, 1996;

Friedrich, 1996; Nader & Mello, 2001; Silberg, 1998; Webb, 2003). Individual parent sessions or parent groups have enlisted the cooperation of parents in the treatment process; have assisted parents to understand their children's responses, to adjust to regressions and other changes in the children, and to establish a rhythm with each child that enhances recovery; and have trained parents in methods of dealing with specific child behaviors and symptoms (Nader & Mello, 2001; Silberg, 1998). Conjoint or family work has helped children and other family members when, for example, (1) there has been intense worry about a family member during the traumatic event; (2) there are differences in the course of response and recovery; (3) cooperation is needed to resolve specific issues; or (4) family dysfunction impedes progress.

Case of Jason, Continued

Jason's mother (Tanya) was frantic when she heard about the shootings. In addition to her response to her son's injury and the deaths of his peers, Tanya began to reexperience symptoms that had followed an assault on her 10 years before. She was referred for individual treatment, and she attended periodic psychoeducational and regular parent group meetings at the school to learn about Jason's traumatic response and how to cope with changes in his behavior. A few conjoint sessions assisted Tanya and Jason with Tanya's sense of being overwhelmed and tendency toward overprotection, and Jason's tendency to be rageful and defiant.

Groups

Whether to make groups a primary or an adjunct treatment method depends on such factors as the number of children affected by the event and the goals of treatment. Group methods have reduced posttraumatic stress disorder (PTSD) and specific symptoms (Glodich, 1999; March et al., 1999). There are advantages and disadvantages of group treatment for traumatized children (Nader, 2001). Advantages include the following: Groups can help to overcome any "conspiracy of silence" (Danieli, 1985); a larger number can be treated; youth learn that others in their situation have experienced similar emotions; youth may accept from peers what they will not accept from adults; members benefit from the work of others; and there are opportunities for listening without participating (Glodich, 1999; Terr, 1989). Limitations of group methods are as follows (Terr, 1989): (1) Courtroom credibility is lost because of group influence; (2) new symptoms may develop after a youth hears new types of horrors from others; (3) some aspects of traumatic experience and response are very personal and private; and (4) the needed examination of internal mental processes stimulated by trauma may not be possible or advisable without the privacy of individual sessions. Youth's inclinations to be strongly influenced by their perceived expectations of others can be both an advantage and a disadvantage of group treatment. Some individual treatment may be essential to prevent the translation of traumatic impressions or symptoms into ongoing undesirable patterns of behavior (Nader, 2001). Following mass traumas, group methods have helped to educate, provide support, resolve differences, and assist recovery. Multiple methods and modalities may be best for traumatized youth.

After mass traumas affecting multicultural populations, consideration must be given to the composition of therapy groups. Assessment must take into account multiple factors. Culture and religion in and of themselves may or may not be issues for young children. For a parent group, however, questions must be asked about how differences affect the group's ability to meet its goals. After September 11, 2001, planned mixed religious groups following specific guidelines have helped individuals to use religion and each other as support systems (Drescher, in press). In contrast, following the 1992 Los Angeles riots, several all-female teacher groups were half Hispanic and half African American. The African American teachers expressed rage and desires for retaliation. The Hispanic teachers were afraid and desirous of protection. Their fears of the African American teachers resulted in reluctance to share anything that might upset the African American teachers (Stuber, Nader, & Pynoos, 1997). The question becomes whether resolving such difficulties is part of a group's purpose or will interfere with it. If the goal is reconciliation, then one of the goals should be resolution of reluctance and fear. If the goal is to gather information or to process the traumatic experience, mixed groups of two cultures experiencing tensions will be ineffective unless these issues are resolved.

Attention must be given to the subcultures that arise from mass traumas. For example, parents of either traumatized, dead, or injured youth may become tightly knit groups. After a tornado, tensions arose between parents of deceased and those of traumatized children, whose separate therapy groups were led by unassociated therapists. Preexisting adult or child groups (e.g., cliques or subgroups) may become less permeable after mass traumatic events. For example, it was important to include part-time teachers in posttornado teacher group meetings, in order to minimize the already existing division between the full-timers and the part-timers (Nader, 1997). Some adult and child groups have benefited from including unexposed, nontraumatized members to provide support and to reduce the reinforcement of a traumatic state of mind.

Case of Jason, Continued

Before Jason was able to return to school, a classroom session was held to prepare his classmates for his reentry. Two additional classroom sessions were held, one of them after Jason yelled and slapped at his hovering peers. Each of the students who had been in the closet with Jason had different traumatic reactions and courses of recovery. It was not until each of them had made some progress in individual treatment that they were brought together for several group sessions regarding their closet experience. If sufficient staffing had been available, Jason would also have benefited from a four-member group with one other grieving student and two nontraumatized peers who had already resolved a previous loss.

TIMING, COURSE OF TREATMENT, AND RECOVERY

Variations in Course of Treatment

Recognizing variations in the course of treatment and recovery is important to effective posttrauma treatment. Individual children and family members will have different recovery rates, trauma issues, and readiness to focus on or resolve specific issues. Part of the treatment process will include assisting differently traumatized and nontraumatized peers or family members to adjust to their varying paces, needs, concerns, and foci. For example, some family or peers will be ready to return to a normal course of activities or to grieve, while some individuals may need to resolve specific trauma issues before returning to the normal routine or grieving. The needs of grieving families to honor their deceased members, or the needs of some individuals for more information about the trauma, may conflict with the needs of traumatized individuals to have periods without being reminded of the event. Scheeringa and Zeanah (2001) tell the story of a child who would cry in a corner until his mother stopped prodding him for details about his experience. Differences in course or needs may become a source of stress for a community group or family. For example, after the tornado mentioned above, parents of deceased children began quarreling angrily with parents of traumatized children over the number and nature of memorials visible in a school.

Across the course of treatment, a child or adolescent may emerge from varying degrees or stages of numbing. When the event is perceived to be over rather than ongoing, or when the numbing wears off, there may be a reassessment of the experience or an aspect of it, its results, and one's role in it; of beliefs and expectations; and of the meaning of events and interactions. In order to cope, the youth may unwittingly intersperse periods of numbing and avoidance between phases of reexperiencing and arousal or between attempts to face aspects of his or her experience and response (Nader, 2003). The child's periodic need for avoidance of traumatic memories and thoughts can be honored across the course of his or her response, while gently assisting the child therapeutically.

Length of Treatment

The length of treatment for traumatized youth varies, depending on a number of factors; these include the method used, the number of traumas, the severity of traumatic response, personality, previous experience, emotional health, and family circumstances (Nader & Mello, 2001). Mildly to moderately traumatized children and adolescents may benefit from 2–16 sessions (Goenjian et al., 1997; March et al., 1999; Nader, 2001). Moderately to severely traumatized youth may need 1–3 years of treatment or more. Exposure to specific experiences (e.g., life threat, multiple bloody deaths or injuries) may prolong the length of treatment needed to fully resolve traumatic reactions. Specific characteristics of a youth or aspects of the trauma may increase the length of treatment, regardless of exposures. Over the course of treatment, additional sessions may be required as a result of developmental factors, trauma factors, or life events, or as traumatic impressions take on new meaning for the youth/adult (Nader, 2001).

In addition to the symptoms of PTSD, intense traumatic impressions may affect a youth's quality of life and may result in undesired patterns of thought and behavior (Nader, 2001). When there have been dual or multiple individual traumas or a trauma and loss, attention to relevant aspects of each event and their interactions may be necessary. Depending on the emotional impact of each event, some children may need first to address a previous trauma before attending to the current event; others may be reminded over time of the previous trauma and undergo symptoms related to each; some may need to address aspects of the trauma before they can grieve. In addition, issues that were of relevance in an earlier trauma or traumatic sequence (e.g., abandonment, betrayal, victimization) may appear as issues in the current trauma or traumatic episode (Nader & Mello, 2001).

METHODS

For people of all ages, following traumatic events, it is important to restore a sense of safety and to meet physical needs prior to other interventions. Some relief is afforded traumatized youths by caring adults providing assessment, preliminary interventions, comforting contact, or routine community service (Friedrich, 1996; Nader, 2003). Specialized treatment methods can provide additional relief, recovery, and prevention of future disturbances in emotional well-being, character, personality and behavior. Although treating a selected range of symptoms may help to alleviate some of the other symptoms (March et al., 1999), multiple treatment foci are needed for a child who presents with a range of symptoms (Friedrich, 1996; Nader, 2001).

Effective treatment requires (1) a good fit among method, clinician, and child; (2) an understanding of childhood trauma and child psychotherapy principles; (3) flexibility; (4) rapport with children; (5) observational skills; (6) knowledge of treatment methods; and (7) skill in child therapy. Some methods require more communication, interpretive skills, insight, and/or empathy than others. Although clinicians have made adjustments for single-incident versus multiple or ongoing traumas (Cohen, 1999; Nader, 2001; Parson, 1996), whether specific methods are best applied for individual child characteristics (e.g., personality, temperament, locus of control) and situations (e.g., specific levels or kinds of exposures, previous experiences, or relationships) has not been clearly delineated.

Most treatment approaches for school-age and older children include single or repeated narratives of the traumatic experience; play is commonly used for young children (Pynoos, Nader, & March, 1991; Webb, 1999). A number of methods (e.g., cognitive-behavioral therapy, psychodynamic psychotherapy) may be successful to the extent that they selectively activate representational processes dominant in each brain hemisphere (right and left) and integrate them (Siegel, 2003). Many treatments include a combination of methods (e.g., cognitive, behavioral, play) as adjunctive methods or method components.

Drawings

Drawings have been used as major or minor components of some treatment methods (Nader & Pynoos, 1991). In their drawings, children invariably signify, in some way, their unconscious preoccupations with trauma memories. The use of drawings (and play) in the assessment and treatment of trauma can (1) display a child's spatial representation of the event; (2) indicate the child's processing and eventual resolution of traumatic elements; (3) reveal elements of the child's continuing internal experience and the details of the event that continue to influence the child; (4) provide opportunities for reexamination of an experience, in order to give it new meaning; (5) permit the child to symbolically complete a desired or fantasied act within a safe therapeutic setting, and (6) permit the interpretation or the linking of depictions to aspects of a traumatic episode. When a youth draws a picture and tells a story about it, a traumatic link is most often identified after completion of the story.

Although some symbols may appear frequently after traumatic deaths (e.g., balloons, flowers), each child's *own* symbolism, history, and personal traumatic experience are the most important factors. For example, after Rashida's therapist recognized that a four-leaf clover represented shared behaviors with her friend who had been killed in a bombing, the changing location and color of the clover in Rashida's pictures were more meaningful to the therapist. Jason's inadvertent smudges on the clothing of drawn figures were reminiscent of the tissue that had stuck to his shirt during the shootings (see the case example presented earlier).

Play Therapy

Play therapy has been adapted for use with single-incident and repeated traumas (Gil, 1991, 1998; Webb, 1991, 1999) and is often a component of other treatment methods (March et al, 1999). Methods of play therapy differ in the levels and nature of their guidelines and structure; in their emphasis on play versus verbalization; and in the amounts of direction from, interpretation by, and participation by the therapist. Approach, sequencing of interventions, and focus on reconstruction of the event or its episodes vary among clinicians, across methods, and by age group (Nader, 2001, 2002). When play therapy is a component of other treatments, techniques such as drawings, stories, board games, or specific rule-guided interactions may be used. When play therapy is the primary mode of treatment, the therapy room usually includes a variety of drawing materials, toys, and other materials that permit the youth to focus on or deviate from focusing exclusively on traumatic themes (Webb, 1991, 2002).

Among the styles of play therapy that have been adapted for traumatized youth (Gil, 1991) are psychoanalytic (Esman, 1983; Freud, 1965), facilitated (Levy, 1939; Nader, 2001, 2002; Pynoos & Eth, 1986; Terr, 2001; Webb, 1999), group (Homeyer, 1999; Leben, 1995), relationship-oriented (Axline, 1969; James, 1994), and sandtray (Gil, 1991; Kalff, 1980) play therapies. Therapists may use an integrated approach—for example, a combination of directive and nondirective methods, of interpretation and silent observation, of relationship and trauma-focused methods (Gil, 1998; James, 1994; Webb, 1999). Selected methods are described below.

Directive Play Therapies

Directive play therapy (Nader, 2001, 2002; Pynoos & Eth, 1986; Terr, 2001) facilitates the abreactive or cognitive reprocessing of traumatic impressions and emotions. In directive play therapy, to one degree or another, the therapist assumes responsibility for guidance of the play. As in nondirective play therapy, the child may direct the action or assign characters. The clinician's direction may be as simple as a request to focus more intensely or in more detail on a scene, or the clinician may assist a child to talk about the unspeakable (James, 1994). Directions may also be more complex. For example, recognizing clues from the child's symbolic drawings or actions, the therapist may establish a rhythm with the child in which he or she follows in the direction the child is moving and then adds, magnifies, redefines, assists, or even carefully pushes the child through processing a set of memories and emotions. Some eclectic (Bevin, 1999;

Nader & Mello, 2001; Pynoos & Eth, 1986), cognitive-behavioral (March et al., 1999), and relationship-focused (James, 1994) play therapies are directive (Nader, 2001).

Nondirective Play Therapies

In non-directive play therapy, the therapist permits the child ample opportunity to direct his or her own play and therapy (Axline, 1969; Gil, 1998). The child is given permission not only to be him- or herself, but also to depict his or her own reality in the child's own way. That self and that reality are completely accepted, without evaluation or pressure to change. Although the clinician may act as silent witness while the child externalizes his or her internal reality, nondirective therapies generally encourage insight and personality development through interpretation (e.g., recognition and clarification or verbalization of emotions and attitudes; Axline, 1969; Gil, 1998). Many psychoanalytic and sandtray play therapies are nondirective; they use the transference relationship and nondirective observation of the child's play and behavior, followed by interpretations or directions of attention designed to elicit insights and subsequent changes (Gil, 1998).

Relationship-Focused Play Therapies

Preexisting disturbed attachment styles affect a youth's level of posttrauma symptoms, interactions with a therapist, and the course of recovery. Single, chronic, and repeated traumatizing events may be characterized by, or may create, faulty attachment relationships. Relationship-focused play therapies address attachment relationships (e.g., the child's ability to engage in healthy child–adult interactions such as interactive play, conjoint problem solving, or healthy touch; Brody, 1994; Harvey, 1994; James, 1994). Emotionally deprived or seriously traumatized young children are often inhibited in their abilities to engage in symbolic play or fantasy; in order to benefit from relationship or other play therapy, some children first must be taught how to play (James, 1994). Relationship-focused therapy may include the individual child or the family.

Group Play Therapy

Group play therapy has been used successfully with traumatized youth, often in combination with individual, family, and sibling therapies (Homeyer, 1999; Sweeney & Homeyer, 1999). Group members may include children with the same gender, similar physical size, and similar developmental age, together with a balanced number of those who internalize versus those who externalize the trauma in behaviors (Homeyer, 1999).

Group play therapy is contraindicated for youth who exhibit the ability to hurt others without remorse, serious psychiatric disturbances, suicidal behavior, nonsuicidal self-mutilation, or severe mood or thought disturbances; it is also contraindicated for youngsters who were recently abused in a group.

In nondirective group play therapy, the children and the play therapist are actors on the stage of each child's design and direction (Homeyer, 1999). When appropriate, the therapist sets limits and enlarges the meaning so that the children can better hear or see the meaning of each child's story. Directive group play therapy sessions may include motivational games and games selected to meet individual objectives for each child or a main objective for the entire group (e.g., learning to "boss back PTSD"; March et al., 1999). Groups may include (sometimes fast-paced) structured and semistructured games. Groups are modified to meet children's ongoing needs and to facilitate discussion. Skills learned in a group are generally transferred to other social situations (Leben, 1995) and may be followed by reductions in other symptoms (March et al., 1999).

Behavioral and Cognitive Therapies

Behavioral and cognitive methods may serve as primary treatment or adjunctive methods. Behavioral therapists strive to change behaviors and thereby reduce distressing thoughts and feelings. Cognitive therapists first change thoughts and feelings, thereby improving functional behavior (March et al., 1999). Treatment may include a variety of behavioral and cognitive techniques, such as exposure, cognitive restructuring, behavior management, psychoeducation, stress management, and safety skills (Cohen, 1999; Silberg, 1998); over the course of sessions, it may include some play therapy methods as well (e.g., the child reviews and adds to a book or artwork).

Exposure Therapy

In exposure therapy (Deblinger & Heflin, 1996; Saigh, Yule, & Inamdar, 1996), fears are confronted in a systematic manner. Confrontation with the feared stimuli (e.g., traumatic reminders) is followed by the introduction of corrective information (e.g., the reminder itself does not represent danger, remembering the trauma is not the same as reexperiencing it, anxiety can diminish without avoidance, and experiencing trauma symptoms does not have to lead to loss of control; see Meadows & Foa, 1998). For example, "gradual exposure" techniques may include encouraging the child to describe a traumatic episode repeatedly and with increasing detail (Bevin, 1999; Cohen, 1999; Cohen, Berliner, & Mannarino, 2000; Deblinger & Heflin, 1996; Nader & Mello, 2001). Recounting a traumatic memory decreases the associated anxiety, thus allowing reorganization of the memory (March et al., 1999). Prolonged exposure (Saigh et al., 1996) and eye movement desensitization and reprocessing (EMDR; Greenwald, 1994, 1998; Lovett & Shapiro, 1999; Pellicer, 1993) therapies are among the exposure therapy methods used with traumatized youth.

Cognitive Therapy

Cognitive appraisals of events and what one already knows can influence reactions to stressful, novel, or traumatic situations (e.g., Gunnar et al., 1996; Howe, 1997). Cognitive therapy is based on the assumption that the interpretation of an event, rather than the event itself, determines emotional states. Accordingly, dysfunctional thoughts (e.g., inaccurate or overly extreme thoughts) lead to pathological emotional responses. Treatment is aimed at changing the pathological thoughts first by identifying the thoughts underlying intense negative emotional states, then by evaluating their validity and challenging erroneous or unhelpful thoughts, and finally by replacing the thoughts with more logical or beneficial ones (Meadows & Foa, 1998). For example, treatment progress may be reflected in an increasingly coherent narrative of the trauma that can be more readily integrated with the victim's existing mental schemas (March et al., 1999; Siegel, 2003). Among the cognitive treatment methods for trauma are individual trauma-focused cognitive-behavioral therapy (Cohen, 1998, 1999; Cohen & Mannarino, 1997) and group trauma-focused coping (March et al., 1999; March, Amaya-Jackson, Murry, & Schulte, 1998; March, Amaya-Jackson, Terry, & Costanzo, 1997). Cognitive restructuring, redefinition, or processing are used as components of some directive play therapies (Nader, 2001; Terr, 2001).

Behavioral Management Strategies

Behavioral management strategies are used for children who are exhibiting inappropriate behaviors (e.g., conduct disturbances, sexualized behavior problems). Contingency reinforcement programs can be used to help such children develop more appropriate alternative behaviors and to reward adaptive behaviors (Cohen et al., 2000). Reinforcement may include active ignoring or time outs, as well as providing desired responses, items, privileges, or situations (e.g., desired time with a specific person).

Psychoeducation

Psychoeducational information (e.g., about trauma, loss, the course of recovery, the nature of specific symptoms or syndromes) can help to prepare for or normalize the child's and parent's reactions. Psychoeducational groups have been used to assist cognitive restructuring regarding specific posttrauma symptoms (e.g., reenactment; Allen, Kelly, & Glodich, 1997) or specific traumatic events such as child abuse (Cohen et al., 2000) or mass traumas (Nader & Mello, 2001).

Anxiety Management Techniques

Anxiety or stress management techniques reflect the view that pathological anxiety results from skill deficits (Meadows & Foa, 1998). Techniques such as deep breathing, progressive muscle relaxation, thought stopping, and positive imagery can add to a child's sense of control over negative thoughts and emotions. A brief massage therapy technique has been used to reduce anxiety, depression, and cortisol levels (Field et al., 1996). Stress management techniques may be especially helpful at bedtime, during school, or with friends. In treatments that do not use the escalation of emotions in the processing of traumas, stress management techniques may be used during sessions (e.g., exposure sessions; Cohen et al., 2000).

Multimodal Treatment Methods

Many treatment methods use a number of adjunct treatments to supplement the main method. Multimodal treatment methods use a combination of methods within a series of overlapping or consecutive treatment phases. For example, a multimodal family therapy method might include these phases: (1) team building, assessment, and restoration of safety; (2) exploration of problematic and alternative behavioral patterns (through individual, family, play, and group therapy); and (3) relapse prevention (review of what has been learned and changed, planning for future difficulties, and recognition of strengths (Trepper & Barrett, 1986, 1989). For multitraumatized inner-city youth, posttrauma child therapy has included these phases: (1) pretherapy (modeling, role play, psychoeducational techniques, focus, and goal setting); (2) stabilization (cognitive and behavioral techniques, and, when indicated, psychopharmacology and/or residential treatment); (3) return to scene (using relaxation, EMDR, cognitive methods, and dynamic procedures); and (4) completion and integration of self (individual and play modalities, as dictated by the child's developmental needs, along with psychodynamic approaches) (Parson, 1996, 1997).

SUMMARY

The nature of the traumatic experience (e.g., intensity, duration, and phase), its meaning to the child or adolescent, and its link to other issues in the youth's life affect the youth's traumatic reactions, as well as treatment and recovery processes. Characteristics of the child or adolescent (e.g., age, personality, coping skills) and of his or her support systems (family, culture, etc.) are also important to response, intervention, and recovery. Because young people's personalities, values, and behaviors can be changed by traumas, more study is needed to determine clearly the association between aspects of the event and the child on the one hand, and aspects of posttrauma symptoms and course on the other. Especially after mass traumas, children and adolescents may benefit from interventions using multiple methods, modalities, and settings. A number of play therapy and behavioral therapy methods have proven effective in treating traumatized youth.

REFERENCES

Achenbach, T. M., & Rescorla, L. A. (2001). *Manual for the ASEBA School-Age Forms and Profiles*. Burlington: University of Vermont, Research Center for Children, Youth, and Families.

Allen, J. G., Kelly, K. A., & Glodich, A. M. (1997). A psychoeducational program for patients with trauma-related disorders. *Bulletin of the Menninger Clinic, 61,* 222–239.

Axline, V. M. (1969). *Play therapy*. New York: Ballantine Books.

Bevin, T. (1999). Multiple traumas of refugees: Near drowning and witnessing of maternal rape. In N. B. Webb (Ed.), *Play therapy with children in crisis* (2nd ed.): *Individual, group, and family treatment* (pp. 164–182). New York: Guilford Press.

Bowlby, J. (1973). *Attachment and loss: Vol. 2. Separation: Anxiety and anger*. New York: Basic Books.

Bretherton, I. (1993). From dialogue to internal working models: The co-construction of self in relationships. In C. A. Nelson, (Ed.), *Minnesota Symposia on Child Psychology: Vol. 26. Memory and affect in development* (pp. 237–263). Hillsdale, NJ: Erlbaum.

Brody, V. (1994). Developmental play therapy. In B. James (Ed.), *Handbook for treatment of attachment-trauma problems in children* (pp. 234–239). Lexington, MA: Lexington Books.

Brodzinsky, D. M., Gormly, A. V., & Ambron, S. R. (1986). *Lifespan human development* (3rd ed., pp. 111–120). New York: Holt, Rinehart and Winston.

Burke, J., Borus, J., Burns, B., Millstein, K., & Beasley, M. (1982). Changes in children's behavior after a natural disaster. *American Journal of Psychiatry, 139*(8), 1010–1014.

Cohen, J. A. (1998). American Academy of Child and Adolescent Psychiatry, Work Group on Quality Issues: Practice parameters for the assessment and treatment of posttraumatic stress disorder. *Journal of the American Academy of Child and Adolescent Psychiatry, 37*(Suppl.), 4S–26S.

Cohen, J. A. (1999). *Treatment of traumatized children* (Trauma Therapy Audio Series). Thousand Oaks, CA: Sage.

Cohen, J. A., Berliner, L., & Mannarino, A. P. (2000). Treating traumatized children: A research review and synthesis. *Trauma, Violence, and Abuse: A Review Journal, 1*(1), 29–46.

Cohen, J. A., & Mannarino, A. P. (1997). A treatment study for sexually abused preschool children: Outcome during a one year follow-up. *Journal of the American Academy of Child and Adolescent Psychiatry, 36,* 1228–1235.

Copping, V., Warling, D., Benner, D., & Woodside, D. (2001). A child trauma treatment pilot study. *Journal of Child and Family Studies, 10*(4), 467–475 .

Danieli, Y. (1985). The treatment and prevention of the long-term effects of intergenerational transmission of victimization: A lesson from Holocaust survivors and their children. In C. Figley (Ed.), *Trauma and its wake: Vol. 1. The study and treatment of post-traumatic stress disorder* (pp. 295–313). New York: Brunner/Mazel.

De Bellis, M., Baum, A., Birmaher, B., Keshavan, M., Eccard, C., Boring, A., Jenkins, F., & Ryan, N. (1999). Developmental traumatology: Part I. Biological stress systems. *Biological Psychiatry, 45,* 1259–1270.

De Bellis, M., Keshavan, M., Clark, D., Casey, B., Giedd, H., Boring, A., Frustaci, K., & Ryan, N. (1999). Developmental traumatology: Part II. Brain development. *Biological Psychiatry, 45,* 1271–1284.

Deblinger, E., & Heflin, A. H. (1996). *Treating sexually abused children and their nonoffending parents: A cognitive behavioral approach.* Thousand Oaks, CA: Sage.

Deblinger, E., Lippmann, J., & Steer, R. (1996). Sexually abused children suffering posttraumatic stress symptoms: Initial treatment outcome findings. *Child Maltreatment, 1,* 310–321.

Drescher, K. (in press). Spirituality in the face of terrorist disasters. In L. Schein, G. Spitz, H. Burlingame, & P. Muskin (Eds.), *Group approaches for the psychological effects of terrorist events.* New York: Haworth Press.

Esman, A. H. (1983). Psychoanalytic play therapy. In C. E. Schaefer & K. J. O'Connor (Eds.), *Handbook of play therapy* (pp. 11–20). New York: Wiley.

Field, T., Seligman, S., Scafidi, F., & Schanberg, S. (1996). Alleviating posttraumatic stress in children following Hurricane Andrew. *Journal of Applied Developmental Psychology, 17,* 37–50.

Fletcher, K. E. (2003). Childhood posttraumatic stress disorder. In E. J. Mash & R. A. Barkley (Eds.), *Child psychopathology* (2nd ed., pp. 330–371). New York: Guilford Press.

Friedrich, W. N. (1996). Clinical considerations of empirical treatment studies of abused children. *Child Maltreatment, 1,* 343–347.

Friedrich, W. N., Gerber, P. N., Koplin, B., Davis, M., Giese, J., Mykelbust, C., & Franckowiak, D. (2001). Multimodal assessment of dissociation in adolescents: Inpatients and juvenile sex offenders. *Sexual Abuse: A Journal of Research and Treatment, 13*(3), 167–177.

Freud, A. (1965). *Normality and pathology in childhood.* New York: International Universities Press.

Garbarino, J., Kostelny, K., & Dubrow, N. (1991). What children can tell us about living in danger. *American Psychologist, 46,* 376–383.

Gil, E. (1991). *The healing power of play: Working with abused children.* New York: Guilford Press.

Gil, E. (1998). *Play therapy for severe psychological trauma* [Videotape]. New York: Guilford Press.

Glodich, A. M. (1999). *Psychoeducational groups for adolescents exposed to violence and abuse: Assessing the effectiveness of increasing knowledge of trauma to avert reenactment and risk-taking behaviors.* Unpublished doctoral dissertation, Smith College School for Social Work.

Goenjian, A. K., Karayan, I., Pynoos, R. S., Minassian, D., Najarian, L. M., Steinberg, A. M., & Fairbanks, L. A. (1997). Outcome of psychotherapy among early adolescents after trauma. *American Journal of Psychiatry, 154,* 536–542.

Goodman, G. S., & Quas, J. A. (1996). Trauma and memory: Individual differences in children's memory for a stressful event. In N. Stein, P. A. Ornstein, C. J. Brainerd & B. Tversky (Eds.), *Memory for emotional and everyday events* (pp. 267–294). Hillsdale, NJ: Erlbaum.

Greenberg, M. T. (1999). Attachment and psychopathology in childhood. In J. Cassidy & P. Shaver (Eds.), *Handbook of attachment* (pp. 469–496). New York: Guilford Press.

Greenwald, R. (1994). Applying eye movement desensitization and reprocessing (EMDR) to the treatment of traumatized children: Five case studies. *Anxiety Disorders Practice Journal, 1,* 83–97.

Greenwald, R. (1998). EMDR: New hope for children suffering from trauma and loss. *Clinical Child Psychology and Psychiatry, 3,* 279–287.

Gunnar, M. R., Brodersen, L., Krueger, K., & Rigatuso, J. (1996). Dampening of adrenocortical responses during infancy: Normative changes and individual differences. *Child Development, 67,* 877–889.

Harvey, S. (1994). Dynamic play therapy: Creating attachments. In B. James *Handbook for treatment of attachment-trauma problems in children* (pp. 222–233). New York: Lexington Books.

Homeyer, L. (1999). Group play with sexually abused children. In D. S. Sweeney & L. Homeyer (Eds.), *The handbook of group play therapy* (pp. 299–318). San Francisco: Jossey-Bass.

Howe, M. L. (1997). Children's memory for traumatic experiences. *Learning and Individual Differences, 9,* 153–174.

Howe, M. L., Courage, M. L., & Peterson, C. (1995). Intrusions in preschoolers' recall of traumatic childhood events. *Psychonomic Bulletin and Review, 2*(1), 130–134.

International Society for Traumatic Stress Studies. (1998). *Childhood trauma remembered: A report on the current scientific knowledge base and its applications.* Chicago: Author.

James, B. (1994). *Handbook for treatment of attachment-trauma problems in children.* New York: Lexington Books.

Johnson, M. K., & Foley, M. A. (1984). Differentiating fact from fantasy: The reliability of children's memory. *Journal of Social Issues, 40,* 33–50.

Kalff, D. (1980). *Sandplay.* Santa Monica, CA: Sigo.

Krakow, B., Hollifield, M., Schrader, R., Koss, M., Tandberg, D., Lauriello, J., McBride, L., Warner, T., Cheng, D., Edmond, T., & Kellner, R. (2000). A controlled study of imagery rehearsal for chronic nightmares in sexual assault survivors with PTSD: A preliminary report. *Journal of Traumatic Stress, 13*(4), 589–609.

Krakow, B., Sandoval, D., Schrader, R., Keuhne, B., McBride, L., Yau, C. C., & Tandberg, D. (2001). Treatment of chronic nightmares in adjudicated adolescent girls in a residential facility. *Journal of Adolescent Health, 29*, 94–100.

La Greca, A. M., Silverman, W. K., Vernberg, E. M., & Roberts, M. C. (Eds.). (2002). *Helping children cope with disasters and terrorism*. Washington, DC: American Psychological Association.

Leben, N. (1995). *Directive group play therapy: 60 structured games for treatment of ADHD, low self-esteem, and traumatized children*. Pflugerville, TX: Morning Glory Treatment Center for Children.

Levy, D. M. (1939). Release therapy. *American Journal of Orthopsychiatry, 9*, 713–736.

Lewis, M. (1995). Memory and psychoanalysis: A new look at infantile amnesia and transference. *Journal of the American Academy of Child and Adolescent Psychiatry, 34*, 405–417.

Lovett, J., & Shapiro, F. (1999). *Small wonders: Healing childhood trauma with EMDR*. New York: Free Press.

Lyons-Ruth, K., & Jacobvitz, D. (1999). Attachment disorganization: Unresolved loss, relational violence and lapses in behavioral and attentional strategies. In J. Cassidy & P. Shaver (Eds.), *Handbook of attachment* (pp. 520–554). New York: Guilford Press.

March, J., Amaya-Jackson, L., Foa, E., & Treadwell, K. (1999). *Trauma focused coping treatment of pediatric post-traumatic stress disorder after single-incident trauma* (Version 1. 0). Unpublished protocol.

March, J., Amaya-Jackson, L., Murry, M., & Schulte, A. (1998). Cognitive-behavioral psychotherapy for children and adolescents with post-traumatic stress disorder following a single incident stressor. *Journal of the American Academy of Child and Adolescent Psychiatry, 37*, 585–593.

March, J., Amaya-Jackson, L., Terry, R., & Costanzo, P. (1997). Post-traumatic stress in children and adolescents after an industrial fire. *Journal of the American Academy of Child and Adolescent Psychiatry, 36*, 1080–1088.

Meadows, E. A., & Foa, E. B. (1998). Intrusion, arousal, and avoidance: Sexual trauma survivors. In V. M. Follette, J. I. Ruzek, & F. R. Abueg (Eds.), *Cognitive-behavioral therapies for trauma* (pp. 100–123). New York: Guilford Press.

Muller, R., Sicoli, L., & Lemieux, K. E. (2000). Relationship between attachment style and posttraumatic stress symptomatology among adults who report the experience of childhood abuse. *Journal of Traumatic Stress, 13*(2), 321–332.

Murray, C. C., & Son, L. (1998). The effect of multiple victimization on children's cognition: Variations in response. *Journal of Aggression, Maltreatment and Trauma, 2*(1), 131–146.

Nachmias, M., Gunnar, M. R., Mangelsdorf, S., Parritz, R., & Buss, K. (1996). Behavioral inhibition and stress reactivity: The moderating role of attachment security. *Child Development, 67*, 508–522.

Nader, K. (1997). Treating traumatic grief in systems. In C. R. Figley, B. E. Bride, & N. Mazza (Eds.), *Death and trauma: The traumatology of grieving* (pp. 159–192). London: Taylor & Francis.

Nader, K. (2001). Treatment methods for childhood trauma. In J. P. Wilson, M. Friedman, & J. Lindy (Eds.), *Treating psychological trauma and PTSD* (pp. 278–334). New York: Guilford Press.

Nader, K. (2002). Innovative treatment methods. In S. Brock & P. Lazarus (Eds.), *Best practices in crisis prevention and intervention in the schools* (pp. 675–704). Bethesda, MD: National Association of School Psychologists.

Nader, K. (2003). *Assessing traumatic experiences in children and adolescents.* Manuscript under submission.

Nader, K., & Mello, C. (2001). Interactive trauma/grief focused therapy. In P. Lehmann & N. F. Coady (Eds.), *Theoretical perspectives for direct social work practice: A generalist–eclectic approach* (pp. 382–401). New York: Springer.

Nader, K., & Muni, P. (2002). Individual crisis intervention. In S. Brock & P. Lazarus (Eds.), *Best practices in crisis prevention and intervention in the schools* (pp. 405–428). Bethesda, MD: National Association of School Psychologists.

Nader, K., & Pynoos, R. (1991). Play and drawing as tools for interviewing traumatized children. In C. Schaefer, K. Gitlin, & A. Sandgrund (Eds.), *Play, diagnosis and assessment* (pp. 375–389). New York: Wiley.

Ochberg, F. M., & Soskis, D. A. (1982). Planning for the future: Means and ends. In F. M. Ochberg & D. A. Soskis (Eds.), *Victims of terrorism* (pp. 173–190). Boulder, CO: Westview Press.

Parson, E. R. (1996). Child trauma therapy and the effects of trauma, loss, dissociation: A multisystems approach to helping children exposed to lethal urban community violence. *Journal of Contemporary Psychotherapy, 26,* 117–162.

Parson, E. R. (1997). Post-traumatic child therapy (P-TCT): Assessment and treatment factors in clinic work with inner-city children exposed to catastrophic community violence. *Journal of Interpersonal Violence, 12,* 172–194.

Pelcovitz, D., Libov, B., Mandel, F. S., Kaplan, S. J., Weinblatt, M., & Septimus, A. (1998). Posttraumatic stress disorder and family functioning in adolescent cancer. *Journal of Traumatic Stress, 11*(2), 205–221

Pellicer, X. (1993). Eye movement desensitization treatment of a child's nightmares: A case report. *Journal of Behavior Therapy and Experimental Psychiatry, 24,* 73–75.

Piaget, J. (1952). *The origins of intelligence in children.* New York: International Universities Press.

Putnam, F. W. (1997). *Dissociation in children and adolescents.* New York: Guilford Press.

Pynoos, R. S., & Eth, S. (1986). Witness to violence: The child interview. *Journal of the American Academy of Child Psychiatry, 25,* 306–319.

Pynoos, R. S., & Nader, K. (1989). Children's memory and proximity to violence. *Journal of the American Academy of Child and Adolescent Psychiatry, 28,* 236–241.

Pynoos, R., Nader, K., & March, J. (1991). Post traumatic stress disorder in children and adolescents. In J. Weiner (Ed.), *Comprehensive textbook of child and adolescent psychiatry* (pp. 339–348). Washington, DC: American Psychiatric Press.

Reynolds, C. R., & Kamphaus, R. W. (1998). *Behavior Assessment System for Children: Manual.* Circle Pines, MN: American Guidance Service.

Roche, D. N., Runtz, M. G., & Hunter, M. A. (1999). Adult attachment: A mediator between child sexual abuse and later psychological adjustment. *Journal of Interpersonal Violence, 14*(2), 184–207.

Rossman, B., Bingham, R. D., & Emde, R. N. (1997). Symptomatology and adaptive functioning for children exposed to normative stressors, dog attack, and parental violence. *Journal of the American Academy of Child and Adolescent Psychiatry, 36,* 1089–1097.

Ruchkin, V., Eisemann, M., & Hagglof, B. (1998). Juvenile male rape victims: Is the level of post-traumatic stress related to personality and parenting? *Child Abuse and Neglect, 22,* 889–899.

Saigh, P. A., Yule, W., & Inamdar, S. C. (1996). Imaginal flooding of traumatized children and adolescents. *Journal of School Psychology, 34*(2), 163–183.

Scheeringa, M. S., & Zeanah, C. H. (2001). A relational perspective on PTSD in early childhood. *Journal of Traumatic Stress, 14*(4), 799–815.

Schore, A. N. (2002). Dysregulation of the right brain: A fundamental mechanism of traumatic attachment and the psychopathogenesis of posttraumatic stress disorder. *Australian and New Zealand Journal of Psychiatry, 36*(1), 9–30.

Siegel, D. J. (1996). Cognition, memory and dissociation. *Child and Adolescent Psychiatric Clinics of North America, 5,* 509–536.

Siegel, D. J. (2003). An interpersonal neurobiology of psychotherapy: The developing mind and the resolution of trauma. In M. Solomon & D. J. Siegel (Eds.), *Healing trauma* (pp. 1–56). New York: Norton.

Silberg, J. L. (Ed.). (1998). *The dissociative child: Diagnosis, treatment, and management.* Towson, MD: Sidran Press.

Silverman, A. B., Reinherz, H. Z., & Giaconia, R. M. (1996). The long-term sequelae of child and adolescent abuse: A longitudinal community study. *Child Abuse and Neglect, 20*(8), 709–723.

Stuber, M., Nader, K., & Pynoos, R. (1997). The violence of despair: Consultation to a HeadStart program following the Los Angeles uprising 1992. *Community Mental Health Journal, 33*(3), 235–241.

Suomi, S. J., & Levine, S. (1998). Psychobiology of intergenerational effects of trauma. In Y. Danielli (Ed.), *International handbook of multigenerational legacies of trauma* (pp. 623–637). New York: Plenum Press.

Sweeney, D. S., & Homeyer, L. (Eds.). (1999). *The handbook of group play therapy.* San Francisco: Jossey-Bass.

Terr, L. (1985). Remembered images and trauma. *Psychoanalytic Study of the Child, 40,* 493–533.

Terr, L. (1989). Treating psychic trauma in children: A preliminary discussion. *Journal of Traumatic Stress, 2,* 3–20.

Terr, L. (2001). Childhood posttraumatic stress disorder. In G. O. Gabbard (Ed.), *Treatment of psychiatric disorders* (2nd ed., Vol. 1, pp. 293–306). Washington, DC: American Psychiatric Press.

Trepper, T. S., & Barrett, M. J. (1986). Vulnerability to incest: A framework for assessment. In T. S. Trepper & M . J. Barrett (Eds.), *Treating incest: A multiple systems perspective* (pp. 13–25). New York: Haworth Press.

Trepper, T. S., & Barrett, M. J. (1989). *Systemic treating of incest: A therapeutic handbook.* New York: Brunner/Mazel.

Udwin, O., Boyle, S., Yule, W., Bolton, D., & O'Ryan, D. (2000). Risk factors for long-term psychological effects of a disaster experienced in adolescence: Predictors of post traumatic stress disorder. *Journal of Child Psychology and Psychiatry, 41*(8), 969–979.

Webb, N. B. (Ed.). (1991). *Play therapy with children in crisis: A casebook for practitioners*. New York: Guilford Press.

Webb, N. B. (Ed.). (1999). *Play therapy with children in crisis (2nd ed.): Individual, group and family treatment*. New York: Guilford Press.

Webb, N. B. (Ed.). (2002). *Helping bereaved children: A handbook for practitioners* (2nd ed.). New York: Guilford Press.

Webb, N. B. (2003). *Social work practice with children* (2nd ed.). New York: Guilford Press.

West, M., Adam, K., Spreng, S., & Rose, S. (2001). Attachment disorganization and dissociative symptoms in clinically treated adolescents. *Canadian Journal of Psychiatry, 46*(7), 627–631.

Williams, M. B. (1994). Intervention with child victims of trauma in the school setting. In M. B. Williams & J. F. Sommer (Eds.), *Handbook of post-traumatic therapy* (pp. 69–77). Westport, CT: Greenwood Press.

Wilson, J., & Raphael, B. (Eds.). (1993). *The international handbook of traumatic stress syndromes*. New York: Plenum Press.

Yule, W., Udwin, O., & Bolton, D. (2002). Mass transportation disasters. In A. M. La Greca, W. K. Silverman, E. M. Vernberg, & M. C. Roberts (Eds.), *Helping children cope with disasters and terrorism* (pp. 223–239). Washington, DC: American Psychological Association Press.

Yule, W., & Williams, R. M. (1990). Post-traumatic stress reactions in children. *Journal of Traumatic Stress, 3*, 279–295.

❧ PART II

Helping Interventions

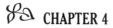

CHAPTER 4

Treatment of Childhood Traumatic Grief

Application of Cognitive-Behavioral and Client-Centered Therapies

ROBIN F. GOODMAN

Human compassion, common sense, and clinical observation all suggest that grieving children and families benefit from bereavement services. Science is striving to confirm this fact and to demonstrate what is needed, when, and for whom. Although the emotional, social, and cognitive functioning of a child is threatened by any death of a significant person in the child's life (Nolen-Hoeksema & Larson, 1999; Silverman & Worden, 1993), the risk is even greater if the death was a traumatic experience (Goenjian et al., 2001; Pfefferbaum et al., 1999, 2000). This chapter discusses issues specific to childhood traumatic grief, with a focus on parental death, and describes and compares two specific treatment interventions.

INTRODUCTION TO CHILDHOOD TRAUMATIC GRIEF

Conceptualization

Childhood traumatic grief in children is still emerging as a variant of, yet distinct from, both trauma and grief reactions. Incorporating characteristic features of both has lead to the current parsimonious conceptualization and diagnostic criteria:

77

(a) death of a child's loved one in circumstances that were objectively or subjectively perceived to be traumatic; (b) the presence of significant PTSD [posttraumatic stress disorder] symptoms, including that loss and change reminders segue into trauma reminders, which then trigger the use of avoidant or numbing strategies: and (c) the impingement of these PTSD symptoms on the child's ability to complete tasks of uncomplicated bereavement. (Cohen, Mannarino, Greenberg, Padlo, & Shipley, 2002, p. 318)

Refinement and elaboration of the definition of childhood traumatic grief are presented elsewhere in this volume (see Chapter 1). Of significance for the current focus on parental death, the cause of death does not have to meet the standard definition of a trauma for a child to experience traumatic grief (Eth & Pynoos, 1985). Rather, it is the child's *perception* of the death as traumatic that is important. Hence a child may have traumatic grief after a parent dies following a long battle with cancer, or after seeing a sibling shot to death. Furthermore, one must keep in mind that traumatic grief does not seem to be the norm for children experiencing a traumatic death (Cohen et al., 2002).

As reviewed in Chapter 2, certain factors have been shown to put children at risk for developing problems following the traumatic death of a parent (or other significant person). These include the prior mental health of the child and surviving parent (or other primary caretaker—see Table 4.1 footnote, below), prior trauma and death experiences, parental functioning, social support for the parent and child, family functioning, and secondary adversities such as loss of income. However, some factors can also be protective for children, thus accounting for those children who are resilient (Haggerty, Sherrod, Garmezy, & Rutter, 1996) in the face of a devastating life experience, or for whom death of a significant person can lead to a positive outcome (Oltjenbruns, 2001).

Goals of Intervention

Successful treatment of childhood traumatic grief depends upon the formulation of the problem. Some treatments focus more on alleviation of symptoms related to trauma (Eth & Pynoos, 1985; Figley, 1989; Goenjian et al., 2001); some address the resulting changed self-concept and world view (Finkelhor & Browne, 1985); and still others stress the acquisition of tasks related to resolution of grief (Baker, Sedney, & Gross, 1996; Oltjenbruns, 2001; Worden, 1991). The theoretical understanding chosen is likely to drive the assessment, to determine which person or people are targeted for intervention, and to guide the choice of an intervention technique itself. In addition, the mediating variables that influence symptom formation and improvement constitute a necessary focus of inquiry. The manner in which these different areas overlap is summarized in Table 4.1.

TABLE 4.1. Overlap among Foci in the Formulation of Childhood Traumatic Grief

Identified person(s)	Tasks/self-concept/ world view	Symptoms	Mediating and risk factors
Child	Understand the death and accept the reality	Depression	Prior mental health (parent/child)
Parent[a]	Cope with the current and future feelings	Anxiety	Prior death/loss experiences
Family	Adjust to the changes in the environment and identity	Disorganization, being overwhelmed	Parent functioning, availability of other (and extended) family members
	Deepen existing relationships and allow for reinvestment in new relationships	Enmeshment, overidentification	Social support (parent/child)
	Maintain appropriate attachment through memorialization		
	Address feelings of betrayal	PTSD: reexperiencing, arousal, avoidance	Family functioning (parent/child)
	Confront sense of stigmatization	Shame, disenfranchised grief	Secondary adversities (parent/child)
	Overcome powerlessness	Guilt	Community response/ resources
	Deal with dysregulation	Anger	

[a]"Parent" is used throughout this chapter to identify a child's primary caretaker.

These different domains do not necessarily operate in isolation from one another. Rather, they can be grouped into categories that follow a pathway over time as follows:

1. *Pre-event factors* related to the child, parent, and family: Pretrauma functioning, individual characteristics, social support, resources.
2. *Event factors*: Characteristics of the trauma and death, perception of the event.
3. *Postevent factors*: Secondary adversities, coping, social support, resources.
4. *Functioning* of child, parent, and family: Symptoms, tasks, self-concept, and world view.
5. *Outcome*: The resulting trauma and bereavement response.

TWO APPROACHES FOR TREATING TRAUMATIC GRIEF IN CHILDREN

Choosing the best—that is, the most effective and efficacious—treatment for traumatic grief in children requires making choices as to (1) the primary person(s) receiving intervention, (2) the presenting problems and cause, and (3) the goal of the intervention. Success is usually determined by the absence of some problem (pain) or the increase in functioning (health). In medicine, this straightforward system is rather clear. However, the end of bereavement or the resolution of grief is tenuously defined, and is hindered by being organized around the medical pathology model of grief symptoms. Therefore, the end is seen as "the absence of" grief, rather than "the existence of" something positive.

Models about the bereavement process, focusing on the impact of bereavement on children, have evolved to a "hybrid model: the life trajectory/developmental cascade model of child and adolescent grief" (Clark, Pynoos, & Goebel, 1996, p. 130). This model accounts for a contemporary view of grief, which is fluid with respect to process and coping. It is also more enlightened, as it allows the possibility of positive change rather than pathology. The most beneficial and accurate view of bereavement, in my opinion, is that coping lasts a lifetime. Hence intervention for childhood traumatic grief must be provided with this long-range view in mind.

The ultimate goal of any intervention is to relieve distress, as well as to help an individual adjust and accommodate to the changes brought about by the death. However, none of the array of interventions provided to children bereaved under various circumstances have been subjected to rigorous scientific investigation, and there are conflicting results from a comparison of others (Scheiderman, Winders, Tallett, & Feldman, 1994; Kissane & Bloch, 1994).

As an illustration of the variability in the assessment of childhood traumatic grief, the PTSD symptom of avoidance of trauma-related themes would be conceptualized and treated differently in the following generic models:

1. *Self-actualization model*: Symptoms are viewed as emerging from the lack of trust and the disappointment resulting from the death, and thus require work in relationship building.
2. *Cognitive-behavioral model*: Symptoms stem from intrusion of unwanted thoughts, feelings, and behaviors about the death, which should be addressed through cognitive work, skill building, and coping strategies.
3. *Family systems model*: Symptoms stem from poor communication and fear of expressing feelings to others; thus family members must be accepting and encouraging of expression about the per-

son who died, and learn to adapt to changes in the family together.

The most common basic treatment formats are these:

- *Traditional family therapy*: All members of a single family are treated together.
- *Group therapy*: Children are seen in age-appropriate groups, while parents are treated separately in an adult group.
- *Individual therapy*: The child and parent are seen separately, with or without coordinated or shared aspects of treatment.

In addition to the pros and cons of the different theoretical orientations, there are pros and cons to each format. Different factors influence choice and feasibility such as the availability of family or group members, the homogeneity or heterogeneity of type of death, the risk of reexposure to the trauma from group members, and the timing of treatment in the bereavement process.

Rationale for Individual Cognitive-Behavioral Treatment and Client-Centered Treatment

The two areas of work having particular relevance to childhood traumatic grief are (1) work with children experiencing natural disasters (e.g., hurricanes) (Goenjian et al., 1997), war (Layne et al., 2001), or violence-related trauma (e.g., community shootings) (Saltzman, Pynoos, Layne, Steinberg, & Aisenberg, 2001); and (2) work with children who have been sexually abused (Cohen & Mannarino, 1996). There is growing evidence that cognitive-behavioral treatment (CBT) is effective in helping children who have experienced these types of trauma or abuse (e.g., Berliner & Saunders, 1996; March, Amaya-Jackson, Murray, & Schulte, 1998). This evidence supports the need to address trauma as well as grief in any traumatic grief intervention (Cohen et al., 2001; Nader, 1997). Not doing so is thought to be ineffective at best, and detrimental at worst. However, because treatment has historically been provided by those who are steeped in either trauma or bereavement theories and interventions, CBT for trauma usually differs from less structured approaches for more traditional grief-related issues. There are as yet no scientific data from randomized controlled trials specifically treating traumatic or nontraumatic grief in children to indicate which type of approach is more effective.

Treatment of traumatically bereaved children in the community, regardless of whether the mode chosen is child, parent, family, or group, typically uses either supportive nondirective techniques or structured skill-building techniques. These can be loosely conceptualized as falling under either a CBT or a client-centered treatment (CCT) model. Although clinicians are rarely exact in their use and application of either approach in practice, Cohen, Mannarino, and their colleagues (Cohen et al., 2001; Cohen & Mannarino, 2001) have developed detailed manualized CBT and CCT protocols to allow for delivery of the purest forms of these traumatic grief treatments. These protocols are based on their ongoing research with children who have been sexually abused and, more recently, with bereaved children. Their work is an application of the basic CBT and CCT models organized around certain core beliefs and strategies.

Elissa J. Brown and I are utilizing the Cohen et al. (2001) and Cohen and Mannarino (2001) protocols in a bereavement program for children of uniformed officers who died in the World Trade Center attack on September 11, 2001. The program provides clinical services; in addition, a randomized controlled treatment trial of CBT and CCT for the families is being conducted. The core components include extensive direct outreach to all eligible widows with available contact information ($n = 225$) and children from infancy through 24 years of age ($n = 533$) of fire department, police department, Port Authority, and emergency medical service personnel who died in the attack. Following personal letter and phone contact, services begin with a comprehensive evaluation of each child (which includes a diagnostic interview as well as self-, parent, and teacher report of functioning at home and in school), in addition to measures of parental functioning. Treatment is provided as prevention or intervention, based on the diagnostic presentation of the child(ren) and parent. The 16-week course of treatment involves individual treatment for each child and companion treatment sessions for the parent. The same clinician treats all the members of the family. The two different approaches, CBT and CCT, summarized below are being administered in the same format (individuals interested in detailed descriptions and protocols should contact J. A. Cohen and A. P. Mannarino at the Center for Traumatic Stress in Children and Adolescents, Department of Psychiatry, Allegheny General Hospital, 4 Allegheny Center, Pittsburgh, PA 15212-5234). Six-month follow-up evaluations are conducted after the initial evaluation for children who have completed treatment, as well as for those who did not want or require treatment. A final evaluation is done 6 months after the time 2 evaluation.

The basic components of these two protocols are now outlined, with a discussion of their similarities and differences. Certain primary questions yet to be answered include the following:

1. What is the major focus of the treatment (e.g., the symptoms, the individual's self-concept, the relationship, the trauma, the grief)?
2. What are the best strategies and techniques to use (e.g., avoidance is allowed in CCT, but is addressed directly in CBT)?
3. What are the best modes of intervention (e.g., art and play can be

used as components in both, but are open-ended in one format and directed in the other)?

Cognitive-Behavioral Treatment

CBT interventions stem from a symptom-focused view of traumatic grief. Thus the therapy attempts to alleviate and manage the PTSD symptoms of reexperiencing, avoidance, and arousal related to the traumatic death, as well as other grief-related symptoms of depression and anxiety. The CBT-specific techniques described by Cohen et al. (2001), and used and adapted by different researchers and clinicians, include gradual exposure, cognitive processing, affect regulation, and stress inoculation. Homework assignments specifically reinforce skill building. The 16-week treatment is divided into two halves; the first portion focuses on the trauma, and the second on bereavement.

The technique of "gradual exposure" has been maintained for the protocol, but the term has been changed to avoid any negative reactions to or misconceptions about reliving the actual death experience. For traumatically bereaved individuals, a more helpful way to understand and present the gradual exposure process has been the alternative description "creating a trauma narrative." The purpose is exposure to traumatic memories through a personalized and guided telling of the traumatic event. This can be done in various ways in CBT, but should include specific details about the event itself. It requires telling of one's individual story, with specific questioning about the worst moment. Anxiety and arousal are carefully monitored throughout the process with the child's report of "subjective units of distress." Specific cognitive techniques are taught to help the child manage any anxiety that accompanies or results from the creation of the narrative, as well as symptoms experienced at other times (e.g., intrusive thoughts and images). These strategies include controlled breathing, guided imagery, and thought stopping. Cognitive distortions and misinformation are corrected when presented in the narrative; however, the child's version of the experience is accepted as truth.

Parental involvement is essential in the treatment. This includes teaching the parent the skill-building and stress reduction techniques being taught to the child, and addressing parenting issues related to the traumatic bereavement. Joint child and parent sessions occur at crucial points in the treatment. At least one joint session is focused on the trauma narrative that has been created by the child. Together, the parent and child engage in a discussion of the narrative; this encourages active questioning and communication about the traumatic event. The parent is carefully prepared for the content of the narrative, and specific questions are developed to help guide the discussion.

Following the completion of the trauma narrative, the narrative technique is then repeated, with a focus on bereavement issues. Exploration of memories of the person who died is the centerpiece of this activity. Making a memory book or box revolves around the detailed telling and preservation of memories. This product is also shared with the parent, who has again been prepared for the activity. Silverman (2000) comments on this technique:

> Simply getting feelings out, as an end in itself, is not sufficient. Once labeled, feelings need to be attached to the child's experience and behavior and his or her expression of his new experience. Children often find it more productive to talk about who died, and to be helped to construct an inner representation of the deceased that is both accurate—with space for negative or ambivalent feelings they have toward the deceased—and that is dynamic and fluid, changing as the child matures. (p. 87)

Client-Centered Treatment

Telling the "story" of death is one way family members can communicate about the death (Baker, 1997), but is not necessarily the only type of useful communication for addressing intense emotions or preserving memories. Use of a nondirective CCT approach based on Carl Rogers's original principles (Patterson, 1979; Rogers, 1951) is well suited to Finkelhor and Browne's (1985) dynamic conceptualization of trauma symptoms. Rogers's belief in the power of the therapeutic relationship to promote change fits a model where the focus is on the child's altered sense of self and relationships. Cohen and Mannarino's (2001) CCT protocol elaborates on Rogers's necessary three core elements: unconditional positive regard, empathic understanding, and therapeutic genuineness. The child and parent are told that the treatment time is for them to use as they choose, and they are free to talk about whatever is on their minds and to do whatever they like. The clinician also conveys that in the time they are together, the goals are to get to know more about each individual, to understand him or her, and to help with whatever is needed. The child and parent sessions are conducted separately, with the clinician focusing solely on the parent's needs when with the parent, and solely on the child's needs during the child session. When the parent inquires about the child's work, this is explored in relation to the parent's perspective (except for providing basic information or addressing any emergent issues of concern).

The clinician actively utilizes specific skills to communicate and enhance elements of CCT. These include listening, paying attention, asking questions, accepting, reflecting, clarifying, paraphrasing, summarizing, probing, encouragement of personal problem solving, and interpreting. Being attuned to the individual requires intense focus and suspension of any agenda except the one presented in the here and now by the client. The clinician's acceptance and support of self-initiated content will promote self-disclosure, self-exploration, and self-awareness on the part of the child and parent. Specific questions in sessions 4 and 8 are used in order to explore the death. However, the topic is pursued at the discretion of the child and parent. Thus, if it is ignored or a preference is expressed to address something else, the clinician respects this preference as well as all other feeling states. Children are also allowed to use play and art materials that foster individuality and creativity. Therefore, cars, trucks, and a dollhouse; toys for imaginative play; and basic drawing, painting, and sculpting supplies are available, together with feeling games and interactive table games.

The CCT therapist provides an environment in which all of the individual's feelings and behaviors are understood and accepted in a nonjudgmental fashion, with the goal of fostering self-acceptance. By supporting previously successful problem-solving strategies, the CCT therapist increases the client's self-efficacy and provides a model for working out future problems. In CCT, the child and parent are the agents of change and they direct the content and flow of the sessions. There is no homework or deliberate follow-up on issues from week to week.

CCT interventions are consistent with what Davidowitz and Myrick (1984) have described as being helpful to bereaved adults. Highly facilitative responses that include questions that clarify or summarize and that are feeling-focused have been perceived as "caring, understanding, warm, respectful, accepting and personal" (p. 4). In contrast, interventions that focus on advice, evaluation, and interpretation/analysis may be experienced by clients as "judgmental, non-accepting, unconcerned and impersonal" (Davidowitz & Myrick, 1984, p. 4).

Similarities and Differences: Core Components

At first glance CBT and CCT appear distinct, and when practiced in their purest form in a research context, they should be delivered as such. However, there may be components that are germane to both. Table 4.2 illustrates some of the many ways both treatments either address the same issues (e.g., powerlessness) or can be seen as using variations of similar strategies (e.g., exposure).

Although some clinicians prefer and adhere to either a directive or nondirective approach to treating traumatized and bereaved children, many practitioners do not use one model exclusively. Rasmussen and Cunningham (1995), for example, present arguments for an integration

TABLE 4.2. A Comparison of CCT and CBT

Core issue	CCT technique/component	CBT technique/component
Symptoms		
PTSD (avoidance, numbing, arousal, reexperiencing), anxiety (anger, irritability), depression (withdrawal)	Exposure to an accepting environment and a corrective relationship Reengagement in personal relationship; support of personal strategies	Exposure to content about death (creating the narrative); cognitive processing; affect regulation Skill building with specific instructions; monitoring of distress
Relational issues		
Mistrust/betrayal	Confidence in ability of the bereaved person; establishing a therapeutic relationship; respect, care, genuineness, listening, empathy Belief in treatment	Confidence in the intervention and clinician; consistency Belief in treatment
Fear re: future loss/death	Providing consistent, stable relationship to allow for new experience	Refuting exaggerated cognitions; developing personal safety plan
Stigmatization	Acceptance of person; respect; clarifying	Normalization; cognitive restructuring
Powerlessness	Giving client ability to choose course of treatment; understanding client	Teaching of portable strategies (ones that can be used anywhere); stress inoculation; monitoring of stress
Behavioral dysregulation	Containing and reflecting; modeling calm	Limit setting
Tasks		
Acceptance of death	Evolves through treatment; addressed as it is revealed; existing state accepted	Addressed through activities, especially through the narrative process
Identity development	Clarification of role as presented; support for current identity; self-exploration	Exploration of relationship to deceased person
Communication	Modeling and acceptance of all feelings and behaviors; facilitating self-expression	Introduction of specific topics; problem solving
Parenting	Exploration of current practice; empowerment; increase in self-efficacy/confidence building	Teaching of basic skills; information giving/psychoeducation
Memorialization	Facilitating self-expression	Creating memory object/container
Future	Supporting use of personal strategies	Encouraging use of learned skills

of both interventions when using play therapy with children who have been sexually abused.

Establishing rapport and building a sense of trust are vital to all therapeutic relationships and are probably key ingredients in both treatments. In CCT, these are promoted through an accepting attitude; in CBT, they are provided through the secure structure. When the world feels as if it has come crashing down, a traumatically bereaved child is in desperate need of a safe and predictable haven. Opponents of CCT would say that the lack of direction can make a child and parent feel uncomfortable and insecure. Proponents would say that the stance lets the individuals know they are in a place where they will not be judged.

One can easily reframe concepts to fit a theory. CCT dictates the approach but not the content. CCT does not explicitly promote avoidance of traumatic content; rather, it allows its presentation to be under the control of the child. Of course it is always possible, and will certainly be accepted, in CCT to explore traumatic material as it is revealed. Once provided, it is managed differently in CCT compared to CBT.

The creative arts can be used in both CBT and CCT. Theories about the processing of traumatic events suggest that nonverbal activities help in the retrieval of traumatic memories that have overwhelmed or disturbed the normal coding, storing, and communication processes (Burgess & Hartman, 1993; Greenberg & van der Kolk, 1987). In fact, the literature contains numerous case examples describing art for accessing, describing, and confronting details about a trauma (e.g., Appleton, 2001; Goodman, 2002; Kozlowska & Hanney, 2001; Murphy, 2001; Roje, 1995). However, it is imperative that the child be prepared for exposure work with ways to manage any anxiety that is generated by the exposure, and CBT offers a wealth of techniques for affect regulation. Play therapy, often the main approach with younger children, is typically used nondirectively. This may result in exposure when children

> enact, often in a repetitive, monotonous, or even dangerous way, the death, the burial, and any other aspect of the loss. [Nondirective play therapy] allows children to express conscious and unconscious themes without having to verbally acknowledge, or even have a conscious awareness of, the painful aspects that older children and adolescents are more likely to deal with in words. (Steinberg, 1997, p. 127)

Because exposure has gained acceptance as a valid component of effective trauma intervention, it is hypothesized that it constitutes a necessary part of traumatic grief treatment. However, an expanded definition of exposure and mastery can include triggers that are associated with the trauma. Thus exposure to the traumatic aspects of the death (e.g., intrusive images), to bereavement cues (e.g., the anniversary of the death), and to the relationship (e.g., feelings of insecurity) may all be integral in treatment (Clark et al., 1996).

Some family- and parent-focused interventions utilize aspects of both CBT and CCT (e.g., Baker, 1997). The most effective treatments may differ for the parent and the child, depending on their experience and symptoms. Most intervention programs recognize the impact of the surviving parent on the child's reaction and adjustment, and incorporate some or all of the following in treatment (Baker, 1997; Siegel, Mesagno, & Christ, 1990): psychoeducation (educating the parent about age-appropriate reactions and expectations of children); support and skill building (exploration and acceptance of the adult's grief reactions and help with coping); and empowerment and management (enhancing the survivor's parenting ability, providing assistance with behavior management).

Cohen and Mannarino (1996), comparing CBT and nonsupportive therapy (equivalent to CCT) for sexually abused children, found that parental emotional distress was related to treatment outcome and that supportive counseling alone was not enough to "address parental cognitions, perceptions, and coping responses with regard to the abuse in order to decrease the child's symptoms" (p. 1409). We do not yet know how such parental responses interact with those of a grieving child, given that the responses and relationship of a bereaved child and parent differ from those of an abused child and parent. Even a parent not directly involved in the cause of death may certainly feel concern about the child and responsible for protecting the child from such a horrific experience. In the case of the traumatic death of a parent, both the child and surviving parent are bereaved as a result of the direct experience; one has lost a parent, the other a life partner.

Contributions of the Therapist

Certain common factors have been identified as contributing to good therapy, regardless of the orientation or need for protocol adherence. Effective CBT and CCT therapists need to possess the same qualities, including interest in helping patients, purity of treatment offered, quality of the relationship, confidence in the method being used, a clear rationale for a particular intervention, empathy, and warmth (Miller, 1993). Miller distilled the disparate literature on therapist variables down to the following: "those who combine the qualities of flexible, reflective, and creative thinking with genuine human relatedness and concern" (p. 15). This may account for the qualitative improvement we have noted in children who have been evaluated but do not engage in treatment; the effects of ongoing phone calls, multiple visits, feedback, and availability of reliable support warrant further exploration for any treatment planning.

CASE EXAMPLES[1]

Over the course of 6 months, both of the children described below were seen in weekly individual treatment with companion parent sessions. In the CBT case, there were joint sessions at specified times as described above.

CBT Case

James, an 8-year-old boy, was referred for treatment 6 months after his father was killed in a restaurant. James, his mother, his father, and his 2-year-old sister were having lunch when a gunman came in and shot six people, wounded three, and fled with money. The perpetrator was later found and arrested. The family witnessed the death and the subsequent attempts by medical personnel to resuscitate the father. James presented with disturbed sleep, anger, and difficulty leaving the house for school. The mother was a competent and resourceful parent, but felt as if she were "going through the motions" of parenting. She kept reliving the day of her husband's death in her waking thoughts, and believed she could have prevented the incident by picking a different restaurant or making lunch at home.

    The beginning of treatment with James involved his identifying feelings as a prelude to his understanding CBT concepts. This goal was accomplished by presenting James with different game-like tasks geared to affect regulation, such as asking him to come up with as many feeling words as possible in 3 minutes. As a follow-up activity he was asked to choose one feeling to further describe. He picked "excited" and drew a picture about being excited when he got his dog when he was 5. The clinician explained the relationship among feelings, thoughts, and behaviors as this applied to his personal experience: feeling happy, not being able to sit still and eat his breakfast while he waited for the arrival of his new pet, and feeling warm inside when he cuddled the puppy. Less pleasant experiences were also discussed, and James was taught how to help himself manage his different reactions. For example, when he identified being scared to go to school because he didn't want to leave his mother and little sister home alone, he was instructed about how to use special breathing exercises to calm his stomach. He created a personal safety plan that included keeping his mother's work and cellular phone number with him, and creating a list of school staff members he could go to when he felt worried.

---

[1]To protect the confidentiality of the children and families, these case synopses are based on composites of actual and hypothetical cases. Any similarity to real cases is coincidental.

Concurrently, via parent training, James's mother was helped with her sudden transition to being a single parent. The clinician asked her to identify what triggered the most stress. Once she realized that the morning routine was the most difficult time of day for her, she was helped to implement a behavior chart system for James, and she arranged for the nanny to arrive 15 minutes earlier in the morning so she could get to her part-time job in a more relaxed state. In the process of explaining the instructions for having James practice relaxation breathing at home, the clinician also taught the mother to use the strategies for herself. Such skill building is a necessary prelude to addressing the traumatic memories of the death scene.

Gradual exposure began with a thorough explanation to James and his mother about the need to confront the traumatic event directly, so that the terrible memories did not fester and create more trouble by staying hidden. The analogy of a bad cut that must be cleaned out with antiseptic so it can heal was used; James remarked, "I squeeze my eyes closed very hard until it stops stinging, and then it's not so bad," indicating that he understood the concept. Confident in his writing, he preferred to write the story about his father's death. He was prompted with specific questions to make it a full story. James reported that the emergency workers had helped the other victims first, when in fact his father was tended to immediately. Various questions elicited more accurate details of where and when helpers arrived to minister to his father. James worked on the story over two sessions, rereading it each time until he was satisfied with the content. Then, as he illustrated the story, he was asked to describe how he felt when different things were happening. James was asked which scene illustrated the worst moment for him. As he pointed to the one showing when his father fell on the floor and didn't talk or move while his mother was shaking his father, he became tearful. James was prompted to use his breathing and describe his feelings as they got stronger; they then subsided, as he stayed on task with the drawing and verbal description. When James described the fleeing gunman, he made reference to a recurring nightmare in which the gunman came to find him. Cognitive restructuring helped James cope with this anxiety by addressing the reality that the gunman had been captured.

Faulty cognitions held by James's mother were addressed and challenged in her own sessions—in particular, the impossibility of her knowing where the gunman would be and her guilt about not making lunch at home as the cause for the fatal outing. Her experience of the day, and details about James's involvement with the police following the event were discussed. She was also prepared for the joint session with James where he would share his book, and she was equipped with answers to specific questions he used to "quiz" her about the content. This structured creation and presentation of the traumatic material allowed for mastery as well as shared communication. It set the stage for ongoing dialogue in the family about difficult topics.

As treatment progressed, James's mother expressed her concern about her son's future development without a father, and particularly, his lack of interest in the children's baseball team once coached by his father. She also struggled with resentment and guilt about wanting to keep working, but knowing her children needed her. Her own feelings of helplessness as a single parent were complicated by continued avoidance of restaurants.

For James, a process similar to the one used for the creation and sharing of the trauma narrative was used for activity focused on tasks of bereavement. James talked about where he thought people go after they die, and was able to say that because his father was a good person, he was in heaven. He eagerly brought into the session special mementos of his father for use in making a memory box. Ideas for the contents were generated from a discussion about things they did together and how he felt about his father. This discussion was the basis for exploring current and future reminders of his father. Thus some of the items included were his dad's favorite baseball cap and a label from the jar of his favorite spaghetti sauce; James also made a small cardboard model of a television remote control to add.

Once the box was finished, its contents and the meaning of the objects were shared with his mother in another joint session. She had been prepared prior to the session by talking about what James had brought in and the meaning behind the objects. Together, James and his mother talked about how the family used to be, what would stay the same, and what would be different. James was encouraged by his mother to become involved in baseball again, and was reassured that his closeness to the new coach would be an example of carrying on with something he enjoyed with his father, rather than a betrayal of his memory. As a final activity, James was guided in making a list of answers to questions about his father, things to tell his sister when she got older, ways to remember his father, and suggestions for how to cope with his or his mother's sad feelings. The list was also used to help James when he would encounter hard times in the future.

At the end of treatment, James's symptoms had diminished, particularly his sleep difficulties and reluctance to participate in outside activities. His mother felt more confident in managing the household, but continued to be distressed by intrusive memories of the traumatic event. Later, she received additional individual CBT to address her specific PTSD symptoms.

CCT Case

Fifteen-year-old Natalie's mother died in a terrorist bombing at her office. Her father and her 19-year-old brother (who lived away at college) first heard of the incident on the news. When Natalie came home from school, her father and maternal grandmother told her that her mother had died. The mother's body was badly burned. Her purse and wedding ring were recovered and returned to the family 2 months later. The father was managing as best he could, but he felt ill equipped for life with a teenage daughter, since he believed she was at an age when she needed a mother the most. Natalie was trying hard to fill in the gaps at home; she made dinner and cleaned the house. She was also keeping up with her grades, but had become more withdrawn from friends. Natalie and her father began treatment 8 months after the death. Her brother saw a counselor at college.

Natalie began treatment reluctantly, but was compliant. Aware that Natalie was struggling to maintain the impression that she was handling things well, the clinician encouraged Natalie to talk about the positive aspects of her life, including the details about her getting good grades and going on outings with friends. Liking art, she drew cartoon-like sequences of herself playing basketball, and described being happy when she made a basket. When a difference was noted in her demeanor as she talked about hanging out with friends, it prompted her to share details about some friends' not being as supportive as she had hoped. The clinician heard the message of her being disappointed when she trusted people with her feelings—a theme probably related to Natalie's guardedness in the new therapeutic relationship. Acknowledging Natalie's observations and experiences permitted her to set the pace. Discussion about practice on the school basketball team and school-related issues such as upcoming tests kept specific content about the death at bay. Natalie alluded to life changes as she talked about visiting her grandmother on the weekends and helping her around the house. At these times, the therapist reflected that the visits brought Natalie comfort.

In the parallel parent sessions, Natalie's father also exhibited caution in the form of being protective of Natalie. His focus on her problems, rather than his own, was some indication of his avoidance of forming a new close relationship himself. Exploring the effects of her behaviors on him and the success or failure he felt in dealing with them, rather than instructing him in what to do, allowed him the room to voice his ambivalence about the best way to parent Natalie and to discover what worked best. The therapist summarized his desire to use the best of what his wife had done, while also developing his own style.

Natalie's mother had been a volunteer in the school library, and the school created a book award to be given to a special student each year.

The week following the dedication of the award, Natalie talked a great deal in session. Although she was proud of her mother, she was uncomfortable at being singled out because of the tragedy. The dedication also brought back memories of all the news reports she had seen about the day her mother died, and various people she didn't even know talking about her mother. Natalie's father questioned how much he should involve her in such ceremonies, and noted the lack of control he felt over what others said and did. The therapist empathized with his ambivalence about wanting to do what he thought others expected, including his wife's family, and his desire to let Natalie have some say in what she did. School was an increasing source of difficulty for Natalie. She was studying hard because school was important to her mother, but she didn't see the point. She would go out to the mall with her friends, but frequently called her father after her curfew to say she'd be late. When she was with her friends, Natalie did not pay attention to their conversations, which revolved around gossip and clothes. When home, Natalie stayed in her room and didn't talk to her friends on the phone.

When not alone in her room, Natalie sometimes cooked and often argued with her father about her bedtime. According to her description, Natalie would be on good behavior for a few days following an argument. When the clinician asked her how this compared to arguments with her mother, she said that she used to be able to go to her father if she didn't like her mother's rules. Now she felt "stuck," even though she realized his requests were not unreasonable or different from what her mother would do. The clinician commented that the rules might be the same, but the person making them was different. When Natalie fought with her father, she felt she didn't have any recourse. Although this was not expressed directly, she was struggling with the risk of being angry with her only surviving parent, and worried that something might happen to him. Natalie's father talked about the same incidents from his perspective. He felt her anger at him for making the rules, and he missed being the "good guy." He talked about how difficult it was to parent a daughter; although he accepted that she needed to find her own way, it was painful for him to see her miss her mother. The therapist acknowledged his wish to take away her hurt, but noted the impossibility of doing so.

Natalie talked about her plans to go to sleep-away camp for 2 weeks in the summer, as she had done for the past 5 years. She was eager to see her old friends and leave her hometown, where she felt as if she were under a microscope. However, she worried about whether her father and brother (who would be home from college) would be able to cook and clean for themselves. Four days before she was scheduled to leave on the bus, her father called the clinician because Natalie was crying and upset, saying she didn't want to go. Her reaction was an expression of the impending separation and her panic and anger about what had happened to her mother. In session, Natalie talked about her mother's always being the one who helped her pack for camp and not being able to do it alone. Her grandmother and aunt took over for her father, taking her shopping and making sure she had clothes that fit. Natalie wondered whether she would tell her friends at camp what had happened or not. The therapist listened as Natalie presented her different options. Her best friend was going to be with her, and since the friend already knew what Natalie had been through, she decided that this was enough.

When Natalie returned from camp, she brought pictures to show the therapist, and made a scrapbook with photos and stories about camp activities and friends. She decorated the pages with colored pencil drawings, adding such things as a canoe or a landscape for background. She talked about a friend at camp whose parents had gotten divorced since the previous summer, and the clinician commented on her feeling a sense of kinship with someone else who was going through a tough time and missing a parent.

Her father talked about how quiet the house was with Natalie away at camp. He found himself up at night watching old family videos, including the one from his wedding. He felt he needed to be sad about the profound changes occurring in his life—from being part of a happy couple to now taking responsibility as a single parent. In their own ways, both father and daughter were adjusting to new roles in the family and with others. Natalie reported that she and her father agreed on rules for her dating, and she would point out when other mothers at the basketball games were asking him questions that implied they wanted to "fix him up." Her father also resumed his weekly pickup basketball game with his high school friends. The change to a renewed focus on his own needs was verbalized by the therapist. In his sessions, he identified his problems with Natalie as stemming from her attempts at independence.

When treatment ended, Natalie and her father were able to talk at home easily about Natalie's mother, rather than avoiding the topic. Natalie's behavior had improved, and she was taking on a leadership role as cocaptain of her basketball team. Both she and her father were hesitant to begin dating, but did not connect this to feelings about the mother and her death. Upon termination, it was suggested that they might want or need to have additional treatment if the father became serious about a new partner, or when Natalie began making plans for going to college.

OVERVIEW OF KEY INTERVENTION CONCEPTS AND OTHER ISSUES

The current thinking in the field of childhood traumatic grief is that both trauma and grief symptoms must be addressed (Cohen et al., 2002; Shear et al., 2001; Stubenbort, Donnelly, & Cohen, 2001), and CBT approaches have yielded positive results in treating trauma. The implication is that CBT techniques should be part of all traumatic grief interventions in order to allow for the child's full participation in bereavement tasks. However, resolving existing trauma symptoms does not automatically imply that they are extinct, or that traversing the tasks of bereavement will be straightforward (Cohen et al., 2002). The reader is encouraged to review the factors in the two case illustrations above that reflect aspects of trauma and grief, and to consider how a particular type of treatment may have been indicated or contraindicated and could potentially have changed the outcome.

Issues in Delivery of Service

Key to providing optimal intervention is knowing who should be treated and when (Stokes, Pennington, Monroe, Papadatou, & Relf, 1999). By some estimates, fewer than 10% of bereaved individuals seek help in any form (e.g., from the clergy to mental health counselors), and some might conjecture that time and spontaneous remission are responsible for improvement in most cases (Exline, Dorrity, & Wortman, 1996). However, such predictions cannot yet be made for bereaved children in general or for traumatically bereaved children specifically. For those who are at highest risk or who are most impaired, it is likely that intervention decreases both the severity and duration of distress (the acuity and chronicity), is preventive, is most beneficial, and is perhaps necessary (Exline et al., 1996).

Basic bereavement services may be worthwhile for all traumatically bereaved children and families as preventive for optimal mental health, with ongoing assessment to reveal those children and families in need of more intensive care. Traumatically bereaved children and parents may benefit most from "serialized treatment" (James, 1989), spaced out and delivered when trauma and/or grief issues are relevant at significant developmental points in the life of a particular child and family.

Future Directions

We are far from knowing whether one type or course of traumatic grief treatment can help parents, children, and families—much less whether "one size fits all." Interventions for traumatic grief should be based on research and knowledge synthesizing both theory and practice. Future work will require the following:

1. Differentiation of traumatic grief from trauma and grief reactions.
2. Clear and concise definition and understanding of the bereavement process.

3. Identification of risk and resilience factors.
4. Thorough description of treatment protocols.
5. Ability to tailor treatment to individuals, based on specific criteria.
6. Understanding and delineation of the distinct intervention components.
7. Ability to replicate treatment through training.
8. Comparison to, and provision of, community programs.
9. Definition of successful bereavement interventions.

Although there are more questions than answers in the field of childhood traumatic grief treatment, the solid foundation of work in the related areas of trauma and bereavement provides a basis for moving the field forward. The stage is set for addressing some of these questions:

1. What are the essential components of effective treatment? Many practitioners and programs are eclectic, but are key elements such as psychoeducation, expression of feelings, exposure, and coping strategies necessary in any or all treatments?

2. What is the best type of treatment? Is a directive or nondirective approach best in all or some situations, or can treatment be fluid? How do supportive counseling and group work compare to treatment in an identified therapeutic context?

3. How long, how often, and when should a child be treated with a given treatment?

4. What are the "correct" dose, duration, and form of intervention (i.e., those that will provide the greatest benefit with the least risk of harm)?

5. When is the best time to begin treatment? How does one adapt an approach, given the tremendous variability in response over time (e.g., from shock to sadness to resolution), which causes treatment goals to vary according to the issues being confronted?

6. How should symptomatic and asymptomatic children and parents be treated, and what happens when there is a parent–child difference in severity and form of the symptoms?

7. Do individuals differ in their bereavement needs, and if so, should treatment be tailored as such? Is a support group of more value for newly widowed parents or bereaved children with less intense symptoms than for more impaired parents/children?

8. Should treatment be modified according to symptom presentation? If a death is traumatic, yet a bereaved child or parent does not show evidence of PTSD symptoms, is it necessary to include exposure techniques in order to achieve success?

9. What are the optimal qualifications for clinicians for a given treatment, and how should they be trained?

Whereas the challenge is great and we are just beginning to define and explore the field, there is the potential for tremendous learning and benefit to children and families experiencing traumatic grief.

REFERENCES

Appleton, V. (2001). Avenues of hope: Art therapy and the resolution of trauma. *Art Therapy: Journal of the American Art Therapy Association, 19*(1), 6–13.

Baker, J. E. (1997). Minimizing the impact of parental grief on children: Parent and family interventions. In C. R. Figley, B. E. Bride, & N. Mazza (Eds.), *Death and trauma: The traumatology of grieving* (pp. 139–157). Washington, DC: Taylor & Francis.

Baker, J. E., Sedney, M. A., & Gross, E. (1996). Psychological tasks for bereaved children. *American Journal of Orthopsychiatry, 62,* 105–116.

Berliner, L., & Saunders, B. E. (1996). Treating fear and anxiety in sexually abused children: Results of a controlled 2–year follow-up study. *Child Maltreatment, 1,* 294–309.

Burgess, A. W., & Hartman, C. R. (1993). Children's drawings. *Child Abuse and Neglect, 17,* 161–168.

Clark, D. C., Pynoos, R. S., & Goebel, A. E. (1996). Mechanisms and processes of adolescent bereavement. In R. J. Haggerty, L. R. Sherrod, N. Garmezy, & M. Rutter (Eds.), *Stress, risk, and resilience in children and adolescents* (pp. 100–146). Cambridge, England: Cambridge University Press.

Cohen, J. A., Greenberg, T., Padlo, S., Shipley, C., Mannarino, A., Deblinger, E., & Stubenbort, K. (2001, September). *Cognitive behavioral therapy for traumatic grief in children treatment manual* (rev. ed.). Pittsburgh, PA: Center for Traumatic Stress in Children and Adolescents, Department of Psychiatry, Allegheny General Hospital.

Cohen, J. A., & Mannarino, A. P. (1996). Factors that mediate treatment outcome of sexually abused preschool children. *Journal of the American Academy of Child and Adolescent Psychiatry, 35*(10), 1402–1410.

Cohen, J. A., & Mannarino, A. P. (2001, September). *Treatment of traumatized children: Client centered therapy (CCT) treatment manual* (rev. ed.). Pittsburgh, PA: Center for Traumatic Stress in Children and Adolescents, Department of Psychiatry, Allegheny General Hospital.

Cohen, J. A., Mannarino, A. P., Greenberg, T., Padlo, S., & Shipley, C. (2002). Childhood traumatic grief: concepts and controversies. *Trauma, Violence, and Abuse, 3*(1), 307–327.

Davidowitz, M., & Myrick, R. D. (1984). Responding to the bereaved: An analysis of "helping" statements. *Death Education, 8,* 1–10.

Eth, S., & Pynoos, R. (1985). Interaction of trauma and grief in childhood. In S. Eth & R. Pynoos (Eds.), *Post-traumatic stress disorder in children* (pp. 171–186). Washington, DC: American Psychiatric Press.

Exline, J. J., Dorrity, K., & Wortman, C. B. (1996). Coping with bereavement: A research review for clinicians. *In Session: Psychotherapy in Practice, 2*(4), 3–19.

Figley, C. R. (1989). *Helping traumatized families.* San Francisco: Jossey-Bass.

Finkelhor, D., & Browne, A. (1985). The traumatic impact of child sexual abuse: A conceptualization. *American Journal of Orthopsychiatry, 55*(4), 530–541.

Goenjian, A. K., Karayan, I., Pynoos, R. S., Minassian, D., Narjarian, L. M., Steinberg, A. M., & Fairbanks, L. A. (1997). Outcome of psychotherapy among early adolescents after trauma. *American Journal of Psychiatry, 154*(4), 536–542.

Goenjian, A. K., Molina, L., Steinberg, A., Fairbanks, L. A., Alvarez, M. L., Goenjian, H. A., & Pynoos, R. S. (2001). Posttraumatic stress and depressive reactions among Nicaraguan adolescents after Hurricane Mitch. *American Journal of Psychiatry, 158*, 788–794.

Goodman, R. F. (2002). Art as a component of grief work. In N. B. Webb (Ed.), *Helping bereaved children: A handbook for practitioners* (2nd ed., pp. 297–322). New York: Guilford Press.

Greenberg, M. S., & van der Kolk, B. A. (1987). Retrieval and integration of traumatic memories with the "painting cure. " In B. A. van der Kolk (Ed.), *Psychological trauma* (pp. 191–215). Washington, DC: American Psychiatric Press.

Haggerty, R. J., Sherrod, L. R., Garmezy, N., & Rutter, M. (Eds.). (1996). *Stress, risk, and resilience in children and adolescents*. Cambridge, England: Cambridge University Press.

James, B. (1989). *Treating traumatized children*. Lexington, MA: Heath.

Kissane, D. W., & Bloch, S. (1994). Family grief. *British Journal of Psychiatry, 164*, 728–740.

Kozlowska, K., & Hanney, L. (2001). An art therapy group for children traumatized by parental violence and separation. *Clinical Child Psychology and Psychiatry, 6*(1), 49–78.

Layne, C. M., Pynoos, R. S., Saltzman, W. S., Arslanagic, B., Black, M., Savjak, N., Popovic, T., Durakovic, E., Music, J., Jampara, N., Djapo, N., & Houston, R. (2001). Trauma/grief-focused group psychotherapy: School based post-war intervention with traumatized Bosnian adolescents. *Group Dynamics: Theory, Research, and Practice, 5*(4), 277–290.

March, J. S., Amaya-Jackson, L., Murray, M. C., & Schulte, A. (1998). Cognitive-behavioral psychotherapy for children and adolescents with posttraumatic stress disorder after a single incident stressor. *Journal of the American Academy of Child and Adolescent Psychiatry, 37*, 585–593.

Miller, M. (1993). Who are the best psychotherapists?: Qualities of the effective practitioner. *Psychotherapy in Private Practice, 12*(1), 1–18.

Murphy, J. (Ed.). (2001). *Art therapy with young survivors of sexual abuse*. Philadelphia: Taylor & Francis.

Nader, K. O. (1997). Childhood traumatic loss: The interaction of trauma and grief. In C. R. Figley, B. E. Bride, & N. Mazza (Eds.), *Death and trauma: The traumatology of grieving* (pp. 17–41). Washington, DC: Taylor & Francis.

Nolen-Hoeksema, S., & Larson, J. (1999). *Coping with loss*. Mahwah, NJ: Erlbaum.

Oltjenbruns, K. A. (2001). Developmental context of childhood grief. In M. S. Stroebe, R. O. Hansson, W. Stroebe, & H. Schut (Eds.), *Handbook of bereavement research* (pp. 169–198). Washington, DC: American Psychological Association.

Patterson, C. H. (1979). Rogerian counseling. In S. I. Harrison (Eds.), *Basic handbook of child psychiatry: Vol. 3. Therapeutic interventions* (pp. 203–215). New York: Basic Books.

Pfefferbaum, B., Gurwitch, R. H., McDonald, N. B., Leftwich, M. J. T., Sconzo, G. M., Messenbaugh, A. K., & Schultz, R. A. (2000). Posttraumatic stress among young children after the death of a friend or acquaintance in a terrorist bombing. *Psychiatric Services, 51*, 386–388.

Pfefferbaum, B., Nixon, S. J., Gucher, P. M., Tivis, R. D., Moore, V. L., Gurwitch, R. H., Pynoos, R. S., & Geis, H. K. (1999). Posttraumatic stress responses in bereaved children after the Oklahoma City bombing. *American Academy of Child and Adolescent Psychiatry, 38*, 1372–1379.

Rasmussen, L. A., & Cunningham, C. (1995). Focused play therapy and non-directive play therapy: Can they be integrated? *Journal of Child Sexual Abuse, 4*(1), 1–20.

Rogers, C. R. (1951). *Client-centered therapy*. Boston: Houghton Mifflin.

Roje, J. (1995). '94 earthquake in the eyes of children: Art therapy with elementary school children who were victims of disaster. *Art Therapy: Journal of the American Art Therapy Association, 12*(4), 237–243.

Saltzman, W. R., Pynoos, R. S., Layne, C. M., Steinberg, A. M., & Aisenberg, E. (2001). Trauma- and grief-focused intervention for adolescents exposed to community violence: Results of a school-based screening and group treatment protocol. *Group Dynamics: Theory, Research and Practice, 5*(4) 291–303.

Schneiderman, G., Winders, P., Tallett, S., & Feldman, W. (1994). Do child and/or parent bereavement programs work? *Canadian Journal of Psychiatry, 39*, 215–217.

Shear, M. K., Frank, E., Foa, E., Cherry, C., Reynolds, C. F., Bilt, J. V., & Masters, S. (2001). Traumatic grief treatment: A pilot study. *American Journal of Psychiatry, 158*, 1506–1508.

Siegel, K., Mesagno, F. P., & Christ, G. (1990). A prevention program for bereaved children. *American Journal of Orthopsychiatry, 60*(2), 168–175.

Silverman, P. R. (2000). Children as part of the family drama: An integrated view of childhood bereavement. In R. Malkinson, S. S. Rubin, & E. Witztum (Eds.), *Traumatic and nontraumatic loss and bereavement: Clinical theory and practice* (pp. 67–90). Madison, CT: Psychosocial Press.

Silverman, P. R., & Worden, J. W. (1993). Children's reactions to the death of a parent. In M. S. Stroebe, W. Stroebe, & R. O. Hansson (Eds.), *Handbook of bereavement* (pp. 300–316). New York: Cambridge University Press.

Steinberg, A. (1997). Death as trauma for children: A relational treatment approach. In C. R. Figley, B. E. Bride, & N. Mazza (Eds.), *Death and trauma: The traumatology of grieving* (pp. 123–137). Washington, DC: Taylor & Francis.

Stokes, J., Pennington, J., Monroe, B., Papadatou, D., & Relf, M. (1999). Developing services for bereaved children: A discussion of the theoretical and practical issues involved. *Mortality, 4*(3), 291–307.

Stubenbort, K., Donnelly, G. R., & Cohen, J. (2001). Cognitive-behavioral group therapy for bereaved adults and children following an air disaster. *Group Dynamics: Theory, Research, and Practice, 5*(4), 261–276.

Worden, J. W. (1991). *Grief counseling and grief therapy* (2nd ed.). New York: Springer.

Creation of a Group Mural to Promote Healing Following a Mass Trauma

IDALIA MAPP
DAVID KOCH

The purpose of this chapter is to describe a group art project created at Big Brothers Big Sisters of New York City (BBBS/NYC). It was begun a month after the attack on the World Trade Center (WTC) twin towers on September 11, 2001. The primary goal of the "Mural Project," as it came to be called, was to provide social, psychological, and emotional support to the youngsters served by the agency—the "Little Brothers" and "Little Sisters," between the ages of 7 and 18 —who were experiencing various responses of fear, anxiety, and posttraumatic stress following the egregious attack.

The rationale behind the Mural Project was that art can serve as therapy for psychological and emotional trauma, and that through the process of creating art in a group, children and youth receive social support that helps them cope with their feelings of stress. Although this particular project was a response to a specific event, we believe that the benefits of art projects and social support can apply to *any* traumatic event.

Over the past several decades, various researchers have conducted studies reporting the benefits both of art therapies (Glaister & McGuinness, 1992; Moon, 1999; Riley, 2001; Walsh, 1993) and of social support (Benard, 1995; Longres, 2000; Rak & Patterson, 1999) for alleviating negative symptoms of traumatic events. According to Riley (2001), for example, distressed adolescents often tend to avoid help from adults or professional therapists. Art therapy, however, offers teens a nonthreatening way to express their inner feelings. Adolescents may "act out" as a cover for their depression, but art therapy is useful in assessing and treating such depression (Cantlay, 1996; Wohl & Kaufman, 1985; Malchiodi, 1998). Art therapy can also offer support to adolescents experiencing abuse, lack of self-regard, or sudden social or academic failure. Art as an expressive language provides an entrée into a relationship with teenagers by tapping into their creativity and offering a form of accessible, friendly communication.

In addition to the potential benefit of art projects for people suffering from traumatic events, social support has been shown to be of great value in helping adolescents and adults cope with and resolve the negative consequences of crises. Longres (2000) defines "social support" as "the comfort, assistance, or information individuals receive through their formal or informal contacts with others" (p. 562), based on the principles of mutual aid. The many positive functions served by social support groups include reducing isolation, instilling optimism about the future, and facilitating friendships among individuals who are experiencing similar problems. In addition, support groups can provide an atmosphere of trust and respect that enables individuals to discuss their fears with role models who exhibit effective adaptive strategies to overcome difficulties. Members of support groups also profit from helping others. As a result, when individuals "leave support groups, it may be with higher self-esteem and confidence and a heightened sense of purpose and belonging" (Longres, 2000, p. 53).

Social support can tap into and nourish an individual's innate resilience. According to Benard (1995), "resilience" refers to a set of qualities we each innately possess in varying degrees that foster a process of successful adaptation and transformation despite risk and adversity. In the literature on stress and coping, social support is defined both as a protective factor and as a recovery factor, in which resilience plays a major part. When individuals or families confront risks or crises, they often draw from a network of relationships to give them strength and direction. On occasions, individuals or families rely on existing sources of support in addition to sometimes seeking other, unique forms of support, such as group gathering, group projects, and other kinds of activities. These may give meaning to the situation, help individuals develop coping strategies, and foster their ability to change.

Most of the benefits provided by social support were evident during the Mural Project at BBBS/NYC, which is described and illustrated in detail in this chapter, and then interpreted within the context of the literature on art as therapy and on social support and resilience. First, however, we describe the background, mission, and structure of the national BBBS organization, since the Mural Project was initiated and implemented in the New York City agency of this organization.

A BRIEF OVERVIEW OF BIG BROTHERS BIG SISTERS

At the beginning of the 20th century, in 1902, Big Sisters was the first "branch" of the BBBS organization to be initiated. It was quickly followed by the Big Brothers movement, in 1904, which eventually led to the organization of a Big Brothers agency in Cincinnati in 1910. Before World War I, the Big Brothers and Big Sisters movements were characterized by many forms of organization, but all of the efforts were united by a single spirit—a desire to help children (generally from one-parent homes) whose moral, mental, and physical development was endangered by their environments and backgrounds. The two organizations grew and changed in many ways throughout the following decades, and in 1977 Big Sisters International and Big Brothers of America merged and became one organization, BBBS of America.

Initial efforts focused on the development and piloting of a set of *Standards and Required Procedures for One-to-One Service* (BBBS of America, 1986, 1996); these were first adopted in 1986 and consisted of both corporate and program management standards. Compliance with these standards and required procedures became the hallmark of an effective BBBS agency and the basis for building consistent services in more than 500 BBBS agencies across all 50 states.

In essence, BBBS is a community mentoring program that matches (on a one-to-one basis) an adult volunteer, known as a Big Brother or Big Sister, to a child, known as a Little Brother or Little Sister, with the expectation that a caring and supportive relationship will develop. The match between volunteer and child is the most important component of the intervention. Equally important are the ongoing supervision and monitoring of the "match relationship" by a professional staff member, who selects and matches each volunteer and child, and communicates with the volunteer, the child's parent or guardian, and the child throughout the life of the matched relationship.

The volunteer intervention in the one-to-one relationship with a child comprises about 3–5 hours per week, every week, over the course of the relationship, which may last a year or longer. The activities that characterize a specific matched relationship relate to the goals that were initially identified by the case manager, based on a lengthy interview with the child and his or her parent or guardian. The primary general goal is to develop a mutually satisfying relationship in which both parties meet on a regular basis; specific goals are more varied, and can relate to the young person's drug behaviors, relationships with other children and siblings, school attendance, academic performance, general hygiene, or learning new skills. Once the goals for a specific match are established, they are then developed into an individualized case plan that is regularly updated by the case manager as progress occurs and circumstances change.

The rationale that has guided BBBS service for nearly a century has been the belief that the consistent presence of a nonfamilial caring adult has a positive impact on the social-emotional development of a child or young person, particularly one growing up in a single-parent family or in an adverse situation. Over the years, the development of the BBBS service has been based on the overriding belief that a consistent and frequent volunteer contact is a powerful influence in a young person's life.

BBBS/NYC annually serves over 4,000 children and their families through its various programs. In addition to the "Traditional Core Mentoring Program," in which the mentor spends at least 4–5 hours biweekly with the young person and is in regular phone contact with him or her, the agency has established a number of regular mentoring programs, including the following:

- The Workplace Mentoring Program
- The Borough Partnership Program
- The Juvenile Justice Mentoring Program

The Workplace Mentoring Program focuses on collaborative efforts between BBBS/NYC and schools and corporations; it requires that students spend 2–3 hours weekly with a mentor at the mentor's work site, where the focus may be on homework, life skills, and an introduction to the business world. The Borough Partnership Program focuses on outreach efforts into underserved neighborhoods in Brooklyn, the Bronx, and Queens, and has enabled BBBS/NYC to recruit and match volunteers with youngsters in their own neighborhoods. The Juvenile Justice Mentoring Program matches specially trained volunteers with youth who have been in trouble with the law.

In the face of the traumatic events surrounding the WTC attack, the BBBS/NYC experienced extraordinary stressors, which led the agency to develop an expanded set of programs that were congruent with its core mission. The days and weeks following the attacks were characterized by strains that affected the functioning of the agency and its ability to provide services to children. Due to the attacks, for example, the Workplace Mentoring Program was in disarray. Staff members and volunteers were disoriented, confused, and frightened, both because of the terrible events and because the agency moved from a financial surplus to a deficit (thus increasing the risk of staff layoffs).

With a sense of institutional resilience and hardiness, BBBS/NYC responded to the trauma of the WTC attack through the development of new programmatic and financial initiatives. One of these was the "Teddy Bear Project," in which the agency collaborated with a radio station in Georgia to distribute over 6,000 teddy bears for the children in New York City affected by the events that soon became known simply as "9/11."

Another project, the "New Americans" program, was designed to help immigrant families who experienced bias after the attack. Other special programs were developed for children who experienced impaired functioning because of fear of terrorism or who lost a parent or relative during the attack. One of these children's programs was the Mural Project, officially called "Our City, Our Children, Our Pride," which represented an attempt to provide children (as well as mentors, staff, and volunteers) with a community project that would enable them to process the stressors and strains associated with the 9/11 attack. As noted earlier, although this project was specific to the events of that day, its approach could be adjusted to traumatic events of various types (such as natural disasters, transportation catastrophes, and situations of community violence).

THE MURAL PROJECT

The germ of the idea for the Mural Project developed after the 9/11 attack when Emil Ramnarine, a BBBS/NY borough network manager who facilitated training in the agency, felt uneasy and helpless, as did all the people who worked with him. These feelings were intensified in part by the sad realization that BBBS/NYC lost a Big Sister during the attack. The news of her death was shocking to all at the agency, even those children and staff members who did not know her.

Looking for a way to be useful in this face of the crisis, Emil went to "Ground Zero"—the site of the attacks, where the WTC twin towers had stood—to volunteer in whatever way he could. When he arrived there, he was told to get in line and sign up as a volunteer. While making several attempts to put his name on the list, he kept receiving the same message: "At this time, we are not accepting any more volunteers. We had a tremendous response, and at the moment we do not need any more volunteers."

Emil therefore went back to the agency and began to think about what he could do to boost his and the agency's morale to help the children, mentors, staff members, and other volunteers to cope with the aftermath of the crisis. He especially thought of doing something with the children that would help them to bounce back. He thought that involving children in an activity that was fun and creative might help them to cope better. That thought process, and Emil's impulse to help the people at the agency, led him to the idea of developing a mural in which everyone could participate.

As Emil was germinating this idea, a volunteer at the agency who was a sculptor became interested in helping. This person created art out of junk, and he invited Emil to his studio to see whether any of his materials might be of use for the development of the mural. Emil looked around and found pieces of plywood about 12" × 12", and immediately thought of having each child join with his or her mentor to work on the plywood. As for the rest of the materials that would be needed for the Mural Project, such as pencils, markers, and brushes, Emil planned to raise the funds through donations from individuals—friends, family members of the children, and the agency staff—since he knew that most organizations and institutions were involved with sending donations to help the cause at Ground Zero directly.

Although both the basic idea for a group art project and the materials for the project existed, the specific idea for the design of the mural had yet to be conceptualized. That idea came from a woman named Cynthia Clark, who by sheer chance contacted BBBS/NYC at that time, in an attempt to offer her services as a volunteer.

Cynthia was motivated to help after she heard Mayor Rudolph Giuliani plead with the public for assistance. Since Cynthia had graduated from the Fashion Institute of Technology in jewelry design and had worked as a jewelry manufacturer in New Jersey for the past years, she thought she would best be suited to help with some kind of art project. At the same time, she saw an ad on TV for BBBS; this made her think of a friend who had become a single mother at 18, and of her friend's 10- year-old son, whom Cynthia had cared for as a baby and with whom she had developed a close relationship over the years. That connection to her friend's child made Cynthia feel that she related well to children and could help with children. She thus felt inspired to contact BBBS/NYC to be a mentor.

When she got to the agency, however, she was told that it would take 6 months to process her application, and she did not want to wait. As she put it, "I wanted to do something *now*; the motivation, the intensity, the interest was *now*, and I did not want the energy to weaken or go away." As fate would have it, Cynthia was at the agency at the same time Emil and others were developing the idea of creating a mural, and they mentioned to her that volunteers were needed for that project. She thus grabbed the opportunity and said, "I am an artist and I love children," and so Cynthia became intricately involved in the Mural Project.

As a result of her artistic sensibilities, Cynthia came up with the idea of using the American flag's red, white and blue for the creation of the mural, as a gesture of patriotism. Cynthia also contributed to the mural's design by drawing a small sample with little people, and suggested that this idea could be executed on a larger scale. Every child, volunteer, and staff member, she further suggested, could use a design area modeled on a "postage stamp," and place a person or people on the underlying "flag," to signify the 50 United States. Emil liked the idea. The mural team members felt that this project would give all the participants an opportunity to express mourning, compassion, and respect for both the people directly affected by the attack and their grieving families and close friends. Even more than this, the team envisioned that the mural would be a tribute to survivors of the attacks who were in the area surrounding the WTC and barely made it out, as well as all people who were forced to live in the shadow of 9/11 and its aftermath—the scary, uncertain, radically changed future.

As envisioned by the creators of the Mural Project, the completed mural would be displayed at the agency as a constant reminder to the many children involved that they accomplished this piece of artwork during a time of crisis, and that they supported each other and were able to commit themselves every weekend to completing it. The creators of the project hoped that if the children became involved in the mural, it would give them something to look forward to doing, keep them engaged in making something creative and meaningful, and provide them with a way to cope with and work through their complex feelings related to the crisis. The initiators of the Mural Project also expected that the display of the mural would give the children, their families, the staff, and the mentors a sense of pride and satisfaction about engaging in a joint effort that was therapeutic and supportive.

Involving the Children and Mentors in the Mural Project

First, the mentors had to be told about the Mural Project. Two social workers from BBBS/NYC contacted them individually and informed them about the project. Each mentor, in turn, contacted his or her matched child and the child's parent(s), to explain the project to them and get them involved. In all, 17 children aged 8–15 years worked on the mural, and there were also 17 mentors, one matched with each child. The mentors were responsible for bringing the children to the center and returning them to their homes.

The participants in the Mural Project (Emil, Cynthia, the mentors, and the children) started on the first weekend in October 2001 and continued every weekend until the end of January 2002. People came at different hours of the afternoon, from about 1 to 5 P.M. Parents were concerned about the safety of their children, but the mentors reassured them that their children were safe. Cynthia was there every weekend for the duration of the project, even though she worked at two other jobs during the week.

To initiate the making of the mural, each mentor–child pair was first given a big sheet of paper on which they were asked to jot down or draw any ideas or any feelings related to the 9/11 crisis. This first step produced many ideas, including expressions of anger, fear, anxiety, and hope, among other feelings. The words then became images that were drawn on the plywood by each child (with the support of his or her mentor, the other children, the staff, and the volunteers), in accordance with the overall design concept for the mural as explained above. The aims were to enable each child to create his or her own artwork, to contribute to the overall mural, and to achieve some kind of closure. Because the pencils, markers, and other material used for this project were limited, each child, mentor, and volunteer communicated with others about various aspects of the artwork being produced, to avoid wasting materials. Eventually, in January 2002, each individual artistic depiction was joined together to create the final mural. On February 13, 2002, the mural began a display tour to corporate lobbies around New York City. Its eventual home will be back at the BBBS/NYC.

Artworks Created in the Mural Project

In this section, reproductions of seven representative artworks created by youth in the Mural Project are shown, accompanied by a brief discussion that highlights the symbolism, cognitions, and emotions depicted in each work. The children and families involved have granted permission to BBBS/NYC to reproduce their art for the purpose of community education and healing.

Figure 5.1, created by Rubin, age 15, is titled "United We Stand." It depicts emergency and health care workers, including a fireman, a policeman, and a nurse. Behind them is the American flag. This is a patriotic picture that also depicts unity, togetherness, and oneness in the face of a crisis, as indicated by its title. In addition, the picture depicts both men and women, and people of both black and white ethnic/racial backgrounds; this conveys the idea that America is a multicultural society, and that people of both sexes work together to help in an emergency.

Figure 5.2, created by Shanna, age 14, is titled "Touching Fingers" and is very optimistic. In the picture, we see two hands reaching out to touch each other, symbolizing the need for human contact and support; on the hands are written the words "The sun will still come out tomorrow." Even after such a horrific attack, this individual child still felt optimistic about the new day to come "tomorrow." Behind the touching fingers are a blazing yellow and red sun, blue sky, and white clouds—which together compose the colors of the American flag. Below the hands there appears to be green grass, which also symbolizes life. The artist of this picture felt no need to show the people attached to the hands, apparently because the hands—which are reminiscent of the "touching fingers" on the ceiling of the Sistine Chapel—symbolize to the artist the part of us that can make contact and give comfort to one another.

Figure 5.3 was done by Sylvia, age 9, with help from Velma, her Big Sister. The picture is an optimistic depiction despite the traumatic events of 9/11, though there is also a sense of great loss suggested by the art-

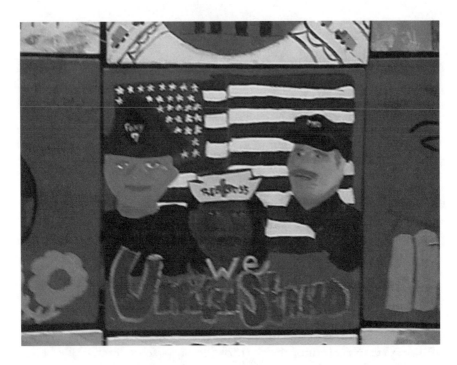

FIGURE 5.1. "United We Stand."

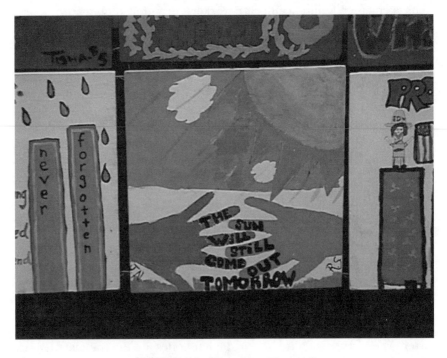

FIGURE 5.2. "Touching Fingers."

work. Most obvious is a large red heart that contains the WTC twin towers in the center, one of which boasts a waving American flag. Sylvia said, "We decided to add words that came out of the heart that are needed for a peaceful world, like 'patience,' 'kindness,' 'truth,' 'tolerance,' 'love,' and 'hope.'" Above the heart is the phrase "Always in our hearts," and below the heart is the phrase "Always remembered." The term "always" in both of these phrases, which symbolizes eternity and invincibility, could reflect the artist's profound feelings of loss attributable to the attack. That sense of loss may also be indicated by the fact that the picture contains no people, which could signify the artist's emotional feeling that people were lost in the attack.

Figure 5.4, created by Tati, age 11, captures both the trauma of the event and the optimism and positive feelings people can experience when they know they are doing a good deed to help out in a crisis. The latter feeling is depicted in the image of the driver, who is smiling while driving the emergency van. The van is mainly black, which symbolizes the darkness and death related to the attack, but on its side is a large red cross, which symbolizes hope, love, and caring. The patriotic spirit of the picture is conveyed by the colors of the word "emergency," which are red, white, and blue; those colors are also prominent elsewhere in the picture—along

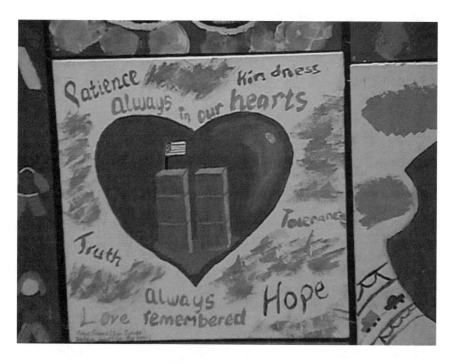

FIGURE 5.3. "Always in Our Hearts."

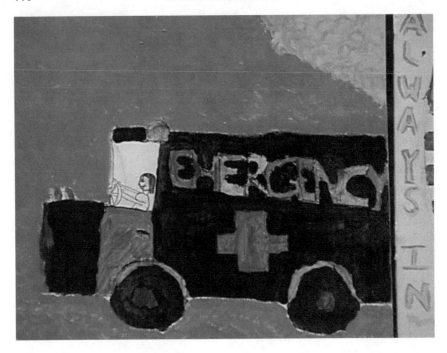

FIGURE 5.4. "Emergency Van."

the tops of the wheels (blue), on the side of the cab (red) and inside the cab (white). The youth who drew this picture apparently felt that no matter how dark and ominous an event may be, there is reason to smile if you know you are helping out both your fellow human beings and your country.

In Figure 5.5, created by Whitney, age 8, two complex feelings and images are given equal prominence: those of love and longing. One feeling—of love, togetherness, and acceptance of differences—is conveyed by the two young women, one white and one black, who are holding hands. Their shirts say "I Love NY" (with the word "love" depicted by a heart). A heart is also attached to the center of the twin towers, but the tower on the right appears to have smoke coming out of its top—which could indicate the damage done by the attack. That idea is supported by the words in front of the twin towers, on the green grass: "We miss you, WTC." The feeling of loss and longing thus coexists with the feeling of love and support in this picture. The patriotic theme is prominently displayed in two ways: The girls are waving flags, and the red, white, and blue colors are prominent in the hearts, the clouds, and the sky. A large yellow sun in the upper left corner of the picture conveys the positive feelings of the young artist who created this basically optimistic artwork.

Figure 5.6 was created by Isella, age 12; its title, "Proud of What We Do," conveys a positive message about Americans and America. In this picture, we see the WTC twin towers prominently in the center, and the two people on top of the buildings display a patriotic symbol, the American flag. The flag's colors are realistic (i.e., red, white, and blue); they are also the colors of the words in the picture, in keeping with the patriotic theme. As in some of the other pictures, the individuals in the artwork are of different skin complexions. In this work, the individual on the left appears to be female, while the one on the right appears to be male—again reflecting the diversity of the people of America.

Figure 5.7 is by Evadney, age 12, assisted by her Big Sister, Mandy. It is full of symbolism, mystery, defiance, hope, remembrance, and love. Mandy said about the number "27" in the picture, "Someone I knew once was 27 and worked at the WTC and is gone now." The rest of the words convey universal expressions of loss. The word "gone" (at the top) indicates loss, and "never again" recalls the slogan of Jews about the Holocaust of World War II. These are words of defiance, indicating that such an annihilation we not be allowed to happen again. On the twin towers themselves are written the words "never forgotten," which indicates that

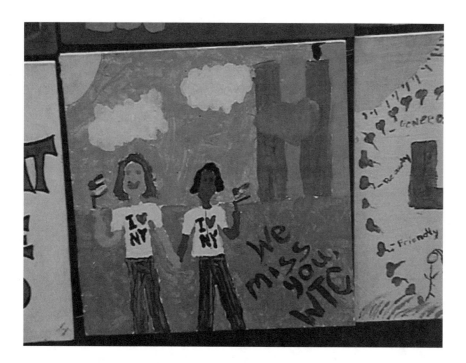

FIGURE 5.5. "Love and Longing."

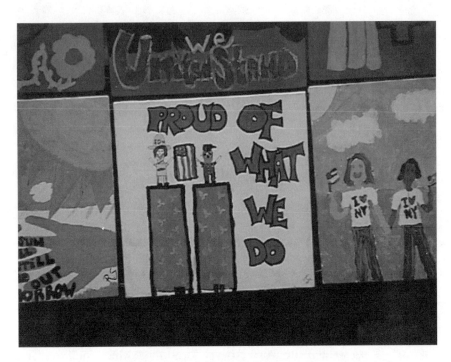

FIGURE 5.6. "Proud of What We Do."

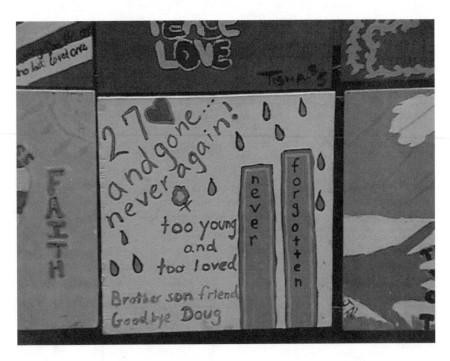

FIGURE 5.7. "27 and Gone . . . Never Again!"

the murdered victims of 9/11 will remain in our minds and hearts—and, at the top of the picture, the heart symbolizes love. Drops are falling from the sky onto the towers, symbolizing tears from heaven. Between the drops is a flower with a "cross" for its stem, which symbolizes either Christianity or the Red Cross—in either case, caring and love. Most startling of all about this picture, however, are the words written at the bottom: "Brother son friend Goodbye Doug." This suggests that the youth who drew this picture lost a friend or a relative in the WTC attack. Above these words is written "too young and too loved," indicating that Doug was himself a youth, and that the artist (and no doubt others) loved Doug very much. Also noteworthy about this picture is that no people are depicted, which could indicate the artist's sense of the complete annihilation of humankind in this egregious attack. This picture is remarkable for the diversity of its symbolism, imagery, words, and emotions.

Overview/Summary of the Mural Project

Interviews with the children, mentors, staff, and volunteers have affirmed that the Mural Project provided important psychological and emotional benefits to help the participants cope with their fear, anxiety, and stress unleashed by the 9/11 attack. The final result of the project—the mural that combined the separate pictures into a single artwork—symbolized the beneficial support the participants received from one another, as they came together to share their contributions. Through their interactions, they received support and strength to go on. In addition, they created a context in which they could process their grief and mourn in their own way. The horrific situation they were memorializing helped them empathize with those directly affected, cope with their own suffering and pain, and at the same time build hope for themselves in the present and for the future.

ART PROJECTS AS THERAPY

Numerous studies have documented positive outcomes for art projects carried out in a supportive environment during a time of crisis by young people in various types of traumatic situations (Deane, Fitch, & Carman, 2000; Gabriel, 2001; Glaister & McGuinness, 1992; Kozlowska & Hanney, 2001; Moon, 1999; Walsh, 1993). For example, Kozlowska and Hanney (2001) described the treatment of five traumatized children (aged 4–8 years) via adjunctive group art therapy, and reviewed the theoretical basis for such a treatment strategy. All the children had been exposed to cumulative traumatic experiences of parental violence. The children presented symptoms of posttraumatic stress, exhibited developmental problems related to trauma, had difficulties with any discussion of traumatic events or family concerns, and reacted with hyperarousal and/or an "emotional shutdown" response to reminders of the trauma. Previous treatments had included a combination of social, family, psychological, and biological interventions.

The group was given a therapeutic intervention developed by a child psychiatrist and an art therapist to facilitate therapeutic change. The therapeutic use of artworks facilitated exposure to traumatic cues in a less direct manner, allowed for desensitization of anxiety and unpleasant body sensations, helped the children recount the story of the parental separation, and enabled them to label and articulate affective states using art and narrative. According to the researchers, the art therapy intervention helped the children by promoting their positive expectations about the future and making overt the coping skills they used to manage ongoing stresses.

According to Glaister and McGuinness (1992), both adolescent and adult survivors of chronic trauma, who may have survived hundreds of episodes of battering and abuse, have no gauge of what is "normal" and continue to live in an emotional climate of fear. Their coping patterns prevent healthy adaptation. Such traumatized individuals can be helped by the inclusion of expressive techniques in therapy, such as therapeutic drawing, which can facilitate the emotional processing of chronic trauma issues.

Walsh (1993) conducted a study to test the effectiveness of an "art future-image intervention" designed to increase self-esteem, improve future time perspective, and decrease depression in hospitalized suicidal adolescents. The intervention consisted of drawing oneself or other people, places, or events at a future time. A pretest–posttest design was used with two groups, an experimental group and a placebo group. The experimental group, although hospitalized for a shorter length of time, showed greater positive changes than the placebo group ($p = .08$). According to Walsh, the effectiveness of the art future-image intervention was demonstrated by participant enthusiasm, shorter hospitalization, and positive comments at follow-up.

SOCIAL SUPPORT AND RESILIENCE

The research literature shows the capacity of social support to enhance coping abilities and to increase resilience and hardiness during times of crisis, trauma, and stress (Dohrenwend & Dohrenwend, 1981; Kessler, Magee, & Nelson, 1996; Longres, 2000; Pearlin, 1989; Rak & Patterson, 1999; Thoits, 1983; Wheaton, 1990; Winfield, 2002). Rak and Patterson

(1999) identified social support as one of four major groups of protective factors in the so-called "buffering hypothesis." This hypothesis holds that certain variables, called "protective factors," may provide a buffer of protection against life events that affect at-risk children. In addition to social supports in the environment (e.g., role models, such as teachers, school counselors, mental health workers, neighbors, and clergy), protective factors include the personal characteristics of the children, their family conditions, and self-concept factors.

The social support literature also often focuses on stressful life events and their relationship to coping outcomes and mental health indices (Dohrenwend & Dohrenwend, 1981; Kessler et al., 1996; Pearlin, 1989; Thoits, 1983; Wheaton, 1990). Specific stress-moderating variables have been identified that facilitate more effective or adaptive functioning in the face of either discrete stressful life events or more chronic strains. These variables have included social support resources (Cohen & Syme, 1985; Cohen & Hoberman, 1983; Wortman, 1984), as well as personality variables such as resilience, hardiness, and dispositional optimism (Saleebey, 1997; Winfield, 2002) (see Figure 5.8).

According to Winfield (2002), "In reality, resilience is an interaction between the characteristics of the individual and the environment" (p. 1). The concept of resilience has been used in health and psychiatric research, where there is considerable interest in understanding the characteristics that enable individuals to survive severely traumatic experiences. Terms often considered to be synonymous with "resilience" include "positive coping," "persistence," "adaptation," and "long-term success despite adverse circumstances." Winfield cautions that the most "meaningful con-

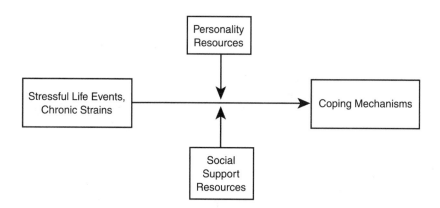

FIGURE 5.8. Stress, coping, and stress-moderating variables. Based on Dohrenwend and Dohrenwend (1981).

ception views resilience not as a fixed attribute, but as vulnerabilities or protective mechanisms that modify the individual's response to risk situations and operate at turning points during his or her life" (p. 2).

Saleebey (1997) claims that resilient youth have taken the opportunity to fulfill the basic human need for social support, caring, and love. Sometimes this need cannot be fulfilled at home, and so it is vital that schools or other organizations, such as BBBS, provide opportunities for young people to develop caring relationships with both adults and other youth.

A stress-moderating factor that is related to resilience and that also varies among individuals is hardiness (Kobasa, 1982; Ouellette, 1993). There is substantial agreement that hardiness moderates stress, such that in the face of highly stressful circumstances, hardiness is predictive of more effective coping; that is, individuals high in hardiness are more able to handle high-stress or strain situations adaptively.

"Hardiness" has been conceptualized as a stance toward self and the world that is defined by a sense of commitment, control, and challenge. "Commitment" is characterized by a purposive connection to what one is engaged in doing, while "challenge" suggests a sense of being in a world where change is expected. "Control" suggests a sense of personal influence over one's life activities. According to the hardiness perspective, it was to be expected that those youth involved in the BBBS/NYC Mural Project who demonstrated a high degree of hardiness would be more apt to channel their coping effectively through the creation of the mural.

CONCLUSIONS: THE BENEFITS OF THE MURAL PROJECT AT BBBS/NYC

The children's Mural Project at BBBS/NYC demonstrates the various facets (discussed throughout this chapter) of coping, art as therapy, social support, resilience, and hardiness. Substantial life stressors and chronic strains are associated with trauma, such as that evoked by the WTC attacks. These stressors and strains require superior coping mechanisms. Categories of coping mechanisms include problem-focused (e.g., direct action, information seeking, reframing, and planning) and emotion-based (e.g., venting, distraction, avoidance, and emotional regulation) coping mechanisms (Folkman & Lazarus, 1980; Moos & Schaefer, 1993; Nerenz & Leventhal, 1983).

Social support mechanisms facilitate effective coping in response to strain and stressors. These mechanisms can include tangible aid, emotional support, and cognitive support; together, they can help ameliorate the negative consequences of any kind of severe trauma. In response to the trauma of 9/11, for example, the children at BBBS/NYC were able to utilize the social support resources of the BBBS/NYC agency. In particular, emotional support was a central feature of the development of the children's mural. Children and mentors came together in the form of a community to provide each other with nurturance.

Through the group process of creating the mural, the children and mentors completed a task that combined images of hope, optimism, and love with those of fear, stress, and anxiety. The mural provided a venue whereby trust and connection to others were intensified. The deployment of social support resources buffered the negative effects of the stressors and strains in the children's everyday life. In keeping with the research evidence, this project showed that social support moderated stress and distress. We believe that those individuals with the most resilience and hardiness would be those who experienced the most positive outcomes.

The experience at BBBS/NYC also demonstrated how organizations may facilitate resilience and hardiness among individuals. What emerged within the children's Mural Project was a combination of the utilization of social support resources and the display of personality features such as hardiness within a highly resilient agency setting. In essence, the children's Mural Project both ameliorated a number of the negative mental health effects of the World Trade Center attacks and revealed a picture of a hardy agency that was able to respond resiliently to the stressors and strains with programmatic innovations (Koch & Mapp, 2002; Luks, 2002). In its response, the agency demonstrated a creative approach to New York City's children in need. We hope that this detailed presentation of an agency in crisis can serve as a template for program development to benefit children in the aftermath of trauma.

REFERENCES

Benard, B. (1995, August). *Fostering resilience in children: ERIC Digest* (No. ED386327) [Online]. Available: http://www.searcheric.org

Big Brothers Big Sisters (BBBS) of America. (1986). *Standards and procedures for one-to-one service*. Philadelphia: Author.

Big Brothers Big Sisters (BBBS) of America. (1996). *Standards and procedures for one-to-one service* (rev. ed.). Philadelphia: Author.

Cantlay, L. (1996). *Detecting child abuse: Recognizing children at risk through drawings.* Santa Barbara, CA: Holly Press.

Cohen, S., & Hoberman, H. M. (1983). Positive events and social supports as buffers of life change stress. *Journal of Applied Social Psychology, 13*, 99–125.

Cohen, S., & Syme, S. L. (1985). Issues in the study and application of social support. In S. Cohen & S. L. Syme (Eds.), *Social support and health* (pp. 3–22). New York: Academic Press.

Deane, K., Fitch, M., & Carman, M. (2000). An innovative art therapy program for cancer patients. *Canadian Oncology Nursing Journal, 10*(4), 147–151, 152–157.

Dohrenwend, B. S., & Dohrenwend, B. P. (1981). Life stress and illness: Formulation of the issues. In B. S. Dohrenwend & B. P. Dohrenwend (Eds.), *Stressful life events and their contexts* (pp. 1–27). New York: Prodist.

Folkman, S., & Lazarus, R. S. (1980). An analysis of coping in a middle-aged community sample. *Journal of Health and Social Behavior, 21*, 219–239.

Gabriel, B. (2001). Art therapy with adult bone marrow transplant patients in isolation: A pilot study. *Psycho-Oncology, 10*(2), 114–123.

Glaister, J. A., & McGuinness, T. (1992). The art of therapeutic drawing: Helping chronic trauma survivors. *Journal of Psychosocial Nursing and Mental Health Services, 30*(5), 9–17.

Kessler, R. C., Magee, W. J., & Nelson, C. B. (1996). Analysis of psychosocial stress. In H. Kaplan (Ed.) *Psychosocial stress: Perspective on structure, theory, life course and methods* (pp. 333–366). New York: Plenum Press.

Kobasa, S. C. (1982). The hardy personality: Towards a social psychology of stress and health. In J. Suls & G. Sanders (Eds.), *Social psychology of health and illness* (pp. 3–33). Hillsdale, NJ: Erlbaum.

Koch, D. E., & Mapp, I. (2002). *Guide for case study week, 2002.* New York: Fordham University, Graduate School of Social Service.

Kozlowska, K., & Hanney, L. (2001). An art therapy group for children traumatized by parental violence and separation. *Clinical Child Psychology and Psychiatry, 6*(1), 49–78.

Longres, J. (2000). *Human behavior in the social environment.* Itasca, IL: Peacock.

Luks, A. (2002). *The big picture.* New York: Big Brothers Big Sisters of New York City.

Malchiodi, C. (1998). *Understanding children's drawings.* New York: Guilford Press.

Moon, B. (1999). The tears make me paint: The role of responsive artmaking in adolescent art therapy. *Art Therapy, 16*, 78–82.

Moos, R. H., & Schaefer, J. A. (1993). Coping resources and processes: Current concepts and measures. In L. Goldberger & S. Breznitz (Eds.), *Handbook of stress: Theoretical and clinical aspects* (pp. 234–257). New York: Free Press.

Nerenz, D. R., & Leventhal, H. (1983). Self-regulation theory in chronic illness. In T. Burish & L. Bradley (Eds.), *Coping with chronic disease: Research and applications* (pp. 13–37). New York: Academic Press.

Ouellette, S. C. (1993). Inquiries into hardiness. In L. Goldberger & S. Breznitz (Eds.), *Handbook of stress: Theoretical and clinical aspects* (pp. 77–100). New York: Free Press.

Pearlin, L. I. (1989). The sociological study of stress. *Journal of Health and Social Behavior, 30*, 241–256.

Rak, C. F., & Patterson, L. E. (1999). Promoting resilience in at-risk children. In L. Shulman (Ed.), *The skills of helping individuals, families, groups, and communities* (4th ed., pp. 368–373). Itasca, IL: Peacock.

Riley, S. (2001). Art therapy with adolescents. *Western Journal of Medicine, 175*, 54–57.

Saleebey, D. (Ed.). (1997). *The strengths perspective in social work practice* (2nd ed.). New York: Longman.

Thoits, P. A. (1983). Dimensions of life events that influence psychological distress: An evaluation of the literature. In H. B. Kaplan (Ed.), *Psychosocial stress: Trends in theory and research* (pp. 33–103). New York: Academic Press.

Walsh, S. M. (1993). Future images: An art intervention with suicidal adolescents. *Applied Nursing Research, 6*(3), 111–118.

Wheaton, B. (1990). Where work and family meet. In J. Eckenrode & S. Gore (Eds.), *Stress between work and family* (pp. 153–174). New York: Plenum Press.

Winfield, L. F. (2002). *NCREL Monograph: Developing resilience in urban youth* [Online]. Available: http://www.ncrel.org.

Wohl, A., & Kaufman, B. (1985). *Silent screams and hidden cries: An interpretation of artwork by children from violent homes.* New York: Brunner/Mazel.

Wortman, C. B. (1984). Social support and the cancer patient: Conceptual and methodological issues. *Cancer, 53*, 2330–2360.

How Schools Respond to Traumatic Events

Debriefing Interventions and Beyond

MARY BETH WILLIAMS

$\mathbf{A}$s the events of September 11, 2001 unfolded, television sets in various locations in school buildings across the United States were hooked up and kept on. Teachers and other staff members had difficulty tearing themselves away to return to their classrooms or offices. At that time, I was the school social worker in Falls Church City, Virginia, a community located about 5 miles from the Pentagon building in Washington, D.C.–one target of the "9/11" attacks. During fall 2002, Falls Church itself was on the national news as the place where the ninth victim of the "D.C. snipers" died, at a Home Depot in Seven Corners Shopping Center. When the first draft of this chapter was written in September 2002, schools in the entire D.C./Virginia/Maryland metropolitan area were on lockdown because of concerns relating to the snipers' threats and assassinations. All field trips, all outside activities, and all football games (including homecoming games) were canceled. At most schools, since one of the snipers said that "no child is safe anywhere," armed police were on duty. Children of all ages were discussing the snipers' attacks; children as young as 7 described the velocity of the .223-caliber bullet and the size of entrance and exit wounds. The mood was actually more fearful and intense, in many ways, than that following 9/11 (or even September 11, 2002, when the country was placed at a higher level of alert, in response to possible new attacks). Before discussing ways in which D.C.-area schools responded to the crisis of the snipers, I discuss the aftermath of 9/11.

THE RESPONSE TO 9/11: WHEN WAS LITTLE ENOUGH?

At the time of the 9/11 attacks, I was directly up the hill from the Pentagon at Immigration and Naturalization Services (INS), getting my fingerprints taken for a federal criminal check as a requirement for international adoption. The first of the World Trade Center's twin towers had just been hit by a plane; initially, it seemed as if someone was playing a sick joke on a talk show. As the TV reports were broadcast at INS, the second plane hit the World Trade Center. Then the Pentagon was struck by another plane, and the guard at the INS took me outside to see the smoke start to billow. I realized that there was a possibility of major disruption at Falls Church schools, and that a variety of organizations would probably need social work and other disaster interventions and services. As a member of the American Red Cross disaster response team; as a certified trauma specialist with the Association of Traumatic Stress Specialists; and as a member of my local critical incident stress management team, the Rapidan–Rappahanock team, I recognized many sources of need. In the meantime, Falls Church provided rescue and public safety units that were among the first to arrive on the scene at the Pentagon, and police and sheriff's departments assisted in traffic control around the building.

A major source of immediate concern in all school systems in the metropolitan area was how to cope with children who might be affected by the death of a parent or other significant person at the Pentagon or on a plane. The first disaster-related event held in the Falls Church school system's central office was a meeting with all the after-school day care providers to talk to them about how children might respond. At this point, school personnel did not know whether any student or staff member would experience a personal loss through death or injury. During this meeting, school student service team members (psychologists and the school social worker, myself) presented information to the staff concerning how to relate to potentially traumatized children. The system did not mobilize the crisis response team immediately to intervene in the schools, nor did the system set up a procedure for immediate defusings. In fact, the decision was to maintain routine and calmness until enough information accumulated to lead to an appropriate response. In this case, doing less was more than enough initially, to avoid overdramatizing or overresponding, without causing concern or even hysteria by the presence of a crisis team. School staff members made a conscious decision to maintain a presence and attitude of calmness and support.

Meanwhile, at the schools, parents who themselves were seriously affected by the events (either directly or through their own personal fears and vulnerabilities) began to come to school to retrieve their children. Even though staff members believed that it would have been better for the children to remain in a routine environment, school personnel had no choice but to let them go. One father, as I stopped for a home visit after learning he had taken all three of his children from school, was frantically throwing things in the back of his car to leave the area as soon as possible for a cabin in North Carolina, so that his children would not "have to smell the smoke from the city burning." His wife was standing by in utter amazement at her husband's frantic behavior, unable to stop him. Trying to calm him down, or to show him that his behavior was scaring both his wife and the children and teaching the children inappropriate ways to deal with stress, was to no avail. He told me emphatically to leave, and then got in the car and sped down the highway. His own terror and mental health issues of compromised trust, safety, and fear were now passed on to his children through his response of panic. In addition, his behavior conveyed to the children that the school social worker was also no longer a safe person, because of my stance of calmness, rationality, planning, and evaluation of details and information. Furthermore, his actions caused his spouse to lose faith in him and his rationality in the face of stress. The family returned about 5 days later when "the world did not end." Since that time, the children have had increasing mental health problems, including overeating, migraines, and sleep disturbances, and the wife has had posttraumatic stress reactions to this and other crises. Similar scenes were repeated in many jurisdictions by many families who wanted to escape and protect their children from possible further attacks.

Simultaneously, both the school system and the Falls Church municipal government implemented measures to safeguard the welfare of students and staff, and to prepare for potential losses of or injuries to family members. Superintendent Mary Ellen Shaw wrote in the local newspaper, the *Falls Church News Press*, on Thursday, September 20, 2001:

> We feared our students and staff members could have family members injured or killed . . . we prepared to take care of students whose parents were not able to get home at their normal time [beyond the normal closing time]. Teachers volunteered to stay beyond the normal hours and bus drivers were alerted to return students to school if parents were not home as planned. The staff of the [after-school] day care programs came in an hour early to meet with the school psychologists and social worker to discuss how to answer students' questions and to support students if they were upset. (Shaw, 2001, pp. 2, 19)

The Falls Church schools were fortunate not to experience any direct impacts of a death, and by 6:00 P.M., all students were delivered safely home or had been picked up. At the end of that fateful Tuesday school day, the school superintendents and city and county executives of the jurisdictions in the greater D.C. area participated in a conference call. Superintendents decided, as a group, to close all schools and cancel all school activities for the following day, so that police, fire, and rescue services could focus their efforts on providing assistance to the Pentagon as well as on dealing with possible additional attacks. Thus all student and parent activities for Falls Church schools were canceled for Wednesday, September 12. Having no school Wednesday also gave me the opportunity to begin to respond to the myriad of calls and to do crisis interventions and debriefings.

The schools reopened on Thursday, September 13. Staff members were on alert, should a need to provide debriefings, defusings, or separate interventions arise. (These terms are defined later in this chapter.) None did. In fact, students returned to the tasks at hand—academic instruction and performance—without a great deal of disruption. It was as if they were glad to have the safety of the school setting around them, in contrast to the sudden lack of safety in the world at large. One of the few aftermaths involved the report about and photos of the actual damage from the explosion at the Pentagon. A child's father had provided her with graphic pictures taken from inside the building. The girl eagerly passed them around to everyone, traumatizing the adults in the elementary school building even more than the children. On 9/11, this child had been afraid that her father had been hurt or killed and had called home (children who were frightened during the first day had been permitted to do so). Her mother had come to get her, once she knew that her husband was safe.

George Mason Middle and High School in Falls Church opened on Thursday morning (9/13/01) with the following announcement:

"Good morning, Mustangs. We are glad to have our school community back together today. . . . The immediate victims of these tragedies in New York, Pennsylvania, and here in Virginia were people of all ages, all colors, and all beliefs. These unfortunate souls number in the thousands. Those of us who grieve over these attacks and feel sad and angry about them are many, many millions. . . . We speak many languages, we hold many different religious beliefs, and we often dress and look different from one another. But we are united in that we are all, in a very real sense, victims of what happened on Tuesday. . . .

"George Mason is a wonderfully diverse school community. . . . It is to be celebrated that we all have come to be in the same school together. In this time of national and international tragedy and mourning, let's count on each other's support and understanding to move forward together. The flags outside our building fly at half-mast this morning to honor the victims and heroic rescue workers who perished on Tuesday. This morning's minute of silence will be extended to honor their memory as well."

Terrorist attacks of any scope are intentional and purposely inflict pain and despair. The world of children, after 9/11, was no longer benign and predictable. The terrorists chose symbols of power, stability, and control to give this message, prophetically summarized by Myers in an August, 2001 paper: "We can get you anywhere, at any time. If we are willing to kill your children, we will not hesitate to kill you. There is no one who can protect you." Such threats became more personal in fall 2002, as everyday citizens from the greater D.C. area to Richmond, Virginia were cut down, whether mowing a lawn, loading building materials into a car, going to school, standing in a bus, leaving a restaurant, pumping gas, or doing other routine activities.

Casualties of mass and individual terrorist attacks are psychological as well as physical. As Sandra L. Bloom stated in a message to the International Society of Traumatic Stress Studies on Sunday, September 16, 2001,

> Our memories literally engrave vivid nonverbal imprints of the sounds, the sights, the body sensations and emotions that haunt us long into the future, triggered by even faint reminders of the terrible pain of mass destruction. Today, we are a traumatized nation, impaired by the overwhelming nature of unimaginable events. . . . Emotional safety can only be restored by giving ourselves time to grieve for our losses, to find meaning in what happened, and, most important of all, to find ways to rebuild a shattered trust.

RESPONDING TO TERRORIST ATTACKS: THE COMMUNITY LEVEL

How can communities respond to such attacks? The following suggestions (based on the work of Everly & Mitchell, 2001) can be potential goals for intervention or rationales for response on the community level. First, we must never lose sight of the fact that, as either a primary or a secondary goal, the terrorist act is designed to cause psychological instability and induce a state of uncertainty, personal vulnerability, and fear. Every community directly or indirectly affected should have crisis intervention hotlines and walk-in crisis intervention facilities to help citizens cope with large or small terrorist activities. Ideally, emergency response personnel should have had preincident training; they also need ongoing psychological support during and after a terrorist attack.

It is essential to provide credible information to all members of a community or communities through the mass media (including letters from the school to parents) to contradict the sense of chaos and combat destructive rumors. Police need to provide this information openly, even if it might cause more fear, without threats of lawsuits or without repeated bombardments by reporters to force a crisis team leader to disclose confidential case-related information.

It is important to try to reestablish as much of a sense of physical safety as possible for the public, with special considerations for children, elderly persons, and infirm individuals. Placing uniformed law enforcement officers in cruisers near schools can be reassuring on the one hand, or stress-producing on the other; the nature of a particular situation should dictate this decision. Trying to maintain a normal routine, with a healthy respect for hypervigilance and attentiveness to surroundings, is important. Parents cannot reassure children of ultimate safety if such safety is a myth. Yet maintaining routines that are as close to normal as possible is one way to modulate emotional overreactivity.

It is also important to enlist the help of local political, educational, medical, economic, and religious leaders to facilitate communications, calm fears, provide personal crisis intervention, and instill hope. Interdenominational religious services (such as those held in the greater D.C. area on October 22, 2002) can be designed to bring solace and to calm fears. Furthermore, normal communication, transportation, school, and work schedules should be reestablished as soon as possible. In the instance of 9/11, this occurred in the Falls Church schools 2 days later, on Thursday, September 13. In the case of the D.C. snipers, until they were apprehended or known to be dead, such routines could not be reestablished for several weeks. Stress continued until October 24, 2002, when John Allen Muhammad and his 17-year-old ward, John Lee Malvo, were arrested on federal firearms charges and identified as suspects in the killings.

The power of symbols can be used as a means of reestablishing community cohesion. Again, the symbol of a police presence can often be calming. The increased use of the American flag on cars, bridges, trucks, homes, and offices after 9/11 gave a sense of "one nation," dedicated to its survival. As part of this symbol making or utilization, organizations, individuals, and governments need to initiate rituals to honor survivors, rescuers, and the dead through donations and ceremonies.

GUIDELINES FOR HELPING ADULTS
TO ASSIST CHILDREN AND FAMILIES

During 9/11 and the days following, most children saw the images of terror on television and the Internet. This media overexposure repeated itself at intervals over the following year, especially at the time of the 1-year anniversary. In the weeks of the 2002 D.C.-area killings, media coverage grew as the snipers expanded their range from Maryland to Richmond, Virginia. Everyone, everywhere, of all ages talked about the lack of safety.

Mothers pulled into gas stations and "hit the dirt" behind open doors to pump gas. Men placed themselves between gas pumps and car doors to do likewise. The entire I-95 corridor of traffic became a potential murder scene. A overwhelming sense of relief spread across the area in the early morning hours of October 24, 2002, for those night owls keeping up with CNN reporting, when news of the arrests of Muhammad and Malvo was broadcast. By 9:00 A.M., as evidence from as far away as Tacoma, Washington and Marion, Alabama was gathered, parents walked their children to school buses rather than drove them warily to the front doors of schools, and children began to anticipate having recess outside and being able to attend their homecoming football games.

During the trying times after 9/11, and during the snipers' reign of terror, adults needed to keep certain guidelines in mind (both as parents and as educators/interveners) as they worked with children or acted as their role models at home and in the community. Such guidelines will be equally necessary as similar crises arise in the future.

Safety

The first goal for parents and other adults in such crises is to establish as much of a sense of safety as possible. In attempting to assure safety, adults should keep calm and maintain a relaxed, calm environment in the schools and in their homes, if at all possible. If they cannot stay calm because of personal involvement, then it is important to explain to children why they are upset. The modeling of calmness and control can serve as an emotional cue for children. Adults should assure children that they are trying to make sure that children are safe at home, at school, and in the community, to the best of their ability. They also need to reassure children that the adults they know and want to trust are safe and in control of their own responses (as much as is possible). Furthermore, they may remind children who is in charge—law enforcement, fire and rescue, the President, the military, teachers—and emphasize that these people are trustworthy.

Monitoring Children's Behaviors and Making Referrals

Parents and other adults should look for signs of behavioral and emotional impacts of the traumas on children, such as sleeplessness, nightmares, generalized anxiety, and misbehavior. It is important for parents, in particular, to be familiar with what emotional states and responses are age-appropriate (National Association of School Psychologists, 2001). Parents should be advised to give their children extra reassurance and care; to ask questions or make observations to open up the possibilities of discussion (while remaining tolerant of their children's responses); and to let their children know that feeling upset after such events is normal and acceptable. Helping children to talk about their feelings can indicate their needs (American Psychological Association Disaster Response Network, 2001; Nader, Pynoos, Fairbanks, & Frederick, 1990; Stevenson, 2002).

If children continue to have emotional and/or behavioral problems 2 months after the disasters, their caregivers need to seek out professional help for them. Children who are socially close to those who experienced a disaster—those whose family members or close friends were directly involved or affected—may be especially vulnerable. Children who knew victims as acquaintances or less intimate friends are usually somewhat less vulnerable. Children who identify with the victims in age or as citizens may also be vulnerable. Responsible adults need to make sure that these vulnerable children receive appropriate interventions.

Mental health professionals can go to local schools and offer to talk to PTAs/PTOs or other organizations about trauma and its healing path. They may also offer to develop and/or lead trauma-specific counseling groups with the students (Nader & Pynoos, 1993; Pynoos & Nader, 1989; Nisivoccia & Lynn, 1999). They may want to offer some sliding-scale services to those who cannot afford them or have no insurance.

Monitoring Media Exposure

Adults/parents should monitor the amount and types of children's television/movie/VCR and Internet exposure, particularly if they have exhibited trauma-related symptoms. It is important to try to restrict adult viewing times to when children are not around or not awake. This may be difficult, particularly if new events occur and adults again succumb to what an Australian colleague of mine, Lenore Meldrum, has termed "CNN syndrome" (personal communication, September 2001).

Finding Meaning

Adults/parents should listen to what children ask and say to them, even when the questions are repetitious. Children, too, are trying to find meaning in what has happened. Providing children with the truth about the extent and seriousness of what occurred, sticking to facts without dwelling on gruesome details, and discussing the event in a developmentally appropriate manner can all help in this process.

During and after a crisis such as 9/11, adults/parents should also encourage children to be kind to all peoples of all ethnic groups and emphasize that violence, hate, and terrorism are senseless acts of individuals or small groups, not of entire peoples. This was done through the morning announcement on September 13, 2001, in Falls Church City's George Mason Middle and High School (quoted earlier). In a series of post-9/11 family/employee meetings held at the World Bank, I discussed the need for tolerance and helped other bank members provide reassurance to their Islamic colleagues. Adults/parents should discuss the presence of good and evil in the world, particularly with older children and adolescents, as part of the context of finding meaning. One way to find meaning is to take some form of action—often action to help others. In this light, parents/adults should encourage children to volunteer in activities to help the victims of violence: doing drawings for *Sesame Street*, collecting money for Afghan children, or (for teens) working as Candy Stripers or participating in other volunteer work.

Parents'/Adults' Responses

Parents and other adults respond to terrorism within the community on the basis of their own psychological, physical, emotional, spiritual, and other traits and characteristics. Parents should look at how the events have affected their own personal lives and activities, and should consider the impact of travel and separations from their children on their families. When parents have made changes in their normal routines (e.g., allowing children to sleep with them), they should be advised to create a timeline for when the children are to return to their own beds, rooms, or routines.

The responses of parents and teachers to a tragedy or terrorist act strongly influence the children's abilities to recover. Those children who experienced direct exposure to the events of 9/11, the D.C.-area snipers' attacks, or any other mass crisis situation are the most vulnerable to longer and more severe impacts. Those who were witnesses or who had a "near-miss experience" are next in vulnerability. Those within hearing, feeling, or smelling range who did not witness what happened fall next on the vulnerability continuum, and children outside the disaster area—in such cases, the whole nation—are typically least vulnerable (Pynoos & Nader, 1989). However, many of those children repeatedly witnessed the events of 9/11, the 1-year anniversary of 9/11, and the snipers' attacks on television and the Internet.

GUIDELINES FOR SCHOOLS

In any crisis, every public and private school aims to be a safe, responsive environment, attempting to reassure children of their own personal safety. As part of that endeavor, school systems have many tasks and obligations. In order to fulfill these tasks, many, if not most, school systems have created crisis response protocols and teams to deal with potential situations, both large and small, that may occur within or affect their environment. As those teams respond, however, it is essential that they not interfere with the tactical assessment and rescue efforts of law enforcement and/or emergency medical service professionals (Everly & Mitchell, 2001).

Roles

Before any plan can be implemented, certain policies and procedures concerning roles and working relationships must be implemented. Those individuals in charge of a school's crisis team (generally members of the administration) must ensure that all personnel can work well together in order to plan and carry out appropriate interventions. The faculty needs to be flexible in allowing crisis team members to come into classrooms as time and availability allow. The superintendent, taking a supportive role with the assistant superintendent, may decide to stand in the halls of the most affected school, as comforting "parental" figures. In some systems, all decisions are made from the "top down"; in others, the building administrator has control, checking with the central office when necessary or when the situation indicates. Usually the school administrator writes letters about crisis responses and events that students take home, and sets the tone for crisis team members' acceptance in the building.

In view of these considerations, before trying to implement any part of a plan, crisis team coordinators/leaders need to make sure that they have the support of administrators in the school and at the central office. It is important, ahead of time, to identify any potential trouble spots or hazards that need immediate intervention and to define roles clearly. Few things are worse than professional infighting and stepping on others' toes in times of crisis.

Any school crisis plan must be adaptable and flexible, designed to meet specific crises as they arise. The roles of persons who belong to the crisis team must also be flexible. Faculty members may colead debriefings, develop appropriate class activities, and express personal grief during these events. Administrators must remain visible, get appropriate information to the school information/media liaison officials, maintain constant contact with the superintendent and the crisis team, be available to family members of deceased students or staff members, set up schedules of debriefings and interventions, and chair a community meeting if needed. Crisis coordinators may need to be on site, to spend time in the community with parents and officials, and to maintain links with the central office and administrative staff.

Safety and Routine

Ideally, schools train teachers and staff members about various aspects of trauma, crisis response, abuse, debriefing, and posttraumatic stress prior to a crisis, so that all school personnel can help students and themselves cope with and adjust to the aftermath of the crisis and can help those most affected to reenter and succeed in the school environment. When such training has not occurred, the crisis points out the need for it.

Although the goal of a school system is first and foremost educating its students, children cannot be expected to perform at their full academic potential shortly after a traumatic event. Creating a sense of safety within the school is the first priority, while maintaining structure and routine to the extent possible. It is best to limit major tests and projects that might be due shortly after a major traumatic event has occurred. Those students who have been most directly affected will often need additional support and leniency in academic requirements. Helping them to return to a sense of normality and routine takes precedence over term papers or scores on examinations. On the other hand, after some interval, students will need to return to class or academic activities, rather than mill around the halls or use a crisis as a reason to get attention or just stay out of class. One advantage to using a team "from within" is that members of the team frequently have more than crisis-based information about the students and are more able to recognize when requests for help and intervention are manipulations rather than true crisis responses.

PROVISION OF INFORMATION AND CREATION OF MEANING

Early Responses

Schools are frequently major sources of information to parents and communities during a time of crisis, particularly if the crisis has occurred within a school's boundaries or otherwise directly affected a school. School personnel, particularly office staff members, may become inundated with phone calls as soon as word of a crisis "gets out." Advanced preparation can help lessen the stress on the staff. For example, all crisis-related phone callers can receive a prepared response such as the following:

> "You have reached [school name] on [date]. [State the general nature of the problem: death of a student/staff member, bomb threat, bus accident, etc.] All staff members are currently working on this situation, and we cannot take your phone call right now. Phone lines must be kept open. [If there is a safety emergency, then add:] All necessary measures are being implemented to ensure student safety, which is our top priority. Please do not come to the school building. Students will be sent home with written information for parents. Thank you for your patience and cooperation. [You might also add:] Each school building has a crisis management plan that will help staff deal with the situation and will maintain student safety. Please turn to cable

channel_ [if such a channel is available] for important information [or to a school Web site]."

Extra staff members may be needed to answer phones. Someone should
be designated to respond to the media.

Information Guidelines

Crisis response team leaders in the schools provide information to teachers (and parents) as to what to say to children and how to answer their
questions; they then give examples of ways to provide that information as
they attempt to resolve children's distress. Within the school system itself,
information needs to be given by school staff members in person, rather
than via public address systems or other media.

Early elementary school children need brief, simple information balanced with reassurances of safety and structure. The extent of family disruption often influences a young child's degree of upset. Older elementary and early middle school children tend to ask questions about safety
and interventions. They are more aware of potential danger around themselves and search for order. They have active imaginations that stir up
fears and anxiety reactions, and may have some difficulty understanding
why humans do such horrible things to other humans. They tend to have
somatic complaints and regressive behaviors or school reluctance. Upper
middle and high school students have strong opinions and may have concrete suggestions for interventions, such as making commitments to do
things to help victims and communities. They need to appear competent
during this time and may lose faith in the adults around them, particularly
if those adults appear weak. They may develop depression and sadness or
may withdraw. In most instances, their symptoms do not last over extended time periods.

TYPES OF INTERVENTIONS

Before crisis intervention activities are implemented, crisis team members
(working with administrators in charge) must decide what type(s) of inter-
vention(s) to use. Possible choices include defusings, debriefings, large-
group meetings, parent information meetings, and others.

Defusings and Debriefings

A "defusing" occurs very shortly after a traumatic incident occurs, in a 1:1
conversation that is designed to help a person "talk out" the incident and
receive some objective support, generally from a peer. When teachers, ad-

ministrators, pupil personnel staff members and other school staff members process a traumatic event prior to interacting with students, they frequently defuse one another. The key aspects of defusing are promptness, proximity (closeness to the incident), positive atmosphere of expectancy of recovery, brevity, and simplicity (Snelgrove, 1998).

An "educational debriefing" frequently takes place prior to intervening with students and/or families. Thus it is important for crisis team members, central office staff, and administrators to meet with school staff members as soon as possible after the trauma. It is important to get the facts straight during this debriefing and plan what to tell students, parents, and others. A "phone tree" can assist with dissemination information.

The word "debriefing" generally refers to a psychological and educational group process designed to mitigate the impact of the critical incident. A debriefing is not a therapy session, an investigation of what happened, or a critique of process or procedure. It is a structured group process designed to help individuals examine and review their personal experiences resulting from or dealing with the critical incident. There are numerous models of debriefing. However, all models have a series of stages that begin with more educational and rationally based information (what happened, what a participant thought about what happened); proceed into a discussion of emotional issues (e.g., the impact of what happened and the worst part of the event) and the symptoms the event might engender; and conclude with a more rationally based stage that includes teaching and closure activities. Guidelines for who should receive debriefing include the following: Debrief those with the greatest need first; try to keep debriefing groups homogeneous (for children, those of the same age or in the same class); do not push everyone to participate; and carefully observe symptoms during the debriefing process (Mitchell & Everly, 1993).

Debriefings may begin with discussion of the students' (and staff's) factual knowledge, their reactions at the time of the event through the present time, and feelings then and now surrounding the crisis event. Other aspects of the debriefing include discussing the meaning of what happened and providing information about future potential reactions. With younger children, the debriefing can include an art activity. Johnson (1993) suggests that preschool and kindergarten debriefings should last between 15 and 30 minutes; elementary debriefings, between 30 minutes and 1 hour; middle school debriefings, between 45 minutes and 1½ hours; and high school or adult debriefings, 1–2 or more hours. The person conducting a debriefing needs to be aware of community aspects of the events—key themes of the event and community reactions, organization issues, power struggles, and interpersonal relationships within the organization and community. Education is a major function of the debriefing. Debriefings can be conducted with the crisis team as well, although outside help needs to be used for this type of debriefing.

Other Interventions

The crisis team needs to identify individuals who are most seriously affected by the crisis and who need a more individualized approach or smaller-group sessions. Some students will require closer attention and supervision, as well as assessment of risk. In some instances, staff members may be assigned to remain in such areas as bathrooms, breakout rooms, the cafeteria, and other key locations for "at-risk" students and/or faculty. "Drop-in" centers for students, faculty, and staff can provide crisis counseling.

Additional interventions need to be offered for students who were absent on the day of the crisis, or who were directly injured or otherwise affected by the event. These students will heal at a different rate than those involved in school activities shortly after the event occurred.

Crisis team leaders and the administration need to develop resources and materials for classroom discussions and other trauma-specific intervention activities. Some activities, for example, might be designed to teach tolerance and prevent stereotyping of specific groups or nationalities, as ways to mitigate the occurrence of later violence against perceived perpetrators. School staff members might also interact with various community organizations to develop community-based activities as outlets, or even as ways to find meaning concerning the traumatic event. Schools also can make age-appropriate reading materials available to persons beyond the school walls through handouts, at parent informational meetings, and at community activities.

NOTIFICATIONS

The school has an obligation to keep parents, students, board members, and community representatives informed. For example, other schools impacted by a crisis at one school need to be informed (e.g., schools of siblings if there was a death of a student; former students if there was a death of a teacher). In addition, "latchkey" children (those who come home to an empty house without parental presence) may need their parents to come home early to provide support if they were directly affected by a crisis. The first day after a traumatic event, the school needs to send a flier to parents describing what happened, what the school did to intervene after the crisis, and what constitutes a normal posttraumatic stress reaction, as well as answering potential questions. The flier can also provide information about what questions to ask, what to tell children, and how to help children (and adults) through the traumatic grief process. School board members, school administration, the district's central office, and community officials also must be fully informed of the school's response about any unsuspected outcomes (e.g., copycat suicide pacts).

POSTEVENT ACTIVITIES AND INTERVENTIONS

Following the death of a student or faculty/staff member, certain decisions need to be made concerning the personal effects of the deceased individual in his or her locker, desk, or classroom. The timing can be very sensitive. In some instances, a "shrine" may spontaneously develop in a classroom or elsewhere. Staff and students may want to plan school-based or school-sponsored commemorative rituals together, or to participate in whatever wake and/or funeral arrangements the family has made. The school must ask family members about such arrangements—in particular, whether or not they want a small private viewing and/or service, or a large wake and/or service that includes students and staff. If the plan includes an open coffin, the school staff needs to try to let parents know so ahead of time, so that they can discuss death and presentation of dead bodies with their children and/or make informed decisions about whether their children will attend. Crisis team members need to be available at the wake or funeral for those who have such intense reactions that they need immediate assistance.

For example, in the case of a suicide of an eighth grader who belonged to a Greek Orthodox church, the church's practice was to have everyone in the congregation come to view the body and touch, kiss, or display affection to it. I learned of this circumstance shortly before the funeral and called the school to let the staff know about this expectation. Many students attending the funeral were overwhelmed and needed crisis intervention immediately following the service, as did some staff and parents who attended. It is also important to have persons available to staff and students who remain at school during a funeral because they cannot, will not, are not permitted to, or do not want to attend, yet nevertheless are affected by the death.

Referrals

Schools are generally closed systems that prefer to determine their own crisis responses. However, if the schools have good working relationships with local mental health professionals or trained trauma specialists, then those persons may be included in school crisis plans or as potential referral sources for traumatized students and staff members. School counselors are generally the first level of intervention for the most distressed students or students with extreme symptoms. Counselors need to have lists of referral sources for parents who are concerned about the level of distress in their children.

When a crisis has been large in scope or in impact, it may be necessary to obtain help from these trusted or known organizations and professionals. Few things are worse than having a "herd" of grief counselors and trauma specialists descend on a school or event when they have not been invited or are not known to school staff.

Review and Evaluation

After the immediate event has passed, additional interventions may be necessary to help process the grief. These might include follow-up debriefings, play therapy, art therapy, writing, or homework activities with trauma-related themes incorporated into assignments. The team's response and its successes/failures also need to be evaluated. The following questions can guide the evaluation:

1. How much disequilibrium still exists in the school?
2. How much organizational confusion still exists?
3. How well did team members do their jobs?
4. How well were emotions defused?
5. Did rumors and myths get addressed and corrected?
6. Was healthy, adaptive coping stressed and then implemented?

School-Based Activities Dealing with Traumatic Grief

It is possible that those most severely impacted by a death—particularly one that has been traumatic in its suddenness, its type, or its impact—may never fully accept their loss. However, dealing with that death in a school system may be one way to bring a sense of recognition and realization that the death is real and final, and may even lead to some sense of reconciliation (Wolfelt, 1987). Thus grief-based groups led by counselors, psychologists, or school social workers can help students achieve Worden's (1991) tasks of grieving:

1. Accepting the reality of the death.
2. Experiencing the pain and anguish of grief.
3. Adjusting to a world in which the deceased person is no longer present in the physical sense.
4. Moving on with life, putting the deceased person into his or her new role or position.

Children who have lost significant individuals through death, particularly a traumatic death, may feel isolated and alone in their grief. Creating a group that gives guidance and provides an emotional outlet, but that is not a therapy group, can be an important way for school personnel to help combat that isolation in a supportive atmosphere. According to Perschy (1997), the objectives of such a group for students in elementary through high school include the following:

1. Provision of information about the process and tasks of grief.
2. Provision of a forum to express emotions and concerns about the grief process and personal experiences.
3. Inclusion of structured activities to assist in working through grief (e.g., activities looking at how the death has changed their lives, anger- and guilt-based activities, commemorative activities, mixed media activities, and others).
4. Examination of current support systems and ways to use those systems or expand them if they are ineffective.
5. Development of a resource base of materials as well as peers.

Young (1996), in the curriculum for working with grieving children that she has developed for the federal Office for Victims of Crime, suggests numerous intervention methods and strategies that can be adapted to a grief group. These include oral storytelling (sometimes initiated by the leader, who provides the initial sentence of the story); discussion based on a particularly poignant photo, poem, or video; creative writing of poems, memory books, or journal entries; creative art projects; dramatic presentations (making a puppet theater for younger children or writing a play for older students); or craft projects such as creating personalized worry beads.

Trauma-Based Groups Oriented to Resilience and Coping

A group counseling intervention for children who have experienced traumatic events gives participants the opportunity to share feelings, thoughts, reactions, impressions, losses, and responses with others who have experienced similar events. In many ways, a trauma-based group is similar to a group that focuses on issues of grief, because grief reactions are part of a traumatic response. However, a trauma-based group goes beyond a grief-focused group to deal with specific symptoms of posttraumatic stress disorder, including intrusive thoughts, nightmares, avoidance activities, startle responses, and others. It provides a venue for children to express fear, share humor (even "black" humor), gain information from others with more factual knowledge of what happened or will happen, and learn about each other's experiences. Ideally, groups have between 6 and 8 members, although a group of 10–12 is feasible. Children may rotate as leaders and/or helpers, choosing the topic for the following week or an activity to use with the chosen topic. Group leaders may or may not ask the students in attendance to share "the story" of what happened to each of them during or after a trauma. Children may also be asked to write out, describe, draw, make a collage of, or otherwise represent the worst aspect of what happened, the best aspect, the losses, or other topics. They may also create "trigger books" of things that they concurrently smell, see, hear, touch, taste or otherwise experience that remind them of the past event(s) (Nisivoccia & Lynn, 1999).

According to their age and developmental stage, students can engage in various feelings-related activities, ranging from making feeling charts to discussing ways to modulate feelings (Gordon, Farberow, & Maida, 1999). Whatever the assignment, children can be given various options for ways to complete it, so that they can experience an increased sense of postevent power (Reiss, 2002).

One possible group format is based on Schab's (1996) *The Coping Skills Workbook*. This 11-week group begins with an introductory session and then uses each of the nine coping skills in the workbook as a topic. Among these coping skills are dealing with feelings, adjusting attitudes, and discovering choices.

Modifying the Curriculum

Initially, after a serious crisis in the school or the community, region, or nation, the primary responsibilities of the school are to ensure safety, disseminate information, and allow for processing of what happened. Alternative activities introduced in the classroom that involve writing or drawing about what happened can facilitate that processing. Drawings, according to Poland and McCormick (1999), can help faculty members understand how students "perceive what happened during the crisis and can facilitate conversation about how they are coping" (p. 184). Asking students to explain what their artwork says offers them the opportunity to ventilate and express emotions, ideas, and impacts. For example, after 9/11, first-grade students at H. Byron Masterson Elementary School in Kennett, Missouri wrote and illustrated a book about how 9/11 affected them. Their artwork depicted the events of September 12, 2001, and indicated that on that day, they knew "everything would be all right" (H. Byron Masterson Elementary School First Grade Class, 2002, p. 6). Students of all ages can portray thoughts, emotions, somatic responses, beliefs, and other traumatic reactions through artwork. Themes of that work may range from their roles or experiences during an event to their perceptions of the victims to what the event means to them and how they wish to commemorate what happened. If students do not want to draw their responses, they might create a collage, a sculpture, or another artifact symbolic of what happened.

Another way to incorporate what happened into classroom activities is to introduce literary passages and works that portray disaster, trauma, grief, reactivity, resilience, and triumph. Various organizations have compiled booklists on topics related to trauma. The Association of Traumatic Stress Specialists is one such organization, and its Web site (http:// www.atss-hg.com) can be contacted for a listing. Students can be encouraged to develop poetry, essays, research papers, journal entries, or other literary works as means to deal with their own traumatic reactions. Students also may be given writing assignments that relate to a traumatic event. Reiss (2002, p. 151) suggests the following possible assignments:

> Write the worst thing that ever happened to you
> Write about your most scary nightmare
> Write about how you felt when you first heard the news of a
>   traumatic event
> Write about how you now feel that the event is over
> Write about your life as it is now
> Write about what others have said about what happened

The rationale behind such tasks is that the writing activity is in itself cathartic. Children who have been seriously affected and who are having ongoing symptoms may require referral to a mental health professional.

Teaching Children to Make Lists

Reiss (2002) notes that "making lists can be therapeutic to those in mourning" (p. 63). Teaching and encouraging children of all ages to make lists (e.g., lists of things to do, lists of things that have been changed by what happened, lists of things that have not changed, lists of things children like about themselves) can build normality and create a sense of focus and grounding. Lists can be future-oriented, thereby focusing children on something beyond the past traumatic event and the pain of the present. Lists therefore can alter the sense of a foreshortened future that many children experience after a traumatic event. Lists can also encourage the search for meaning as to what happened or can help build a child's sense of resilience. A list of "things for which I am thankful" can help develop a more positive postevent attitude. Children can take the assignment to make a list home and share it with parents/caregivers, as a way to encourage positive thought in families.

WHAT MIGHT SCHOOL PERSONNEL FEEL DURING AND AFTER A CRISIS?

School staff members often feel a variety of emotions and have a variety of responses after a school crisis. They may feel helpless, realizing there is little they can do to change the situation, to bring back the deceased individual(s), or to heal the grief of witnesses or those closely connected to the person(s) who died. They may feel fearful or anxious as well as vulnerable after they have been exposed to the trauma and its impact. Seeing the death of a child can shatter illusions of invulnerability, lower self-efficacy, and decrease the belief in an internal locus of control. Some teachers and staff members become fearful that something similar could occur in their own families or in the families of their loved ones.

Some staff members experience rage and anger toward those who may be seen as responsible for what happened. This rage and anger may lead to intolerance and a lack of trust in others. Others feel intense sorrow and grief. They may have intrusive images of the traumatic events, particularly surrounding the death of a child. Mental images of various scenes (e.g., a memorial on a street corner, a wake, a funeral, the collapse of the twin towers on 9/11) come back intensely and often unbidden.

Other staff members may feel some degree of self-reproach and shame, particularly if they are questioning whether they could have done something differently to prevent the event from occurring. More positively, they may experience a change in values or an increased appreciation of their own families. They may come to appreciate life more. However, finding escape in humor is less useful when children are involved and does not seem to reduce tension, keep emotional distance, or build cohesion and morale in situations where a child has died; thus there is less availability of this defense mechanism (Dyregrov & Mitchell, 1992). My colleagues and I have experienced many of these feelings during our work with school crises.

FINAL THOUGHTS

One thing is clear to all of us more than ever: The next school crisis that occurs could be ours. School crises of various types can happen anywhere, at any time; no two crises are ever alike. The mental health of U.S. children is of utmost concern. Too many children still have no health insurance. Mental health clinics still have long waiting lists. Finding qualified traumatologists is not an easy matter—particularly those willing to operate on a sliding-scale fee system or even to do some *pro bono* work.

And finally, regardless of professionals' roles in the school system, they will not be able to escape the impact of trauma on themselves. As emphasized in Chapter 15 of this book, it is essential for helping personnel to take time for themselves and to talk about their feelings.

We all will go on with our lives, but we may be forever changed by such events as 9/11 or the D.C.-area killings. Yet out of darkness comes light; out of horror come hope and resilience. Although survival after a traumatic event does not always follow a straight path and can be hard, it can be done.

REFERENCES

American Psychological Association Disaster Response Network. (2001, September). *Guidelines for helping children deal with terrorism.* Washington, DC: APA.

Bloom, S. L. (2001, September 16). *Message to the membership of the International Society of Traumatic Stress Studies.*

Dyregrov, A., & Mitchell, J. T. (1992). Working with traumatized children: Psychological effects and coping strategies. *Journal of Traumatic Stress, 5*(1), 5–17.

Everly, G. S., & Mitchell, J. T. (2001). America under attack: The "10 commandments" of responding to mass terrorist attacks. *International Journal of Emergency Mental Health, 3*(3), 133–135.

Gordon, N. S., Farberow, N. L., & Maida, C. A. (1999). *Children and disasters.* Philadelphia: Brunner/Mazel.

H. Byron Masterson Elementary School First Grade Class. (2002). *September 12th we knew everything would be all right.* New York: Scholastic.

Johnson, K. (1993). *Trauma in the lives of children: Crisis and stress management techniques for teachers, counselors, and student service professionals.* Alameda, CA: Hunter House Books.

Mitchell, J. T., & Everly, G. S., Jr. (1993). *Critical incident stress debriefing: An operations manual for the prevention of trauma among emergency services and disaster workers.* Ellicott City, MD: Chevron.

Myers, D. (2001, August). *Terrorism as a special type of crisis.* Paper presented at the annual convention of the American Psychological Association, San Francisco.

Nader, K., & Pynoos, R. (1993). School disaster: Planning and initial interventions. *Journal of Social Behavior and Personality, 8*(5), 299-320.

Nader, K., Pynoos, R. S., Fairbanks., L., & Frederick, C. (1990). Children's PTSD reactions one year after a sniper attack at their school. *American Journal of Psychiatry, 147,* 1526–1530.

National Association of School Psychologists. (2001, September). *Guidelines for parents: Helping your children deal with terrorism.* Bethesda, MD: Author.

Nisivoccia, D., & Lynn, M. (1999). Helping forgotten victims: Using activities groups with children who witness violence. In N. B. Webb (Ed.), *Play therapy with children in crisis* (2nd ed.): *Individual, group, and family treatment* (pp. 74–103). New York: Guilford Press.

Perschy, M. K. (1997). *Helping teens work through grief.* Washington, DC: Accelerated Development.

Poland, S., & McCormick, J. S. (1999). *Coping with crisis, lessons learned: A resource for schools, parents, and communities.* Longmont, CO: Sopris West.

Pynoos, R. S., & Nader, K. O. (1989). Children's memory and proximity to violence. *Journal of the American Academy of Child and Adolescent Psychiatry, 28,* 236–241.

Reiss, F. (2002). *Terrorism and kids: Comforting your child.* Newton, MA: Peanut Butter and Jelly Press.

Schab, L. M. (1996). *The coping skills workbook: Teaches kids nine essential skills to help deal with real-life crises.* King of Prussia, PA: Center for Applied Psychology.

Shaw, M. E. (2001, September 20). Superintendent reports on schools crisis response. *Falls Church News Press,* pp. 2, 19.

Snelgrove, T. (1998, March). *Managing acute traumatic stress: Trauma intervenor's resource manual* (11th ed.). West Vancouver, British Columbia, Canada: Easton-Snelgrove.

Stevenson, R. G. (2002). Sudden death in schools. In N. B. Webb (Ed.), *Helping bereaved children: A handbook for practitioners* (2nd ed., pp. 194–213). New York: Guilford Press.

Wolfelt, A. (1987, Winter). Resolution versus reconciliation: The importance of semantics. *Thanatos, 12,* 10–13.

Worden, J. W. (1991). *Grief counseling and grief therapy* (2nd ed.) New York: Springer.

Young, M. A. (1996, August). *Working with grieving children after violent death: A guidebook for crime victim assistance professionals.* Washington, DC: U.S. Department of Justice, Office for Victims of Crime.

CHAPTER 7

Ongoing, Long-Term Grief Support Groups for Traumatized Families

CHARLOTTE BURROUGH
DANNY MIZE

THE TRAUMATIC EVENT: APRIL 19, 1995

April 19, 1995 seemed like any other sunny, midspring morning in central Oklahoma. Adults were at work, children were in school, and life moved forward as usual. At 9:02 A.M., however, a bomb exploded inside a rented Ryder truck in front of the Alfred P. Murrah Federal Building in downtown Oklahoma City. In a moment . . . in one heartbeat . . . everything changed forever for those of us who live in the heartland of the United States. *All* members of our community suffered loss! Two hundred nineteen children lost at least one parent; three of these children became orphans. The Murrah Building bombing took the lives of 168 people, injured over 500, and destroyed our illusion that we in the heartland of America lived beyond the reaches of terrorism. As Webb (2002, p. 366), quoting Kastenbaum (2001, p. 236), has stated, "The psychological effects of terrorism include an overall weakening of the sense of security," with resultant "changes in the way a society thinks about itself and the rules it enforces."

At this writing, almost 9 years have passed since that first horrific act of terrorism on U.S. soil occurred—about 25 minutes away from the location that is now The Kids' Place, a group support center for grieving children. Although other acts of terrorism have occurred, the end of the

Oklahoma City story has not yet been written, because grief lasts a lifetime.

THE LONG-LASTING EFFECTS OF CHILDHOOD GRIEF

Imagine the life of a 5-year-old girl after losing her father in a terrorist bombing. After the initial shock and suffering, "life goes on" for the adults around her. No, life doesn't return to normal, but life goes on. A year or two or three pass, and adults comment, "She seems to be doing so well." Most of them aren't aware of the roller coaster of emotions she will ride for the rest of her life.

Our imaginary little girl will suffer waves of grief during her grade school years every time a parent–child activity is announced. School plays and music recitals will not be the same, for one proud parent will be missing, one less camera will be flashing. Sporting events will be played under a cloud, since the stands will hold one less cheering father. High school graduation will be a little somber as she walks across the stage. Yes, she'll bask in the attention of family and friends who have helped her grow up and reach this milestone. The glow of the moment, however, will be dimmed by the thought of how it could have been if Dad had lived (Krementz, 1981). Dad will not be walking her down the aisle, nor will he say, "Her mother and I give this woman in marriage." Tears of joy will mingle with tears of sadness on that special occasion.

Then the day will come when another child is born into this rough, loud world. A new life will begin, a reminder of hope for the future. The baby may be dedicated to the memory of a grandfather he'll never know. He may even bear the name of our little girl's absent father. "Dad would have been so proud!" the young mother will think.

Just like our imaginary little girl, 219 Oklahoma children will experience life without at least one parent, because these parents died violent deaths in the Murrah Building. Many adults lost parents or other relatives as well. Even after quite some time, one person who lost a parent in the bombing said, "I am really tired of my heart aching so badly, and I wish someone would tell me how to stop it. This whole thing has almost ruined my life and the lives of my children" (quoted in Kight, 1998, p. 287). Will the children of Oklahoma City, and those affected by other terrorist acts, ever "get over" their losses? How long does the process of grief go on?

With help, families are finding answers. Out of the ashes of our local tragedy has risen The Kids' Place, a grief support center that serves the needs of families with bereavements of any kind. The purpose of The Kids' Place is to provide a safe and supportive environment for children and their adult family members who are mourning the death of a family member or friend.

THE CREATION OF A GRIEF SUPPORT AGENCY

The Kids' Place, founded in 1996, started with one group of families experiencing various losses. Within 5 months, three additional groups were formed. Later that first year, a loss-specific group was developed to meet the needs of numerous families with children who had experienced the death of a parent. Due to an increased demand for grief support in our area, a fifth set of groups was made available to grieving families in September 1998.

We believed that through open and ongoing support groups, children would find comfort as they experienced the hurt following the death of anyone important to them—whatever the cause. Children suffer losses of loved ones for a variety of reasons.

Even though the Murrah Building bombing was the catalyst for the launching of The Kids' Place, services of the center have always been available to families mourning a death from any cause. Children need to feel a sense of safety and security within certain boundaries, whether physical or emotional (Bluestein, 1993).

Zambelli and DeRosa (1992, p. 485) have noted that "bereaved families may need additional means of social support in order to provide the assistance and care a child requires for a continuing healthy development." Wolfelt (1996, p. 209), in discussing the realities of the bereaved family, states that the death of a family member results in special needs for the family as a unit. He goes on to say that the death of any family member results in the reorganization of adult–child relationships in the system, and that healthy reconciliation of grief has long-term implications for the child's and the family's continuing growth.

According to Siegel, Mesagno, and Christ (1990), parents often believe that by avoiding both discussion of the loss and the display of their own grief, they are protecting their children from the pain and other effects of the death. Herz (1991, cited by Shapiro, 1994) suggests that a necessary factor in a positive outcome for the family mourning a death is the establishment of more open communication within the family constellation, helping the family balance the focus on death with a focus on hope for life and living. Shapiro (1994) notes that families who have suffered the death of a family member are especially vulnerable to isolation. Like most others in the field, Shapiro stresses the importance of open communication of feelings between family members; it should be taken into account that family members may be out of phase with each other's grief.

Structure of the Program

To facilitate the need for uninhibited self-expression, family members do not all participate in the same group at The Kids' Place. Children are assigned to one of three groups according to their chronological or developmental age, while their adult caregivers receive support from their peers in a separate group. When the need of surviving parents or other caregivers for support in resolving their loss goes unmet, they are less likely to perceive their children's needs and to provide necessary support for their mourning (Kliman, 1979; Raphael, Field, & Kvelde, 1980; Siegel et al., 1990). Unless caregivers' *own* needs are acknowledged, and they feel supported in expressing their *own* grief, they cannot be expected to engage effectively with their children.

Because of the nature of our ongoing or open groups, a family may choose to participate in the program for a few months or a few years. Therefore, a child may move into the next developmental age while the family is still attending the groups at The Kids' Place. Cook and Dworkin (1992) explain that an open group seems to meet clients' needs best because of the ongoing support, the ability of longer-term members to assist newer members, and the chance for those who stay on to resolve universal issues more fully as new members bring them up.

Content of the Program

One element of the program is an educational component that is paired with group activities. Themes are developed for each group session at The Kids' Place, with appropriate activities for each of the four age groups. Since the entire family has experienced the same focus on that evening, a strong potential exists for communication to develop later in their own environment.

The following themes and coordinated activities illustrate examples from the Younger Group (children 5–8 years old; see below) over a 10-session period (Sessions are usually held twice a month):

- *Session 1*: Introduction of concept of grief; watching a video demonstrating grief; sharing photos of persons who died and telling their stories.
- *Session 2*: Focus on all feelings being acceptable; activities to develop awareness of the presence of many different feelings, such as reading a book about feelings one may have on different days; game matching feelings with times children felt those specific feelings; decorating a tree drawn on paper with different-colored dots, each representing a specific feeling.
- *Session 3*: Identifying changes occurring in the children's lives; reading a book discussing normality of life changes; planting seeds in a small soil-filled peat pot; making bags of a cornstarch mixture tinted yellow and blue, which will change to green when kneaded (demonstrating that changes are not always bad, just different).

- *Session 4*: Discussion acknowledging sadness because of the importance of the persons who died; using helpful items from a decorated container when feeling sad; reading and discussing books about feeling sad; focusing on ways to obtain support when sad.
- *Session 5*: Making masks demonstrating confusion about feelings; using puppets to discuss confusing situations; reading a story about a caterpillar's confusing feelings as he was changing into a butterfly.
- *Session 6*: Normalizing fears that result from the death of an important person by drawing those fears; storytelling about conquering fears; learning relaxation skills to deal with fears.
- *Session 7*: Focusing on reasons for feeling guilt about a death; reading a book to understand that the persons' deaths were not the responsibility of group members; activity with balloons to release negative feelings; making chains from construction paper loops and then breaking them (symbolizing breaking the chain of guilt).
- *Session 8*: Making net from yarn in order to express loneliness, as well as to reinforce the importance of group support; watching a video clip about loneliness; reading a book acknowledging the emptiness that can occur following the death of a loved one.
- *Session 9*: Commemorating the lives of the persons who died by making memory boxes; art activity with a wheel on which to draw special memories; using musical instruments to play and discuss reminders of their special persons.
- *Session 10*: Focus on empowering the group members to feel hope for the future; using a string of paper dolls to demonstrate uniqueness of each person's grief; reading a book demonstrating ways to conquer negative feelings; writing a note to each loved one, attaching it to the string of a helium balloon, and releasing the balloon.

The children and their adult caregivers in the groups develop coping skills to deal with other losses in their lives, not just the specific losses that have brought them to The Kids' Place. The overarching goal of the program is for families to understand that positive outcomes can result even from painful events.

Group Membership

The backgrounds of those who seek our support services are quite diverse in geography, socioeconomic status, and religious and cultural orientations. Some of the families who come to The Kids' Place are able to pay for services, while others may have difficulty buying gas for their cars to travel to the center. Families from a broad area of central Oklahoma are served by the center. Some drive 1½ hours each way in order to attend the support groups.

Staffing

The grief support groups at The Kids' Place are primarily staffed by volunteers. Volunteers constitute the heartbeat of The Kids' Place. Over several years, more than 180 volunteers have been trained, each serving for at least 1 year as a group facilitator. Some facilitators have participated for more than 7 years. In order to ensure adequate attention to the individual needs of each child within each group, a minimum of four facilitators work with the Younger Group (ages 5–8), while three volunteers are assigned to the Middle Group (ages 9–12). The Older Group (ages 13–19) and the Adult Group (caregivers of the children) have two facilitators each (male and female). The use of multiple facilitators in the Younger and Middle Groups permits one or more volunteers to attend to children who may be emotionally distraught or disruptive to the remainder of the group, while the other facilitators continue with the group process (Webb, 2002).

Volunteer group facilitators all complete the same series of training meetings. This ensures that team members will be able to substitute for each other, since each of the five groups function in the same way and follow the same principles.

Volunteers are referred to the agency by current volunteers, through contacts with area churches, and by helping professionals (e.g., teachers, social service workers, and mental health care providers). Some desirable characteristics we look for in a volunteer group facilitator at The Kids' Place include the following:

- Being a good listener from the time the group members arrive until they leave.
- Having the ability to maintain confidentiality outside the group, unless information falls into our list of "Seven Exceptions to Privacy."
- Being aware of individual differences and sensitive to mood swings.
- Being able to function in the group as a facilitator of sharing, not as a teacher of facts.
- Being able to identify safe behaviors, to restrict unsafe ones, and to enforce our rules for safety as necessary.
- Being willing to note and discuss individual group members' needs with the group coordinator.
- Being able to hold to time limits.

Volunteer Training

The 36-hour volunteer training series includes the following: an examination of our video on The Kids' Place, our model, and our policies; an examination of the basics of grief and mourning, including specifics about children's grief; a presentation of developmental information about children, preteens, and adolescents; a presentation about using play with grieving children; an introduction to facilitating adult groups; instruction, practice, and testing in first aid and cardiopulmonary resuscitation; a demonstration about using art with grieving children; a presentation about storytelling and reading to children; instruction in group dynamics and effective listening skills; a presentation on cultural influences, cremation, and the value of rituals and ceremony; an exercise identifying attitudes about death and dying; a role-play experience (see below); and an exploration of the workings of The Kids' Place in detail.

Guest presenters include local university professors, funeral directors, an art therapist, an early childhood specialist, and other resource people who specialize in the training areas listed. The training fee paid by the volunteers provides them with a copy of the book *Healing the Bereaved Child* by Alan Wolfelt (1996).

The final weekend of the four-part training series incorporates a role-play experience, called "The Best of The Kids' Place," into the volunteers' learning opportunity. A team of veteran facilitators helps the trainees experience a "typical night" at The Kids' Place. The trainees become the group members (playing assigned roles as children, teens, or adults) as the veterans guide them through an evening plan. Volunteers in training observe a presession and a postsession meeting in progress (by sitting around the perimeter of the room as the mock meetings are conducted). Trainees report that "The Best of The Kids' Place" experience helps them make sense out of all the information they had previously learned in the training series.

THE FAMILY PROGRAM

The Application Process

When a family has experienced a death and has expressed an interest in the services provided at The Kids' Place, an application packet is mailed to the family's home. Family members bring their completed packet to an orientation meeting, held once a month. During that orientation, they are given a tour of the facility and detailed information about the support program. Two handouts—"Rules for Safety" (i.e., rules that are followed in the children's groups) and "Principles Which Guide the Adult Groups"—

are reviewed in order for participants to understand what is expected of them as group members. The concept of confidentiality is emphasized both in the orientation and at the beginning of each support group session. Assignments to a specific night are based on availability and each family's needs.

Structure of the Groups

The basic structure of each of the five sets of support groups is identical, although a separate set of volunteers and families is assigned to each set of groups. A presession team meeting begins at 6:00 P.M., during which the volunteers reconnect with each other, discuss and clarify details of the activities for the evening, and receive information about new families entering the program. The facilitators of the Adult Group give updates on participating families' attendance and situations, based on the telephone calls the facilitators have made the evening before the group session. With this information, facilitators of all groups can prepare themselves to respond to the group members who will be attending, and can inform the other group members about the reason for nonattendance of any group members.

Curriculum

The decision was made for The Kids' Place support groups to be curriculum- and topic-oriented. At the same time, the groups are fluid and flexible, responding to the needs of the individuals within the groups. The Adult Group and the three children's groups focus on a common theme, with activities in each age-level group related to the topic or theme of the evening. This provides the family members something in common to discuss when they return home. As mentioned previously, themes dealt with by The Kids' Place curriculum include confusion, loneliness, sadness, guilt, regrets, questions, changes, anger, and memories.

A grief author and therapist, Linda Goldman, has told us (personal communication, August 2, 2002):

> I think the family approach to grief used at The Kids' Place in Oklahoma is a unique model for working with grief support groups for children. Joining several families together on a given evening for age-level grief support groups encourages all members to work through their grief process together. The family-centered grief support groups at The Kids' Place help to create an open family system which promotes the expression of feelings and thoughts in a safe and nurturing environment.

A complete plan of activities for each age group is either mailed in advance or made available on our Web site for volunteers to access. Even though such structure might appear to be rigid, the program director strongly emphasizes that flexibility is essential in working with grieving individuals. Each facilitator understands that once the opening ritual is completed, the intent is to stay on the topic as much as possible, but the leader can allow the group to "go where the group members need to go" to address their needs. At times, every activity on the plan is completed. Other times, the needs of the group take them on a different path after introductions.

Although the directors of The Kids' Place do not apply the stage theory of death and dying made popular by Elisabeth Kübler-Ross (see Hagman, 2001), we do incorporate some of the elements associated with her research. For example, in a group session focusing on the theme of anger, a variety of activities would be employed to help group members explore and understand the relationship of anger to loss.

GAMES AND ACTIVITIES

Because playing games enables children to practice new ways of coping and relating (Schaefer & Reid, 2001), various games related to feelings or grief are used in all three children's groups. Since a game is "only a game," children can allow themselves the luxury of feeling emotions and expressing beliefs that would otherwise be taboo. In this way, game playing opens up opportunities for verbal discussions about deaths that might otherwise be difficult to stimulate (Zambelli & DeRosa, 1992).

A report by Roberts (2001) of a study performed by the SandCastles grief support program on the efficacy of children's bereavement support groups indicated that the study found play to be the primary coping strategy used by children in dealing with grief-related emotions. This finding is consistent with many of the current theories about ways children cope with grief (Silverman, 2000; Grollman, 1995; Jarratt, 1994; Glick, 1974; Webb, 2002). The plan for activities of the Younger Group at The Kids' Place emphasizes "free-play time," during which children have choices to play at various centers—a child-size kitchen unit, a construction wrecking ball, or a dress-up corner (where they can find clothing similar to that worn by their special person who died, or where they can engage in fantasy play). Books related to the theme for the evening are read, and all sizes of puppets are enjoyed by all. A rice box (a sandbox filled with rice) is available for scenes to be constructed. At times, a child may set up a scene depicting the accident that killed his or her special person. At other times, the child may simply be playing with small figures in the rice box because it is fun.

Numerous art activities are also available for all age groups. For instance, on one of the evenings during the year when the focus is on memories, memory boxes are created. Group members are invited to bring something that reminds them of their special persons to place into their boxes, which they decorate during the session. Curry (2002) reported that a child whose parent had died experienced her group as a time of healing, because she could share activities with other children who had also lost a parent. During the meetings, the kids not only talked about their experiences, but made memory albums and created memorial ornaments at Christmas. The child looked forward to attending her support group each time.

Activities designed for the adolescent and adult groups serve as catalysts for conversation. At times, the group or individuals make feelings or memory collages. At other times, an activity sheet such as "Defenses Faces" helps participants identify coping skills. Group members may create a "grief map," depicting areas such as "The Grief Fog" or "Question Mountain" to help group members recognize where they are and where they have been (Dawson & Harris, 1997). One 18-year-old female group member whose father had died by suicide when she was 14 years old came to her group at The Kids' Place with new reflections about her grief following the terrorist attacks of September 11, 2001. She stated that the enormous impact these acts had on the country had triggered new needs for her in her grief process. Her response was that she could now cry and connect with friends and family in a different way. She allowed herself to be thoughtful about her father at times other than while participating in the group at The Kids' Place. At about the time of the terrorist attacks, the group members were given disposable cameras to photograph images and places that held memories for them of their loved ones. The photographs allowed her to give pictorial meaning to her new feelings. (A later section of this chapter describes in more detail how The Kids' Place responded to the 2001 attacks.)

The Roberts (2001) report on the SandCastles program indicated that both parents and children in their support groups reported feeling the same negative emotions of sadness, loneliness, anger, and annoyance. However, the parents reported higher frequencies of those emotions than did their children. We believe that the intensity of these negative emotions can be ameliorated through providing group activities and other opportunities for adults who have experienced loss through death to relate to one another.

Rituals

"Rituals provide ties to others as well as providing continuity and security" (Weeks, 2001). Some time ago, we noticed that some members of the children's groups seemed to forget the reason they were attending The Kids' Place. Therefore, we decided to begin each group meeting for children, teens, and adults with a ritual in the form of an "introduction time." Each participant takes turns holding a laminated piece of paper that says, "My name is _____, and the death of _____ is what brought me to The Kids' Place. My feeling I have now is _____." Each person fills in the missing words orally for him- or herself each week. Except for the Younger Group (ages 5–8), the following optional statement is added to the introduction: "What I have done since our last group meeting to mourn or heal is _____." Following the implementation of the introduction ritual, a change in group dynamics was immediately evident in both the Middle Group (ages 9–12) and the Older Group (ages 13–19). Concerning this ritual, one parent said, "I used to get bored with the same introduction of every person each time. I finally realized this is a great 'icebreaker' and is a good way to know where each person is, emotionally, that day. It helps to know how each person is feeling that day." One of our facilitators commented, "Our opening ritual encourages and allows group members to acknowledge the death which brought them to our program."

Songs

Another tradition whose effect has been more far-reaching than initially imagined is singing The Kids' Place song, "Hold My Hand," to close each evening's activities. As the families meet together in a large room following the individual support groups, the evening coordinator informs families of any upcoming activities, then invites anyone who has a birthday that month to go to the center of the circle so the combined groups can wish them a happy birthday in song. Next, the participants are invited to hold the hands of the persons next to them, if they are comfortable doing so, and everyone sings "Hold My Hand" before leaving for the evening: "When you hold my hand, you can touch my heart. In this house, this Kids' Place, I can wear any face—angry, mad, happy, glad, even sad, and you can touch them all when you hold my hand." One mom told of an evening at home when she was quite tearful and very sad about the death of her husband. Her 5-year-old, the youngest of three boys, came to the couch where she was sitting, took her hand, and began to sing The Kids' Place song.

STAFF REVIEW

After the families leave for the evening, the facilitators gather together for an hour-long postsession meeting. This meeting serves several purposes:

- The events and activities of the evening are evaluated from the perspective of every facilitator. Typed copies of the meeting notes are sent to team members prior to the next meeting.
- The volunteers become their own support group, making sure that no one is going home carrying the burden of unresolved feelings stirred up during the evening.
- Cards are written to the children in the groups and mailed a few days later. One dad said, "The Kids' Place has been very important to our son. He enjoys the letters he gets from the volunteers. He doesn't get much mail, and I think it has been one of the things that has moved him forward."

LENGTH OF CONTACT

When families ask to join a grief support group at The Kids' Place, we tell them, through our printed materials and in our family orientation meeting, that the length of their stay in our program is up to them. Some families stay with us for several months; some stay a year, 2 years, or longer. Each person and each family are unique. The length of time that families stay involved with a support group depends on many factors, including the nature of their loss, the relationship they had to the deceased person, the amount of support available to them from other sources (church, family, community), and each person's own coping skills based on life experiences. We help families consider their progress at The Kids' Place by providing each family with a self-evaluation form during the spring of each year. Each family member is asked to respond to questions and topics such as the following:

- Since coming to The Kids' Place, I feel (circle one):

  Much better   A little better   The same   A little worse   Much worse

- Tell about your experience with The Kids' Place:
  - What has helped me the most is:
  - What has been least helpful is:
  - What would help me most now would be:
  - In my journey through the grieving process, I still need to:

When a family informs us of its intention to leave our program, the support group leaders and fellow group members conduct a goodbye ceremony in each age-level group that contains a departing member. For our goodbye ceremony, we have adapted the "rock ceremony" established by Beverly Chappell founder of The Dougy Center in Portland, Oregon. A small cloth drawstring bag containing one rough and two polished rocks is given to each departing group member. A group facilitator explains to the group, "The rough rock reminds us of the roughness of our grief as we entered The Kids' Place. The smooth stones remind us that many of the rough edges of our grief have been knocked off and smoothed out by our group interaction. The stones represent our wish that the road ahead may be smoother for us all, but the rough stone is evidence that there will likely be rough times in the future." One by one, fellow group members are then allowed to hold the rocks and tell the one who is leaving what they appreciate about the person, what they have learned from the person, how they will miss him or her in the group, and what activity they remember doing with the person. Each member also makes a silent wish for the person. After the last group member speaks, the person leaving is given the bag of rocks and shares with the group his or her experiences at The Kids' Place, feelings about leaving, and/or feelings toward the others in the group. A child departing from one of the children's groups may also do a drawing to illustrate his or her feelings (see Figure 7.1).

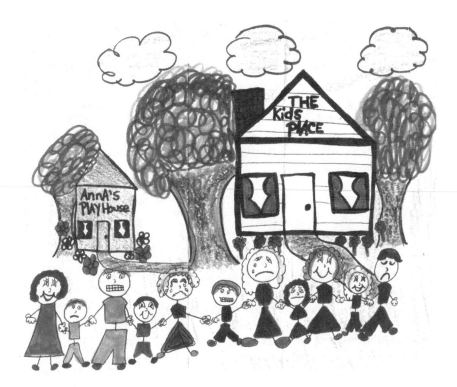

FIGURE 7.1. Drawing by an 11-year-old as she and her family said goodbye to The Kids' Place. The faces in her drawing represent some of the feelings she learned were OK to have, including "happy," "sad," "angry," and "mad."

BENEFITS OF GRIEF SUPPORT GROUPS SUCH AS THE KIDS' PLACE

- They offer a setting where coping skills can be observed and learned for present and future application. Group members often find that the coping skills taught or modeled in our support groups apply to other situations in their lives at home, at school, or in the community.
- They provide an emotionally safe setting for processing or expressing thoughts and feelings. Our "Rules for Safety" promote confidentiality and respect for self and others.
- They give group members opportunities to work on their grief issues in a confidential environment, separated from other family members.
- They provide open, ongoing sessions that allow people whose grief is recent to observe "veterans" and gain hope from those who have progressed beyond them.
- They validate grieving families through the knowledge that the 15 volunteers on "their night" have invested considerable time in training and dedicate 7 hours each month to serving their groups. The families realize that they are important to the team of helpers, and that their thoughts, feelings, and experiences matter.

RESOURCES FOR FAMILIES

Additional resources supplement the support groups. These include a lending library in which the books are divided according to age appropriateness, from young children through teens and adults. Various feelings-related and grief-related books are available, in addition to a resource shelf containing free booklets, articles, and pamphlets. We also make referrals to local counselors whenever families ask for such services or when our leaders feel that it is appropriate to suggest counseling services as a possible addition to the support families are receiving from the program.

SPECIAL OPPORTUNITIES

For each set of groups, one evening in the fall and another in the spring is designated as "meal night," when we serve a simple meal. The mealtime and the other activities on meal nights give families and team members the opportunity to get better acquainted and promote a large-group connection not available in our age-divided groups.

Holiday parties in December provide a time for families and facilitators to visit, snack on finger foods, and make memorial ornaments to be hung on a tree. In a ceremony, the members of each family are encouraged to tell whatever they wish about the ornament and/or the person it commemorates.

June picnics conclude the regularly scheduled group meetings, which roughly coincide with the school year. Following the fun and food outdoors, participants gather in their age-level groups and prepare notes to attach to helium-filled balloons. The evening ends with a memorial balloon release.

CASE STUDY: THE JONES FAMILY

This section describes a family who lost a loved one in the bombing of the Murrah Federal Building in Oklahoma City on April 19, 1995. This was the first family to seek support from The Kids' Place when it opened its doors in 1996.

Family Information

> Mrs. Jones, age 38 and divorced 1 year as of 1995. Occupation: Administrative assistant.
> Mrs. Blair, age 60. Occupation: Office worker. Mother of Mrs. Jones. Died in the Murrah Building bombing. The family waited 10 days before Grandma's body was found.
> Mr. Blair, age 65. Occupation: Builder. Father of Mrs. Jones.
> Mary, age 15 at time of most recent contact, age 8 at the time of Grandma's death.
> Bob, age 11 at time of most recent contact, age 4 when his grandmother died.

First Interview with Mrs. Jones

"The dissolution of our marriage was very hard on the kids and me. By January 1995, things were finally starting to get better for us. Then the bombing hit on April 19, 1995. Prior to that day, the children and I had a weekday morning routine that included getting ready for the day, then driving to drop my daughter off at school and my son at the babysitter. We would stop by to say 'Hi' to Mom many mornings before our other stops. She was always there for me if I needed anything. Someone would take Mom to work, then I'd pick her and the kids up in the late afternoon, and we'd go to her house. We'd eat together or go out to eat, then get involved in activities together. On weekends, Mom would come out to our place for picnics, wiener roasts, and other fun family times. On some workdays, I would go with my friend to the Murrah Federal Building, where I would visit with Mom while my friend conducted her business at the Federal Credit Union. I would always drop in to visit with my mother. We were very close.

"On April 19, 1995, we stopped by Mom's to pick up some books to return to the library. She waved to the kids from her front door. Many mornings, I would call her at work. I didn't make a call to her that morning. Soon after 9:00 A.M., a coworker came to tell me that the YMCA next to Mom's building had blown up. She soon returned to tell me that she'd learned that it was actually the Murrah Building—Mom's building that had blown up! I called Mom's office number, but the phone just rang and rang. I called my brother and sister, and we arranged to meet and go to the area together. The police escorted us up close, and we could see where Mom's office *used to be*.

"During the 10 days before they found my mother's body, I felt like I cried all the time. I didn't even want to eat, but the volunteers at the church where we waited made me eat. I don't know how my children made it through those days. I couldn't take care of myself, much less my kids. One of my best friends stepped in to make sure my son and daughter were cared for. The impact on my daughter was immediate. The next time I took her to school, I had to pry her off my leg to leave her; she was so scared that something was going to happen to me next.

"Our daily routine was changed forever on April 19, 1995. I lost my mother; the children lost their grandmother. We no longer had a reason to stop by her house in the mornings, but we did go there many evenings to check on my dad, the house, the dogs, and to water the plants. It was quite a while before someone bought the house and moved in. In the coming months, I would find myself picking up the phone and dialing Mom's number. I just wanted to say, 'How are you?'—but she wasn't there. The kids would say at times 'Call Grandma and ask her about _____.' Or one of them would ask, 'Are we going to Grandma's house today?' My son might say, 'Grandma's oatmeal would sure taste good today.' My daughter went through our picture albums and pulled out all of the pictures with her grandma, and she is holding on to them to this day."

Facilitator: How did the three of you react to your mother's death as a family?

"More than ever, we did everything together. We weren't involved much in a church back then, and our extended family wasn't really able to help us in all the ways we needed. Some people labeled me as 'the strong one' who could take care of everyone else. I cried myself to sleep at night, because I didn't have anyone to listen to me and to understand what I was going through. I felt alone. My children and I went to many of the meetings of the bombing survivors' support group, but there was so much anger there—and we weren't dealing with the anger like they were.

"During the first few months, I became very concerned about my children. The attitude of everyone seemed to be 'Hey, they'll be OK; kids bounce back easily.' Even counselors told me, 'Watch your children for a few months, and if they seem to have problems adjusting to Grandma's death, then let us know.' No one seemed to understand that *the kids* were grieving, and *I* was grieving, and we all needed someone to help us as a family. Fortunately, we received a letter telling us about plans for the establishment of a family grief center called The Kids' Place. I called; then we attended the dedication ceremony in April 1996. When the support groups started in October of that year, we were there! That was a year and a half after the bombing."

Facilitator: How did Grandma's death affect your son?

"My son, a preschooler at the time of his grandma's death, reverted to wetting the bed. He would wake up during the night with bad dreams, jolting right up out of bed. It wasn't until after he started participating in support groups at The Kids' Place that the bad dreams began to go away. The thing about The Kids' Place that seemed to help my son the most was having other kids his own age to talk with, regardless of the reason for their loss. He was more open with his feelings all along."

Facilitator: How did Grandma's death affect your daughter?

"My daughter, who was in grade school at the time, immediately became fearful, clingy, and withdrawn. She wouldn't talk about anything she was feeling. It wasn't until at Camp KidsPlace that she opened up to anyone. She began to gradually share some at home after that camp experience. Since she was so quiet, the benefit of The Kids' Place for her was just being with other kids and the facilitators. For a long time, she just listened, and she was taking it all in. It has really helped her in the long run. Her involvement in the support groups helped her deal with her grandma's death on a personal level. She didn't 'get over it' like some seemed to think you should. She's still very sensitive to the emotions of what happened."

Facilitator: How did your mother's death affect you, Mrs. Jones?

"I'd had some health problems for years, but I started having more difficulties beginning April 19, 1995. The doctors passed it off as the stress of the situation. All they wanted to do was give me drugs. Later, a new doctor finally discovered that I had a tumor. I had surgery—an event which triggered more fear in my kids. They were afraid that I was going to die. At that point, however, we had been going to support groups at The Kids' Place for several months, and the kids wanted to attend the groups with another family member even when I couldn't go.

"I cried so much during the 10 days before Mom's body was found that I just sat there when her boss came to tell us that she'd been found in the rubble. I was 'cried out' at that point. I had serious emotional problems following my mother's death, but the counselors made me feel like it was my problem—that it was my fault that I was depressed. No one seemed to want to help my children. I was told by counselors, 'Just wait and see if your children develop any serious problems; then we'll see what they need.' Fortunately, I had a best friend I could go to any time and cry all I needed to. She accepted me where I was at the time.

"Physically, I had trouble taking care of myself at first. Intellectually, I had trouble concentrating and staying focused. Spiritually, even though we weren't regularly involved in a church in the early days, I felt strongly that God was with us. I wrote poetry and songs, and I encouraged my son and daughter to write in their journals, too. We learned songs and sang them together. The kids and I especially latched onto the song, 'Angels Among Us,' and that helped keep us going.

Subsequent Interview with Mrs. Jones

"On the first anniversary of Mom's death, I opened up to my dad and insisted, 'You need to listen to me!' I was feeling so low that I was having suicidal thoughts—thinking about killing my children and myself so we could all escape the terrible pain. Instead, I found professional help. Some family members seemed to think that I was going to be fine since I'd had the strength to recognize my problems and get myself some help!

"During the fall after Mom's death, people would tell us that the first Christmas would be the hardest. Well, they were wrong. That first December, just 8 months after the bombing, we were still numb, just going through the motions of life. It was the *second* Christmas that we were devastated!"

Interview with Mrs. Jones 7 Years Later

Facilitator: What was it about The Kids' Place that helped you the most?
"We learned so many helpful things at The Kids' Place, including:

- Nobody is alike in their grief, but being in a support group with others who have had a loss through death allowed us to learn from their experiences. I learned that I was not alone in my grief reactions. I was not overreacting, as some would have had me believe.
- There were many times I would try something with my children that I had heard another adult in our group talk about. It helped me tremendously as a parent!

- The children and I learned about journaling. Writing things down helped each one of us in our own way.
- My children were able to be with other kids who were grieving and know that they were not alone in the world of pain and sadness. We learned that one thing we had been told about grieving children was not true. All children do *not* 'automatically bounce back' after a death in the family.
- After we had been in The Kids' Place support group program for a while, my children became more open to helping others. They even talked on camera for a public television grief special.
- The children and I all experienced the joy of being able to use many of the coping skills we learned at The Kids' Place in other situations in life.
- I've concluded that the family model of grief support used by The Kids' Place is a must! Since April 19, 1995, all three of us have seen individual counselors at times. But grief affects the whole family. I can't imagine it working as well if you didn't have the entire family coming at the same time."

Facilitator: What was it about The Kids' Place that was the least helpful?
"The only challenging thing about my time at The Kids' Place was when, due to the growth of the program, some changes were made in the facilitators staffing my group. It worked out for the best, but it was hard to give up those special folks who guided our group in the early days."

Facilitator: How did you know when you were ready to leave the support groups of The Kids' Place?
"It was just like the directors had told us when we first started in the program. Other activities started pulling us in other directions, making it harder and harder to find the time to attend the support group meetings, even though they were only twice a month. We finally knew that it was time to move on. What we missed the most were the strong relationships we had built with other families and the group leaders at The Kids' Place."

Facilitator: What else do you remember about The Kids' Place?
"It worked! It seemed like, over the course of time, that we dealt with every conceivable topic and need a grieving person might have. It helped me to be a better parent to my children. I learned from The Kids' Place model to not push and pry so much. I'm more available to my kids than ever before. I listen a lot more. I learned to let them be who they each need to be."

Interview with Mary, Age 15, 7 Years after Her Grandmother's Death

Facilitator: Describe the nature and date of your loss.

"My grandmother died while at work in the Murrah Federal Building during the bombing on April 19, 1995. I was 8 years old and told of her death by a school counselor while my mother was on the way to the school to tell me herself. My first responses were shock, fear that others would be dead, and then sadness that my grandmother died. I remember crying a lot."

Facilitator: Describe your personal mourning, your feelings, and actions you took related to your grief.

"I remember crying a lot. I felt confused, but I remember having friends and family to talk to about my grandmother's death. My friends seemed to understand."

Facilitator: How did the loss affect you physically, socially, intellectually, and spiritually?

"I don't think the loss affected me physically. I don't remember feeling sick or not doing something because I didn't feel well. The loss affected me socially because sometimes I didn't want to be with my friends. Sometimes I did want to be with my friends when I couldn't. The loss affected me intellectually because I hadn't thought much about death before, since no one in my family had died. I thought a lot about life and death and a lot of things I'd never considered before. The loss affected me spiritually in that it made me think about who God was and how he could allow death. At times, I was mad at God for allowing my grandmother to die."

Facilitator: Why did you decide to try The Kids' Place support group?

"We decided to try The Kids' Place because my mother said we needed help. I don't remember exactly what my mother said, but Mom was the one who decided we should start attending The Kids' Place."

Facilitator: What helped you the most in your support group experience at The Kids' Place?

"What I remember most are the things we did at The Kids' Place, like the dramas and the memory boxes. I don't remember specific lessons, but that it just helped me to deal with death. I learned to talk in groups, to relate to others my age, and to learn how to help others who have had family members who have died. What helped me the most were the journals we wrote in and the memory boxes we made. I still use them."

Facilitator: What was least helpful or most uncomfortable?

"The least helpful or most uncomfortable thing for me was sharing in small groups. Once I realized I wasn't going to be forced to share, it was OK. Now I know that it was good for me."

Facilitator: What else, besides The Kids' Place, helped you (or continues to help you) as you grieve?

"Family is the only thing besides The Kids' Place that continues to help us. I think things are better now, but I can't really put my grieving on a timeline. I feel that my brother is still having the hardest time dealing with the death because of his problems at school and having to go to the hospital. I remember feeling responsible to take care of him and even my mother."

Facilitator: Describe how you are doing now. How have things progressed with your grief?

"I believe that I am doing OK now. My experiences at The Kids' Place helped me to mature in general, to develop a better self-esteem, and to not be as afraid of death as I used to be."

Interview with Bob, Age 11, 7 Years after His Grandmother's Death

Bob was 4 years old in April 1995 when his maternal grandmother died in the Murrah Building bombing. His favorite memories of his grandmother were her taking him to a local fast food place for lunch and making pancakes or oatmeal for his breakfast. On April 19, 1995, he was with a babysitter and found out about the bombing on the evening news when he heard his grandma's name. "Mom didn't want us to know about it, but we found out anyway."

Facilitator: How did the loss affect you?

"We did stuff differently. Mom would cry a lot, and that would make me cry. I had lots of nightmares about somebody dying. The nightmares turned into good dreams after starting at The Kids' Place."

Facilitator: Why did you decide to try The Kids' Place support group?

"We needed help, emotionally. Mom said it would help us get through life easier."

Facilitator: What helped you the most in your support group experience at The Kids' Place?

"Mostly, it was coming and giving everybody hugs and getting hugs from everybody. I liked coloring, hearing the stories, and seeing my new friends."

Facilitator: How were those friends at The Kids' Place different?
"They had also lost somebody they really cared about. It made me feel closer to them because we had all lost somebody. We got to talk about our losses."

Facilitator: Looking back, what do you wish you could have had or done in group?
"I can't think of anything that we didn't get to do that I wanted to do."

Facilitator: What else, besides The Kids' Place, helped you (or continues to help you) with your grief process?
"Mostly, my mom and my sister help me because whenever we cry, we cry together. We're dealing with it together. One thing we enjoy doing is looking at picture albums of Grandma and us."

Facilitator: What do you remember about how you were doing 2 years after your loss?
"I started feeling like I was being helpful to others."

Facilitator: If you had a friend whose grandma died, what would you tell him?
"That it will be all right. I will help you deal with it on the way. If he would cry I would cry, too, and make him feel he is not alone. I would help him understand that he shouldn't forget her."

RESPONSE BY THE KIDS' PLACE TO SEPTEMBER 11, 2001

A few days following the terrorist attacks of September 11, 2001, and accompanied by several area counselors, Charlotte Burrough (Family Services Director of The Kids' Place) and Gary Woodbridge (a volunteer facilitator whose wife had been killed in the Murrah Building bombing) left for a week of helping in New York City at the request of a church in Queens. Since "9/11," staff members and volunteers at The Kids' Place have assisted more than 75 children's grief programs in the Northeast by phone, fax, mail, and e-mail. Information that helped The Kids' Place support grieving families in the aftermath of the 1995 Oklahoma City tragedy was shared with the leaders of grief programs in New York, the District of Columbia, Maryland, Pennsylvania, New Jersey, Massachusetts, Connecticut, and Virginia. In March 2002, we two authors (Danny Mize, Executive Director of The Kids' Place, and Charlotte) were invited to present information at the 2-day New Jersey Self-Help Clearing House seminar for families who experienced a loss on 9/11, and for professionals working with the families. We spent the remainder of a week offering additional seminars, consulting, and encouragement to grief care providers in New York City; Washington, D.C.; and Fairfax County, Virginia. In June 2002, at the 6th Annual National Symposium on Children's Grief Support in St. Louis, Missouri, the two of us participated in a panel presentation that included some grief practitioners from the Northeast and others from across the United States. The presentation attempted to educate audience members to the challenges and successes of efforts to respond to the tragic events of 9/11.

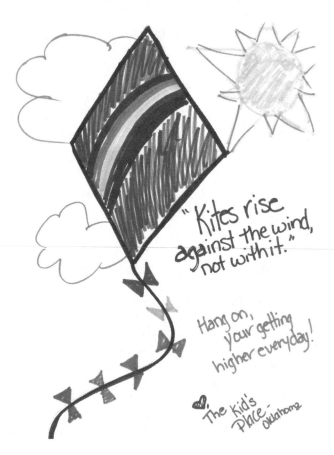

FIGURE 7.2. Drawing by a participant at The Kids' Place in response to the 9/11 tragedy.

Families at The Kids' Place, as well as staff members and volunteers, have responded to those affected by 9/11. Figure 7.2 is a drawing by a child participant that was sent to children who lost parents in one of the 9/11 attacks. Adult participants have reached out in various ways as well.

The connections between the 1995 bombing in Oklahoma City and the 9/11 tragedies in the Northeast have been highlighted in a new educational exhibit at the Oklahoma City National Memorial Museum. The work The Kids' Place has done to encourage programs in the Northeast has been included in that display.

REFERENCES

Bluestein, J. (1993). *Parents, teens and boundaries.* Deerfield Beach, FL: Health Communications.

Cook, A. S., & Dworkin, D. S. (1992). *Helping the bereaved.* New York: Basic Books.

Curry, C. (2002). *Keeping your kids afloat when it feels like you're sinking.* Ann Arbor, MI: Servant.

Dawson, S., & Harris, L. (1997). *Adventure in the land of grief.* Wilmore, KY: Words on the Wind.

Glick, I. (1974). *First year of bereavement.* New York: Wiley.

Grollman, E. (1995). *Bereaved children and teens.* Boston: Beacon Press.

Hagman, G. (2001). Beyond decathexis: Toward a new psychoanalytic understanding and treatment of mourning. In R. A. Neimeyer (Ed.), *Meaning reconstruction and the experience of loss* (pp. 13–29). Washington, DC: American Psychological Association.

Jarratt, C. (1994). *Helping children cope with separation and loss.* Boston: Beacon Press.

Kight, M. (1998). *Forever changed.* Amherst, NY: Prometheus Books.

Kliman, G. (1979). Childhood mourning: A taboo within a taboo. In I. Gerber, A. Weiner, A. H. Kutscher, D. Battin, A. Arkin, & I. K. Goldberg (Eds.), *Perspectives on bereavement* (p. 169). New York: Arno Press.

Krementz, J. (1981) *How it feels when a parent dies.* New York: Knopf.

Raphael, B., Field, J., & Kvelde, H. (1980). Childhood bereavement: A prospective study as a possible prelude to future preventive intervention. In E. J. Anthony & C. Cluland (Eds.), *Preventive child psychiatry in an age of transitions* (p. 169). New York: Wiley Interscience.

Roberts, R. (2001). *The importance of bereavement groups in teaching healthy coping strategies for children ages 10–13.* Detroit, MI: Wayne State University.

Schaefer, C. E., & Reid, S. (2001). *Game play: Therapeutic use of childhood games.* New York: Wiley.

Shapiro, E. (1994). *Grief as a family process.* New York: Guilford Press.

Siegel, K., Mesagno, F. P., & Christ, G. (1990). A prevention program for bereaved children. *American Journal of Orthopsychiatry, 60*(2), 168–175.

Silverman, P. (2000). *Never too young to know.* New York: Oxford University Press.

Webb, N. B. (Ed.). (2002). *Helping bereaved children: A handbook for practitioners* (2nd ed.). New York: Guilford Press.

Weeks, O. D. (2001, June). *Rituals.* Paper presented at the World Gathering on Bereavement, Columbus, OH.

Wolfelt, A. (1996). *Healing the bereaved child.* Fort Collins, CO: Companion Press.

Zambelli, G. C., & DeRosa, A. P. (1992). Bereavement support groups for school-age children: Theory, intervention, and case example. *American Journal of Orthopsychiatry, 62*(4), 484–493.

CHAPTER 8

Bereavement Groups Soon after Traumatic Death

BETH HARTLEY

The traumatic death of a family member or other significant person is a time of chaos and crisis that sends a wave of emotions throughout the entire extended family and friendship network. Traumatic death wounds both the psyches and the bodies of survivors. Yet, sadly, the death of a family member and/or significant person is often disregarded and misunderstood by the very people who are trying to help, as they too are forced to face their own fears about death. Often people don't know what to say to traumatized survivors, so they say nothing, further complicating feelings of isolation, despair, and loneliness among those desperately needing support. Or the best-intentioned people may make statements such as "It's been a year . . . isn't it time you moved on with your life?" or "At least he didn't suffer." This minimizes a bereaved person's grief and often exacerbates the person's pain. For these reasons, families may often feel abandoned in times of grief, particularly in instances of trauma, as friends and even other family members are too frightened or uncomfortable to offer support.

If handled with compassion, love, and support, however, even the most traumatic experience of death can eventually become an important process of personal growth. The Den for Grieving Kids—a nonprofit program of Family Centers, Inc., of Greenwich, Stamford, Darien, and New Canaan, Connecticut—is a peer support center for children and their families who are enduring a significant bereavement. We believe that by providing a safe atmosphere in which families are allowed to grieve, we can help families to create their own meaning as they navigate their individual grieving process. Our program incorporates the following principles within its peer support therapeutic model:

- Grief is a natural reaction to the loss of a family member or other significant person for children as well as adults.
- Individuals possess the natural capacity to heal themselves.
- The duration and intensity of grief are unique for each individual.
- Caring, mutual support, and acceptance assist in the healing process.
- Giving and receiving are the same; by extending love, we can achieve self-love, attaining personal healing and inner peace.

The Den for Grieving Kids also serves as a preventive program: Grieving children are helped to feel, name, and own the thorny feelings with which they are coping, and are provided with a safe and healthy channel for those complex, agonizing emotions. The emotional confusion and anguish that people mourning the death of a family member or significant person experience may be exacerbated by Western culture's denial of death and its denial of the importance of the grieving process. Because unresolved grief can play a major role in the development of adult psychopathology, as well as sociopathic and suicidal disorders, the sharing of emotions proves to be a very beneficial process even when the negative aspects of an intensely emotional experience are stirred up (Pennebaker, Rime, & Zech, 2001). When children are supported in what they are experiencing, this may reduce subsequent damaging, self-destructive forms of grief, such as depression, antisocial behaviors, and physical/somatic complications.

FAMILY BEREAVEMENT CENTERS

In 1990–1991, the Project Research and Development Committee of the Junior League of Greenwich studied the Greenwich community to assess the availability of and need for child- and family-focused bereavement services. Research indicated that although fragmented services were available primarily through churches, there was no known holistic approach to grief for children and their families available in the local community. Further study was conducted to determine whether any organized service had been established elsewhere in the United States. We discovered that successful programs were in fact operating; one of the most successful ones was The Dougy Center of Portland, Oregon, which continues to serve as a national model.

The Dougy Center

Beverly Chappell, a registered nurse who had worked in the area of death and dying since 1974, founded the pioneering program called The Dougy Center for Grieving Children in 1982. Through her attendance at workshops, seminars, and lectures with Elisabeth Kübler-Ross, a long-lasting friendship developed between the two women. In 1979, Chappell heard from Kübler-Ross about a boy named Dougy Turno, who was diagnosed with an inoperable brain tumor. Kübler-Ross asked Chappell to work with Dougy and his family when they came to Portland in August 1981 to seek experimental treatment. While hospitalized, Dougy made rounds at the hospital to visit dying children, saying that he understood their feelings because he too was dying. Chappell saw in Dougy an unquenchable thirst for life, clarity, and love that many people older in years and experience never attain. Dougy's spiritual wisdom went far beyond his physical years and was an inspiration to all who met him. Dougy died in December 1981, but through the work of the Dougy Center, his wisdom prevails. To date, The Dougy Center has provided training and support to over 140 grief-focused programs across the United States and worldwide. (This history and other information are available from The Dougy Center for Grieving Children, P.O. Box 86852, Portland, OR 97286; http://www.GrievingChild.org.)

The Den for Grieving Kids

In the fall of 1991, the Safe Haven Committee of the Junior League of Greenwich was formed to determine whether the Greenwich community would benefit from a program similar to The Dougy Center. In response to the overwhelming need for bereavement services, a pilot program was established in the fall of 1992 as a collaborative effort between the Junior League of Greenwich and Greenwich Hospital. The pilot program was initially called The Den—A Support Group for Grieving Children and Their Families. The program continued under the leadership of the Junior League of Greenwich through 1996, at which time The Den became part of Family Centers, Inc.—a multiservice, family-focused agency serving four Connecticut communities.

By 1998, The Den had doubled in numbers of both facilitators and families. In response to this growth, The Den divided into two sections, each continuing to meet bimonthly, and moved to a new location to allow for continued expansion of the program. Both sections continued to meet the needs of families mourning losses that had occurred primarily through illness and/or accident. Also at that time, the name of the program was officially changed to The Den for Grieving Kids. A "no-waiting-list" policy was established at this time, so that no grieving child and/or family would ever be turned away.

Recognizing that The Den model lent itself well to other populations of families, Family Centers established a program for inner-city children and their families who had experienced multiple losses (e.g., separation/divorce, unemployment/underemployment, poverty, incarceration, and/or substance abuse), as well as the death of one or more family members. Other programs include a summer group for bereaved college students and graduating high school seniors, and a Young Adults Group for people ages 20–30 enduring the loss of a family member, a spouse/partner, or a close friend.

Immediately following the terrorist attacks of September 11, 2001, the Den team set in motion the implementation of an additional "night of service" to address the specific needs of World Trade Center victims' families and those grieving for traumatic deaths caused by terrorism. We realized that because of the severe psychological trauma of this tragedy—namely the violent, destructive nature of the attacks and the fact that they had been carefully organized and orchestrated by foreign terrorists on U.S. soil—we were encountering a level of grief that was unprecedented in U.S. society. Furthermore, we understood that the media attention and the subsequent invasion of personal privacy among the victims' families would be of monumental proportions. We felt obligated to exercise a level of sensitivity and consciousness about possible revictimization among the families as the level of media coverage increased. The magnitude of September 11th, for the families in the New York City and Washington, D.C. areas, and also across the nation, suggested that this picture of grief was going to look far different from anything we had previously witnessed.

Prompt emotional support was provided to all employees who were on site the morning of September 11th at the nine agency locations of Family Centers, Inc., in order to give staff members opportunities to make personal phone calls, watch the news, and debrief. Within hours, the agency contacted all off-site employees in its 28 programs, advising them to return to their homes if possible (due to security, transportation in the three-state Greater New York area had come to a grinding halt) or stay where they were, as the effects of this atrocity were creating an atmosphere of unparalleled confusion, anxiety, and rampant fear.

Within hours, Family Centers contacted local chapters of the American Red Cross, the United Way, local town halls, emergency response agencies/departments, and schools, to ascertain what agency services in terms of emotional crisis support were needed immediately. Family Centers then organized an agency-wide "critical response/crisis intervention" meeting for all clinicians and executive administrators, outlining a strategy for identifying vulnerable individuals and groups and for implementing outreach treatment and community-wide interventions. In the days and weeks that followed September 11th, the critical response team was divided and deployed to a variety of settings (i.e., schools, businesses, churches, and mental health groups), to provide information and help relevant to the tragedy. This included basic advice (such as encouraging parents to turn off their televisions to avoid repeatedly exposing family members to the trauma), as well as assistance with submission of DNA samples and follow-up with the New York City Coroner's Office, and provision of psychosocial care within the local communities.

In the sorrowful weeks that followed, victims' families and the entire country hoped against hope that survivors would be rescued from the rubble of the fallen twin towers. As each day passed, and as desperate hope faded into late September, the nation came to realize that no remaining victims would survive. At the end of September, Mayor Rudolph Giuliani formally announced that "rescue" efforts had been officially redefined as "recovery only." As families, communities, the nation, and the rest of the world struggled to grasp the reality of the terrorist attacks and their traumatic impact, Family Centers staff members, stunned and heartbroken as well, continued to provide intense emotional and therapeutic services to anyone in need. These same services continue to be provided at this writing.

SUPPORT GROUPS

Supportive group work provides a framework that orients members toward helping one another and coping with various life challenges. Because identifying and relating with other grieving individuals are often difficult or impossible outside the group milieu, a grief support group often becomes a "safe haven" where healing can occur. Within the confidential group milieu, grieving individuals often find comfort in connecting with others experiencing similar grief-related emotions—anger, confusion, loneliness, resentment.

The paralyzing effects of trauma can be frightening and overwhelming to those closest to traumatized and grieving individuals. Yet what these individuals require most is to tell their "stories" repeatedly, in order to work through their fears, anxieties, and grief. Within the support group, as members tell their scary truths, identify with others, and extend sympathy and compassion, they ultimately experience the profound sense of being understood; this is vital to the healing process. Supportive therapy groups mobilize the strengths and competence of group members to reduce or control interference from symptoms and trauma-based symptoms that may interfere social, emotional, occupational, recreational, and health-related functioning (Foy et al., 2000).

Family Orientation Meetings

At The Den for Grieving Kids, prospective families are referred through schools, therapists, physicians, hospitals, clergy, and friends. Because of the intensely public nature of the September 11th attacks, referrals to our bereavement groups were swift and forthcoming. Grieving families customarily make the initial contact with the Den staff, as this is an important step and often a first explicit acknowledgment by the grieving persons of the desire to heal. Only the grieving family members can judge when they are ready to deal with the death in a peer support group setting. After an initial phone intake with a parent and/or adult caregiver, each family is asked to attend an orientation/intake meeting with at least two Den staff members/social workers. At times—as is the case with our September 11th families, and depending on the emotional status of the grieving persons in response to their loss—our staff also provides intake/orientation meetings at families' homes. Our hope is to alleviate a small portion of the anxiety and anguish that family members are already enduring by going to them. Such a meeting serves an important function in reducing anxiety and offers an opportunity for a family, as a cohesive unit, to ask questions and share concerns. Families are repeatedly told that confidentiality is of utmost importance at The Den for Grieving Kids; all participants know that what is said in a group stays in the group. It is only when persons are in danger of harming themselves and/or other human beings that an exception to this policy is made.

The family orientation meeting allows the staff to understand the specific nature and complexities of the traumatic death. Certain aspects of the trauma itself can influence the severity of children's reactions. Speculatively, some of the features of childhood trauma that may contribute to the severity of a child's reactions include the following (as discussed in Chapter 1 of this book): the duration of the traumatic event, the presence of interpersonal violence or threat of harm, the degree to which the child experiences a situation as immediately life-threatening, the exposure to traumas involving loved ones as the victims or perpetrators of terrifying harm, the involvement of temporary or long-term physical injury to the child, and the child's perception of the outcome of the trauma (Monahon, 1997; Webb, 2002). In describing each experience, families are offered undivided attention to tell their own stories; individuals' perceptions of the experience can appear quite different even within the same family.

The nature of the relationship between the survivor(s) and the deceased person is also explored during the initial meeting, in order to understand and be open to each particular experience. For example, did the dead person have problematic relationships with other family members? Was he or she a parent who was the sole nurturer within the family? Was the person an ex-spouse? A partner/companion? And so on. Each type of relationship raises different issues, and when a family is massively disrupted emotionally or physically, a child's recovery can be complicated by this chaotic loss (Masten, Best, & Garmezy, 1990)

It is essential to assess each family's support system, so that additional support may be provided or recommended to the family if this seems warranted. It is common for traumatized families to require assistance in exploring concrete services as the result of a death, such as changes in their living/housing situation, immediate employment services, and communication with teachers and school administrators regarding the emergence of a traumatized child's behavioral/emotional changes. Referrals are often made, depending on individuals' needs.

The family orientation meeting also serves as an educational opportunity: The Den staff provides information that can help "normalize," to the extent possible, the mere concept of death for traumatized parents and caregivers. We remind adults that it is important to incorporate the words "death" and "dying" into their vocabulary with children at this time. Also, we remind parents/adult caregivers how concrete children are in their thinking, and we emphasize that they want to know the truth. Moreover, adults are reminded that children's ability to understand death depends on their developmental level. They begin to think abstractly as they develop (e.g., they begin to understand that the significant person is never coming back); their grief is cyclical; and as they reach each new developmental stage, their grief adapts accordingly (Webb, 2002).

New families often ask us how long they need to attend group sessions and when they will know it's time to end. There is no definitive answer, as the individual nature of each person's grief journey varies. The Den for Grieving Kids is an open-ended program. Some families attend for several months, while others attend for up to 5 years or longer. Other families stop attending after an extended period of time, only to return years later as the nature of grief changes with developmental changes in children, and/or with the emergence of future life events or loss and trauma. On average, families tend to attend for a period of approximately 2 years.

Den "Nights of Service"

Upon completion of the orientation meeting, the Den staff determines which "night of service" (program) will best serve the needs of each individual family. When families arrive in the evening, they are greeted by volunteers and served dinner. For busy parents/caregivers, this provides a reprieve from having to prepare the family's nightly dinner. This is also a time to unwind from the day and socialize with other families. Staff members and facilitators meet privately and unwind from their own hectic days—first engaging in a meditation exercise, followed by daily reflections with one another. These two exercises aid in focusing on the tasks of empathic listening, presence, and availability. This time is also used to discuss information on new families; to acknowledge significant anniversaries, dates, and relevant current events; and to distribute pertinent grief- and trauma-oriented articles and literature. Finally, facilitators utilize this time to discuss and organize activities for the evening and to set up their group space before welcoming the families.

Opening Circle

Following dinner, all family members, staffers, and volunteers convene for our "opening circle." This is an important time in which we go around the circle, identify ourselves, and state who has died in our families. For those choosing not to speak at this or any other time during a night of service, the "I pass" rule (see below) is exercised and honored. In the opening circle, we also welcome all new attendees to The Den for Grieving Kids; our welcoming ritual is to ask a child already familiar with the program to present a heart-shaped rock to each new person. Staff members remind the group and inform the new attendees, "Each rock symbolizes the beginning of an often bumpy, rough, and imperfect journey, but we will be there alongside you every step of the way, with open hearts."

Different Groups

Directly following the opening circle, all Den attendees break into age-appropriate peer support groups that are facilitated by our trained facilitators and supervised by Den staff members. The group sessions last 55–75 minutes, depending on each night of service. For those dealing with complicated grief and trauma, shorter sessions (approximately 60 minutes in length) and more frequent group meetings have proven more effective in the healing process. The groups are divided as follows: babies and toddlers, for whom child care is provided; Littles (ages 3–5); Middles I (ages 6–9); Middles II (ages 10–12); Young Teens (ages 13–14): Teens (ages 15–17); Young Adults (ages 18–mid-20s); and one or more Adult Caregivers/Parents Groups.

Children's Groups. The children's groups traditionally begin with a second "opening circle," in which a teddy bear is passed among the children and facilitators, and each person states his or her own name and that of the person who has died. This ritual enhances the focus on the purpose of the session. The second circle may also be a time to review the rules of The Den, particularly if new children are in attendance:

1. *Stop rule*: "Stop, and I mean it." When someone is doing something that feels unsafe to anyone, that child needs to stop immediately.
2. *Throwing rule*: Hard objects may not be thrown. Soft objects may be thrown only in the Volcano Room (a cushioned room in which anger can be expressed via punching bags, boxing gloves, and "bouncy balls," under the supervision of a facilitator on a one-to-one basis).
3. *Put-down rule*: No one should hurt other people's feelings through ridicule, name calling, or put-downs. People should respect each other and themselves.
4. *Hitting rule*: No one should hit another person.
5. *Adult rule*: Children must be with an adult at all times while at The Den for Grieving Kids.
6. *Blood rule*: Do not touch blood. Adults must be told immediately if anyone is hurt and/or bleeding.
7. *Privacy rule*: What is said at The Den for Grieving Kids is private and confidential, except if someone is in danger.
8. *"I pass" rule*: Children and adults can pass if they do not want to talk.

Facilitators then present grief-oriented activities through symbolic play to the children. Each child's level of engagement tolerance (which typically lasts for approximately 20 minutes for children under the age of 6) is always respected. The play permits children a needed distance from traumatic memories, which may remain quite painful and unspeakable if approached directly. Play therapy works in part by changing the usual expectations for children. Within the context of safety, children are encouraged to express their feelings in ways that could not, and should not, be tolerated at home or at school. Children who feel guilty and ugly inside following a trauma (death) may need time to enact their ugly feelings through play. These children may identify with the monsters or "bad guys" in their play; children who have been traumatized often do not want to identify with the helpless and "nice" play figures, as they want power they themselves lacked when victimized by trauma. Helping such children find new solutions and a renewed sense of power following a trauma is most relieving when they can count on the rules in the groups to remain predictable and constant (Monahon, 1997).

Art and play therapy activities and techniques include drawing (e.g., self-portraits and family pictures), clay/sculpture, mask making, play with "magic wish" wands, storytelling, building with blocks, sandtray play, puppets, dress-up games, and theatrical productions (Webb, 2003). For examples of art therapy, see Figures 8.1 and 8.2. Facilitators also offer games such as "feelings" Bingo, word games, and grief-focused board games, to

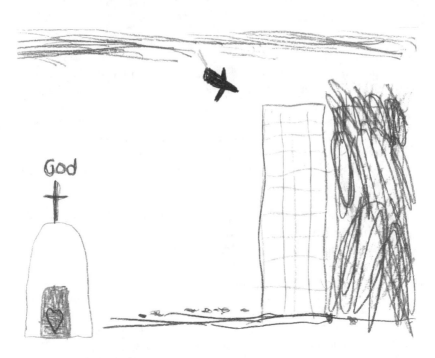

FIGURE 8.1. "September 11th," by Julie, age 8.

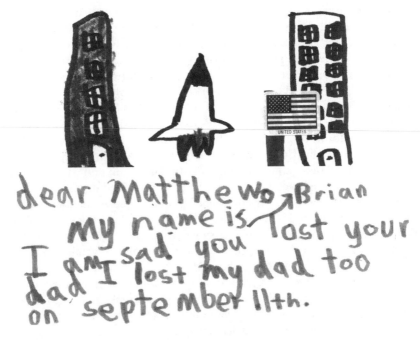

FIGURE 8.2. Condolence card from Brian, age 7, to a child of an astronaut killed in the Columbia space shuttle disaster; front of card (top), inside of card (bottom).

encourage the release of painful and prickly feelings. Facilitators utilize short and honest interactions, frequent repetition, consistent routine within the group, and intensive nurturing and reassurance.

Children between 6 and 9 years of age have a clearer understanding of death, and exhibit an increased interest in its physical and biological aspects. However, they too respond well to age-appropriate grief-focused art activities (including drawing, collage, sculpture, and multimedia sculpture) typically talking and sharing with one another while engaged in a hands-on project.

It is always customary at The Den for Grieving Kids that following grief-focused "work," younger children are encouraged to go about the business of being children and simply play, without direction from the facilitators. Games, toys, and outdoor activities are provided for the remainder of the session—a time in which facilitators continue to provide intensive support.

Older children, between the ages of 9 and 12, continue to enjoy participating in art therapy and grief-focused games. They also particularly enjoy talking and sharing ideas with one another and their group facilitators. Talking is a powerful technique. The talking can help an older child to abreact; to accept the world's randomness; and to develop more flexible, more self-enhancing coping skills. Children with concerns about the randomness of events, their own sense of helplessness, distrust in the future, and ongoing distortions of perceptual and cognitive functions often benefit from "talking it out" (Terr, 1990, p. 302).

By the ages of 9–12, children's awareness of the possibility of personal death is more developed, although they consider themselves invincible or believe that death "won't ever happen to me." Children are also developing an individual sense of self and self-confidence, and they require a safe environment in which they can ask specific objective questions (e.g., "Was the body mangled?" or "Did my mom get out of the building?"), for they are starting to have the ability to understand the concept of death. Children this age have a desire for complete detail in their questioning, as they are becoming more logical in their thinking. Therefore, at The Den, we assign a higher number of facilitators to this age group in order to provide vital "personal" time within the group—that is, to encourage the expression of ideas, thoughts, and feelings and thus empower each individual child.

Groups for Adolescents/Young Adults. Adolescents between the ages of 12 and 17 are very often more willing to speak and share abstractly and subjectively, especially with people outside their immediate families. They often still see death as something that happens to others, however, because they are egocentric and generally continue to consider themselves immortal at this age. Therefore, it is of paramount importance for facilitators to be fully present and to exercise active, empathic listening skills. Adolescents and young adults also need to know that what they are sharing will remain confidential in order to establish trust. The facilitators in a teen group must establish a climate of trust and safety early in the process; set rules, limits, and protection to ensure safety; demonstrate a caring, understanding, and mutually respectful environment; initiate and encourage interactions among peers; deal with barriers to communication; and be directly involved by intermittently clarifying and summarizing what is occurring between the group members. Attempts by adults/facilitators to establish control and/or exercise authority within the group will consistently be met with rejection, acting-out behaviors, and possible rebellion. Therefore, it is critical for facilitators to avoid presenting themselves as "experts" on the topic of grief.

Adolescents and young adults like to engage in journal and poetry writing, watch grief- or feelings-related videos, and (most importantly) talk and identify with one another. The group serves as a safe forum in which young people are reassured that strong feelings—particularly anger, shame, guilt, embarrassment, and sometimes even revenge—are completely normal following a trauma. In turn, each session serves as a time for problem solving, enhancing ego strengths, and connecting with peers who are enduring similar circumstances.

Adult Caregivers/Parents Groups. As the children are attending to their own grief work under the supervision and support of facilitators, parents and adult caregivers convene to discuss their own grief-related issues. Group members share equally in "ownership" of a group. Along with the profound feelings centering around trauma and the loss of a significant person, discussions regarding secondary issues may surface (e.g., the ways children grieve; common behaviors and developmental changes in children; the mundane practicalities of single parenthood; memorials; feelings of guilt, panic, resentment, or unreality; new relationship concerns/difficulties; etc.). Within this peer support model, strong friendships are forged, and these very often continue outside the group.

Closing Circle and Debriefing

At the conclusion of the group sessions, all families reconvene for the "closing circle." Den families, facilitators, and staff hold hands and sing together ("Count on Me" or "Lean on Me", depending on each night of service) to bring a unified closing to the evening. It is common for families to continue talking and sharing for several minutes after each Den session—a time we encourage and acknowledge as also therapeutic.

After the families leave, the cofacilitators of each group meet for approximately 10–15 minutes to discuss the dynamics within their particular group. All facilitators and staff members then reconvene for a formal group debriefing, during which time is allotted for each person to "download" on the stressors and demands of the evening, as well as any countertransference issues stimulated within the group.

Immunization against "vicarious traumatization," sometimes termed "secondary victimization," involves ongoing education regarding trauma syndromes and their treatment, the normalizing of responses, the recognition of the impact of the material on the personal schema, and ventilation in a supportive environment (McCann & Pearlman, 1990; see also Chapter 15 of this book). It is within the debriefing that self-care is practiced, as traumatic material is reworked and processed in the containment and safety of the facilitator/staff group. Facilitators and staff members attend to one another in this "postsession" debriefing by using the same skills they utilize with the families—specifically, empathic listening, skills of awareness of self and others, and the skills of reflection.

CASE STUDIES: FAMILIES DIRECTLY AFFECTED BY SEPTEMBER 11TH

The Johnson Family

Family Information

Molly, age 47, Japanese American, a writer and homemaker.
Jack, age 19, a freshman in college.
Pete, age 16, a sophomore in high school.
Sammy, age 14, an eighth grader.
George, age 49, European American, a bond trader, killed in the World Trade Center attacks of September 11th.

The family had minimal contact with extended family members.

Background

George worked as a bond trader in the North Tower of the World Trade Center. After the planes hit on September 11th, he left a message at home that he was evacuating and would call back when he reached safety. By evening, Molly realized something was seriously wrong, at which time Jack (who was in college out of state) drove home to be with the family. Like all of the victims' families of that tragic day, the Johnsons anxiously waited for word of rescue; finally, on September 25, Molly concluded that there was no hope. A memorial service, in the absence of any physical remains, was held for George at their local church on September 30. At the urging of Molly, Jack returned to college in early October.

Presenting Problems (1 Month after George's Death)

Molly felt numb while grieving for the loss of her husband and trying to cope with the emotional aftermath of the terrorist attacks. She was extremely distressed regarding the emotional well-being and safety of her children, the financial ramifications of her husband's death, and the daunting tasks of paperwork and bureaucracy required of her. She was having difficulty concentrating and sleeping. She was also anxious regarding the pending DNA identification of her husband's remains, should any be found.

In particular, Molly was very worried about her sons. At his mother's insistence, Jack was attending a support group for grieving young adults at college, along with individual psychotherapy. However, he was very irritable and angry, and remained detached from friends and his new college community. Pete was also very irritable and exhibited persistent avoidance of stimuli associated with the trauma—all thoughts and feelings, as well as people, places, and activities, that brought the experience or his father to mind.

Sammy complained of chronic headaches and stomachaches, and was spending a lot of time in the school nurse's office. He was also having difficulty concentrating in school and exhibited periods of panic and crying at school and home, which were a tremendous source of embarrassment for him. He was also having difficulty sleeping and usually crawled into bed with his mom in the middle of the night.

Referral

Molly contacted The Den for Grieving Kids in mid-October 2001, as suggested by her pediatrician, whom she had taken the two younger boys to see in regard to their anxious emotional states. Within 24 hours of her phone call to The Den, an intake was scheduled with the family. Following this emotional in-home intake/orientation session, attended by Molly, Pete, Sammy, and two Den staff members, Molly stated that she would like the family to begin attending The Den immediately. This decision was met with intense resistance from the two younger sons, both of whom told Molly that they would "refuse to go" and would "not get out of the car even if you try to make us." They vehemently complained and whined. Molly cried and ignored them; the Den staffers responded with reassurance and encouragement, though with little effect. After the boys left the room, the Den staffers provided intensive emotional support to Molly for an extended period of time.

The Den Sessions

The Johnson family began attending The Den for Grieving Kids in late October 2001. Molly appeared traumatized, and was very depressed and cried throughout their first several sessions. Pete angrily and repeatedly stated, "I don't want to be here," and "This is so stupid." Sammy remained very quiet, consistently complaining that he had a headache and didn't "feel good." He often lay on the floor by himself during group sessions.

Teen Group: Session 5. In attendance were Pete, Jill (a 15-year-old girl who lost her 28-year-old brother on September 11th), and two facilitators.

Content of Session	Rationale/Analysis
PETE: (*Addressing the group*) Why do I have to come here? It's so stupid and such a waste of time.	Pete initially expresses his grief through rage and denial.
FACILITATOR 1: Sounds like you're upset that you had to come here tonight.	
PETE: Yeah, my stupid mom is making me. She's insane.	Pete finds exploring the loss of his father unbearable and is shifting the focus to his mother.
FACILITATOR 2: It seems that you're pretty angry with your mom.	
PETE: She thinks that (*mockingly*) I'm upset and that I have to work through this, but she doesn't know what she's talking about. I'm not upset about anything. There's nothing to be upset about. (*Long silence*) Nothing has changed in my life. I don't even care. She's the one with the problem. (*Long silence*)	Pete's resistance is directly proportional to his internal pain. His life will never be the same.
F1: This seems very hard for you.	
PETE: No, not really. I don't think so. I don't know why everyone is making such a big deal out of everything. I hate this. I just want things to go back to the way they	

used to be . . . back when everyone just left me alone and I
didn't have to deal with my
mom. (*Puts his sweatshirt hood
over his head and ties it so tight
only his mouth is showing. Rocks
back and forth in his chair.*)

F2: Tell us what that was like.

PETE: *No*! This is all so stupid!

JILL: (*Meekly*) I wish things would go   I am deeply moved by Jill's
back to the way they were when   heartache and courage.
my brother was alive, too.

PETE: Can I have something to eat?
(*Stands up and looks around for
food in the room.*)

F2: In a minute, Pete. The food is
out in the kitchen, and we can
eat again in a little while. Come
back and join us. Jill, can you
tell us again what you just said?

JILL: I just wish things were the way
they were.

F1: It sounds as though both of you   I am pointing out similarities
are wishing that things were the   between Pete and Jill.
way they used to be. Or at least
what was normal for your family.

PETE: Yeah. Whatever. I don't care.   Pete now utilizes humor, via
(*Sarcastically*) My family has   sarcasm, to mask his feelings.
never been normal, though.
(*Elicits a tiny laugh from the
group.*)

JILL: Everything is just so weird at   I want to hug and reassure Jill
home. All my parents do is ob-   as she shares her intense
sess about my brother. I mean,   emotional pain, but refrain
I'm sad, too.   from doing so to encourage
          further verbalizations. It is
          important to validate and
          acknowledge Jill's pain.

F1: It sounds as though things are
very hard for you at home.

JILL: Yeah . . . I . . .

PETE: (*Interrupting Jill*) I want something to eat.

Pete finds this honest sharing intolerable and is desperate to change the subject.

F2: Pete, you just interrupted Jill as she was talking.

PETE: Oh. Sorry. Whatever. (*Laughs.*)

F2: (*Looking directly at Jill*) Go on, Jill.

JILL: (*Looking down*) I forgot what I was going to say. (*Pete looks away, ashamed.*)

Pete exhibits remorse for his avoidance behavior.

F1: We're listening when you're ready, Jill.

JILL: OK.

It is important to convey to Jill that her presence and her feelings are vital to the group.

Pete's resistance was indicative of his chaotic struggle with the intense feelings of doubt, fear, and anger that he was experiencing. His tremendous fear of the group process—as evidenced in his overt, distracting physical behavior and his negative, cynical comments—are not unusual behaviors among grieving teens. Pete was doing everything in his power to avoid the pain related to his traumatic experience. Because teens need time to build a level of trust and security within the group, facilitators must be particularly patient and flexible with this population. In this case, direct support, offering hope, and affirming the work being done would be vital to help the group, and Pete, move forward productively.

Teen Group: Session 11. In attendance were Pete, Jill, Rachel and Gina (two sisters, ages 17 and 15, respectively, whose father died on September 11th, and two facilitators. This was Pete and Jill's 11th session, but only the 2nd for Rachel and Gina.

Content of Session

JILL: All my friends are acting so weird around me now. It's like they don't know what to say, so they don't say anything at all.

Rationale/Analysis

I feel sad for Jill as she expresses her feelings of loss on multiple levels, yet grateful that she has the safety of the group in which she can express herself honestly.

GINA: Yeah, me too. One of my friends started crying because she was talking about her dad and then remembered that I

The girls have connected and require no acknowledgment from me as the process unfolds.

don't have one any more and got all embarrassed. She felt so bad, but, you know, it's not her fault that my dad died.

JILL: Yeah. My friends and I used to hang out with my older brother, you know, like when he was home from college . . . he took us out once in the city and they really liked him. They used to talk about him when he was alive, about how cool he was, but now they don't even mention him. It's so weird.

Jill and Gina identify with their losses and feelings of isolation and confusion regarding their friends. This is very powerful.

GINA: Do you try to talk about him with them?

JILL: No. It's too weird. Everyone is, like, pretending, and I don't want to bring it up.

I take note of the fear involved among teens in taking social risks.

RACHEL: Yeah, I don't either. Sometimes I wish my friends would ask me about it though. (*Long silence*)

F1: It sounds like it would be very helpful if you could talk about your special people with your friends. (*Jill, Rachel, and Gina all nod in agreement.*)

I am reflecting their feelings.

PETE: Hell, no. I don't want to talk about it with my friends. What good would that do? It would be so stupid.

Pete remains stuck in his anger toward his father for dying.

RACHEL: Better than pretending nothing happened, though. *That* totally sucks. (*Pete stares at the floor, hunched over. He remains silent for the rest of the session.*)

This statement touches a nerve in Pete. He is forced to sit with the truth and his own discomfort, and I purposely do not intervene.

Following this session, the Den staff recommended individual psychotherapy for Pete (in addition to regular Den attendance), sensing that he might experience an improved comfort level and willingness to voice his feelings regarding the traumatic event in a private setting. Although Pete only reluctantly agreed to individual treatment, he now exhibits an improved level of willingness to cooperate with treatment, refrains from masking his feelings with constant cynical and negative remarks, and subsequently presents an improved willingness to participate within his Den group. He has also evolved into an active listener with his peers.

The Johnsons continue to attend The Den for Grieving Kids weekly. Sammy also exhibits less erratic behavioral and sleeping patterns. Their attendance helps Molly in knowing that while she is attending to her own grief-related needs, she is also ensuring that her children are receiving the help and reassurance they need. By acknowledging her own vulnerability, she knows her children will benefit also. She occasionally comments that the family has "setbacks," but she remains very grateful that she can bring those issues directly to The Den and talk about regressions with people who "completely understand what we're going through."

The Norton Family

Family Information

Kate, age 35, a full-time mother and attorney (on leave).
Annie, age 10, a fifth grader.
Jack, age 7, a second grader.
Dan, age 38, a banker, killed on September 11th.

Background

Dan called Kate from the stairwell of the North Tower while evacuating and told her that he loved her and their children very much, and that he didn't think he was going to make it out alive. Kate and Dan had been high school sweethearts. Both of them had large, supportive families, whose members all lived locally and were desperately struggling with their loss.

Presenting Problems and Referral

Kate brought her family to the Den in early December 2001, upon the recommendation of her children's school principal, after Jack's teachers and his school social worker reported that he was acting out in school and having difficulty concentrating and sitting still in class. Jack also quit his soccer team and exhibited erratic sleep patterns, accompanied by frequent nightmares. He had been sleeping with Kate on a nightly basis since the terrorist attacks. Annie also seemed worried about and agitated around her mom, asking her repeatedly to "stop crying so much."

Jack's Fourth Session

In attendance were eight children who lost their fathers on September 11th—Jack (age 7), Jessie, Maeve, and Samantha (girls, age 7), Timmy and Courtney (brother and sister, ages 9 and 6, respectively), and Luke and Sam (boys, age 8)—and four facilitators.

Content of Session	Rationale/Analysis
(*Jack is withdrawn and sullen. The children are sculpting clay, and a conversation begins about their late fathers' hobbies.*)	
TIMMY: My dad loved all sports.	It is heartbreaking for me to listen to the children share their fond memories of their dads. Yet I am grateful, as the sharing of memories is important to their grief work.
LUKE: Mine did, too. Mostly he liked to play golf and watch football on TV. He coached my soccer team, too.	
SAM: So did my dad! (*Jack begins pounding a ball of clay on the table, grunting loudly with each hit.*)	Jack expresses his anger while listening to the other children.
JESSIE: Jack, stop it! You're making the table shake! (*Jack continues.*)	
F1: Jack, please listen to Jessie's words.	
JACK: (*Stops pounding the table, becomes very quiet, and pushes his chair back from the table.*) I don't want to do this any more. This is dumb.	
F2: Jack, would you like to go to the Volcano Room?	The healthy expression of Jack's anger is required at this juncture.
JACK: I guess. (*A facilitator takes him to the Volcano Room, during which time he aggressively and continuously punches the wall with boxing gloves. Exhausted, Jack and the facilitator return to the group 10 minutes later; he reclaims his seat at the table with the other children, who are still discussing their fathers. Jack remains somber.*)	

TIMMY: The morning the planes hit, my dad played basketball in his league in the city. Sometimes he got up at four in the morning to go play basketball with the guys he worked with near his office.

Timmy is working through his traumatized feelings by retelling the events of September 11th.

JACK: (*Stops fidgeting.*) Your dad played basketball in the city? So did my dad. Where did he play?

TIMMY: I don't know. Near the twin towers somewhere.

JACK: (*Staring at Timmy*) So did my dad! He played that morning, too. You know, on September 11th. Maybe they played together that day.

Identification allows for the safe expression of what occurred the day their fathers died.

TIMMY: Yeah, maybe. I'll ask my mom. She knows the name of the gym he went to. He went there all the time.

JACK: (*Picks up a piece of clay and starts molding it in his hands.*) I bet if my dad had stayed home and taken us to school that day, he wouldn't have died. But he played basketball instead and went to work. I wish he would have taken us to school. There were other dads who didn't die, just because they took their kids to school that day. (*The children all become silent and introspective.*)

"If only . . . " I am deeply moved by Jack's struggle to comprehend and rationalize what transpired on September 11th. I wish I could take away their pain.

TIMMY: (*Purposely changing the subject*) My dad was a really good basketball player.

Timmy needs to talk about his dad when he was alive, rather than his death.

JACK: Yeah, so was mine. (*Briefly smiles for the first time since attending The Den.*) He used to put me on his shoulders so I could slam-dunk!

F1: Tell us more about your dad, Jack. (*He proudly goes on to describe his father's athletic endeavors.*)

This session was a breakthrough for Jack, as he connected with the children in his group by sharing his perception of what happened the tragic morning of the attacks. This was his first acknowledgment of his loss. Within the shelter of the group, Jack continues slowly to work through his feelings of profound loss and anger. His behavior has stabilized in school, with far fewer outbursts, and he is able to engage in classroom work with minimal need for redirection. He continues to sleep with his mom every night, though his nightmares have subsided considerably. Kate continues to provide him with the time and support he needs to be able to sleep alone in his own room once again.

ORGANIZATIONAL AND PERSONAL PRESSURES AT THE DEN FOR GRIEVING KIDS

As is true of any nonprofit organization or agency, the pressure to raise funds for The Den for Grieving Kids is always at the forefront of all our minds—administrators, staff, and volunteers included. To date, we have been the grateful beneficiaries of both private and corporate donors for over 10 years. Along with all programs at Family Centers, The Den has also been the recipient of numerous grants, enabling us to keep our doors open without having to charge our families.

The work we do is often very painful and distressing and therefore it is of paramount importance that Den staff consistently attend to the psychological and emotional needs of our facilitators. Although support is offered in all of our postsession debriefings, as well as through separate debriefings for facilitators working with September 11th families, we consistently remind facilitators that staff members are available should personal concerns arise that need to be addressed and supported privately.

All those working in the field of bereavement and grief understand the personal pressures involved. This is also true for all mental health professionals, who often are asked, "How can you do that kind of work?" Like most of us, I take pride in this work and feel I am doing what I was meant to do at this point in my life. I appreciate that I must be fully attentive to my own self-care, on a daily basis, in order to survive in this field. Alan Wolfelt (1996) believes that good self-care is critical for three reasons: First we owe it to ourselves to lead joyful, whole lives; second, our work is draining, and we need relief from such challenging work; and, third, we owe taking care of ourselves to our clients themselves, as it is an essential foundation of caring for the grieving.

In the spring of 2002, while attending a symposium on trauma and grief in New York City, I had the privilege of meeting Diane Leonard—a woman whose husband, a U.S. Secret Service agent, was killed in the Oklahoma City bombing in 1995. Since that time, Diane has worked tirelessly as a victims' family advocate, traveling back and forth among Washington, D.C.; Denver, Colorado (site of the Timothy McVeigh trial); and Oklahoma City over a 3-year period. She came to Manhattan immediately following September 11th to extend emotional support to hundreds of victims' families in the tristate area.

After a brief conversation, Diane asked me, "How are you doing?" I very calmly replied, "Fine." She again asked, "How are you doing?" Puzzled, I again said, "I'm fine." She took a step closer to me, looked me directly in the eye, and pointedly asked, "How are *you* doing?" In that moment, I finally understood what she was asking and stopped. Strangely, I felt on the verge of tears. I took a minute to think and finally replied, "OK, I think." I was faced with my truth—namely, that this work is often very grueling and heart-wrenching, and that without self-care I would not be able to continue. Diane smiled, took a deep breath, and reminded me that I had to take extremely good care of myself. On a daily basis, I had to stop and enjoy my family, my friends, and my life, and not get buried in the sadness of my work, or it would "get the best and take all of me." Since then, I have worked very hard to remember Diane's words on a daily basis, sometimes several times a day. For me, taking care of myself includes paying close attention to and enjoying all that is joyful in life; telling the people I love how much I love them, and saying this often; and consistently nurturing my spiritual condition.

I have also learned that I must remain cognizant of my own past traumas, which include the 1971 San Fernando earthquake in Los Angeles, the 1989 earthquake in San Francisco, and a carbon monoxide poisoning in my home in 1990. The latter two events immediately retriggered the familiar feelings of total loss of control and fear of future trauma that I had experienced as a 10-year-old child following the 1971 earthquake. The reemergence of anxiety, hyperarousal, and erratic sleep patterns also returned. It was only through a trauma-oriented support group following the 1989 earthquake, and individual treatment after the poisoning, that I was able to reenact what had occurred through "talk therapy" and to experience a renewed sense of balance and trust. I could not have endured these later traumas without assistance.

Most importantly, my greatest professional support comes from the Den team—an amazing group of social workers with whom I can share my stress, who hold me up whenever necessary, and who help me maintain balance in regard to our work. Without the mutual support of this incredible team, I know I would be ineffective in my work. This connection is what sustains me.

REFERENCES

Foy, D. W., Glynn, S. M., Schnurr, P. P., Jankowski, M. K., Wattenberg, M. S. Weiss, D. S., Marmar, C. R., & Gusman, F. D. (2000). Group therapy. In E. B. Foa, T. M. Keane, & M. J. Friedman (Eds.), *Effective treatments for PTSD: Practice guidelines from the International Society for Traumatic Stress Studies* (pp. 155–175). New York: Guilford Press.

Masten, A. S., Best, K. S., & Garmezy, N. (1990). Resilience and development. *Development and Psychopathology, 2*, 425–444.

McCann, I. L., & Pearlman, L. A. (1990). Vicarious traumatization: A framework for understanding the psychological effects of working with victims. *Journal of Traumatic Stress, 3*(1), 131–149.

Monahon, C. (1997). *Children and trauma: A guide for parents and professionals.* San Francisco: Jossey-Bass.

National Center for PTSD. (2001, October). *Effects of traumatic stress in a disaster situation: A National Center for PTSD Fact Sheet* [Online]. Available: http://www.ncptsd.org

Pennebaker, J. N., Zech, E., & Rime, B. (2001). Disclosing and sharing emotion: Psychological, social, and health consequences. In M. S. Stroebe, R. O. Hansson, W. Strobe, & H. Schut (Eds.), *Handbook of bereavement research: Consequences, coping, and care* (pp. 517–539). Washington, DC: American Psychological Association.

Terr, L. (1990). *Too scared to cry: Psychic trauma in childhood.* New York: Harper & Row.

Webb, N. B. (2002). (Ed.). *Helping bereaved children: A handbook for practitioners* (2nd ed.). New York: Guilford Press.

Webb, N. B. (2003). *Social work practice with children* (2nd ed.). New York: Guilford Press.

Wolfelt, A. D. (1996). *How to care for yourself while you care for the dying and bereaved.* Batesville Management Services.

CHAPTER 9

Music Therapy to Help Traumatized Children and Caregivers

JOANNE V. LOEWY
KRISTEN STEWART

Music has been utilized by humanity virtually since the beginning of time. The Bible portrays David soothing Saul with a harp; ancient tribes integrated music into shamanistic ritual healing practices; and the Kahum Papyrus, our oldest historical documentation of medicine, reflects that chants were essential to the treatment of illness.

In today's world, music is used to heal, educate, and entertain. Music can consciously unify an audience or gathering, as in the singing of the national anthem prior to a sports event. Music helps people to pray, as in hymns sung during a religious or spiritual service. Music easily provides a sense of community in our everyday passages, and particularly in times of need.

The purpose of this chapter is to introduce the reader to music therapy and to illustrate its application with both children and caregivers who are experiencing posttraumatic stress reactions. This model is based on a concept of trauma rooted in a medical perspective of physical compromise, in which feelings of fear and loss become expressed through interactions of the mind and body. Specifically, the later sections of the chapter describe a program combining music psychotherapy and trauma training that was conducted at a New York City (NYC) hospital in response to the events of September 11, 2001.

In this chapter, we present several music therapy approaches used to help individuals coping with the events and aftermath of a traumatic experience, as well as case descriptions illustrating different approaches. The first full-length case is a music psychotherapy process description of a child who was being seen in a medical music therapy setting and required special help on the day of "9/11." The second case addresses the use of music within a self-selected group of adult caregivers seeking support in relationship to their experience of the traumatic events of 9/11. The group began 6 months after 9/11 and focused on the impact of the traumatic events on participants' current day-to-day functioning.

DEFINITION OF MUSIC THERAPY

Broadly defined, "music therapy" is the use of music to restore, improve, or maintain health and well-being. The roots of music therapy as a profession go back to World War II, when music was used to relieve the anxiety and stress of hospitalized veterans. This led to formalized study of the effects of music in medicine, and in 1950, music therapy became a profession. Today, music therapy serves a broad range of patients and clients in both child and adult settings. There are approximately 6,000 music therapists in the United States and 74 academic training programs at colleges and universities throughout the country.

MEDICAL MUSIC PSYCHOTHERAPY

The field of music therapy has made an impact in health care and medicine within the past decade, particularly in the areas of rehabilitation (Thaut, Rice, & McIntosh, 1997), anxiety reactions to illness (Edwards, 1999), pain management (Loewy, MacGregor, Richards, & Rodriguez, 1997), and neonatology (Caine, 1991). Music and music therapy have been shown to be effective in neonatal intensive care units, where the sound environment has become quieted through the selective application of music (Stewart & Schneider, 2000). Music has had a direct effect upon specific physical components of functioning as well. In patients with Parkinson's disease, for instance, increased walking speed has been associated with rhythmic programming (Thaut & McIntosh, 1992). Also, pain associated with needle aspirations has been reduced when the procedure has been accompanied by music therapy (Turry, 1997; Malone, 1996).

A growing number of music therapy programs in the medical arena focus on the biopsychophysical aspects of disease. The role of the mind, and specifically the area of affect, may be significant in the healing process. This relationship has been addressed by doctors and surgeons (Dossey, 1982) and is gaining acceptance within the field of medicine as an influential factor in prognosis and healing.

Children often experience less pain and other discomfort when music therapy accompanies their plan of care in the hospital. This has been found to be true for procedural pain (Loewy et al., 1997), chronic pain (Robb, 1996), and anxiety reactions to illness, such as the loss of breath control experienced by patients with asthma (Griggs-Drane, 1999). Music therapy has also found to be effective with children who are dying (Brodsky, 1989). Lullabies, in particular, can provide the youngest of children with a safe transition from life to death. A melody can serve as a transitional object (Winnicott, 1965) in helping a child navigate from what is familiar to the fear and uncertainty that may lie ahead.

The underlying philosophy of a medical music psychotherapy approach is that music and music therapy interventions can provide a safe means of accessing an individual's unconscious process and offer a way to learn about his or her inner coping capacity as it relates to illness. What patients believe about their illness often directly affects how they recover or cope with treatment. Children project their fears, fantasies, understandings, and questions into music in a variety of ways, allowing a music therapist to assess and enhance aspects of coping, integration, and healing. Specifically, the therapist can expand the child's means of self-expression through an individually designed music therapy treatment plan. This is demonstrated in the case of Scotty to follow.

Music therapy also often provides the treatment team with valuable information about family members, especially their style of support and way of coping. In music therapy, children can easily improvise or write songs describing the significant issues they are confronting. As they select specific musical instruments and develop themes relating to their lives, significant issues can unfold. For this reason, it is useful to perform a music therapy assessment, when possible, with a child alone. It is then beneficial to see how the child relates to his or her parents, both inside and outside the context of a musical relationship; this provides diagnostic information about the parent–child relationship.

The various dynamics that characterize a child and family prior to illness or hospitalization change and become more intense when the child becomes ill. The elements of stress implicit in the hospitalization of a child can bring about fears and many unknowns for the child and the family.

THE CHILD IN TRAUMA

A hospitalized child is often admitted immediately after a traumatic event. Whether this event is a dog bite, a parental beating, or climbing and subsequently falling out of a tree, such a situation presents unique clinical challenges. While the medical staff addresses the physical aspects of the accident and injury, the music therapist addresses the emotional aspects of the trauma and issues of the situation. It is important that the team respond in a unified manner, so that the child and family do not receive mixed messages. If, for instance, a parent has been deemed by child protective services as unfit to take a child home (as in cases of abuse or failure to thrive), it is essential that the social worker and music therapist maintain daily contact. They must clinically coordinate the treatment plan to reflect similar outcome objectives, which may include grief work, focus on separation anxiety, and improved self-expression.

Traumatized children must be treated according to the cultural, religious, and personal belief systems of their families. This can be reinforced and supported from a music therapy perspective, where traditions, musical themes, and rituals may be revealed through musical expression. Such understanding provides a unique perspective and can enhance how children synthesize aspects of their illness and/or trauma into their personal belief systems.

ASSESSMENT

Assessment is a critical aspect of evaluating the significant issues, wants, and needs of the child and family. In music therapy assessment, the child is greeted by the therapist through a personalized, live, musically performed "warm-up," which includes the child's name and an introduction to the many musical instruments that the child is invited to play. The music therapist has an assortment of instruments that provide the child with a broad range of expressive opportunities. These instruments typically include harmonic (piano, guitar), melodic (marimba, bells, flutes, xylophones, keyboards), and rhythmic (drums, woodblocks, tambourines, gato drums) instruments, as well as ones with interesting timbres (ocean drum, windchimes, rainstick, spring drum).

Art and play materials are available for the child's use as well, since sometimes children want to move away from the music and choose to process their feelings in another medium. In some cases, music can take a child to an emotionally challenging place. Puppets and art materials provide other means of creative expression for a child who wishes to move into another modality. Some music therapists train and practice in tandem with art, dance, or drama therapists. The National Creative Arts Therapies Association provides opportunities for such learning. The Hahnemann Creative Arts Therapies Program at Drexel University in Philadelphia offers "cross-training" to art, dance, and music therapists. This is one of the few graduate programs in the United States that offers an advanced degree in creative arts therapy, rather than exclusively in art, dance, or music therapy.

Ideally, sessions are conducted in a music therapy studio that is located in a separate space, away from the child's hospital room. If the child is not mobile, a cart of instruments can be wheeled to the bedside.

The musical instrument a child selects and the way he or she chooses to play it can be significant (Loewy, 2000; Priestley, 1975). For example, choosing the smallest triangle in the room and playing very softly may be a metaphor for a child's feelings of insignificance, or it may reflect fear or shyness. Conversely, the child who chooses to set up many drums and uses two mallets to beat them as fully as possible may have issues of self-control or a need for his or her feelings of hostility to be heard. Or a child longing for what is natural and familiar may not play at all, but may ask the therapist to play a song from his or her school or church. The succession of activities in a music therapy assessment may lead to collaborative play between the therapist and child, which can create a feeling of trust that leads the child to feel comfort in risk taking and exploration. The dynamics (loud and soft expression the child chooses to use while playing); the ability to play in rhythm with a family member; or the resistance a child shows by avoiding contact with a therapist, parent, or sibling may be reflective of a range of possibilities. The music therapy assessment provides the team with important information, which is considered in the context of other information about the broad psychosocial parameters affecting the child at the point of admission. The selected musical instruments, the range of affect reflected in the child's style of musical play, the spontaneity/motivation to play (or avoidance of collaborative music making), and the themes created through structured songs and free improvisation all constitute important elements of the assessment.

The music therapist must be deft at sensing, reflecting, and holding the mood of the music or sound that the child presents once an instrument has been selected and explorative musical play has begun. The child leads the exploration, and the therapist supports and questions the child's intention. This is generally accomplished through the therapist's playing a similar instrument and reflecting the beat pattern a child has selected, or it can be achieved when the therapist frames a child's musical play by playing a chord on the piano or guitar in the same harmonic key that the child is playing in. Asking questions such as "What does that instrument sound like?" or "Who taught you that song?" will yield important information about the child's preferences, which often leads to specific interests and information related to everyday life.

The therapist can also gain a sense of a child's ability to relate to others by giving the child choices. The therapist may ask, "Would you like to select an instrument for me to play, or would you prefer to try that instrument by yourself?" The therapist assesses each musical experience and learns about the child's manner of relating to objects and the therapist. The musical relationship will reflect how and if a child's affect is limited or broad, how the self is experienced, and perhaps some key themes derived from the improvisations and/or selected songs.

A central part of the music therapy assessment is providing space for the child to offer up a song. The music therapy room is equipped with a wide variety of songbooks, and the therapist is trained to be able to play any song at a moment's notice. A child's favorite song may be selected in the moment, or it may present as a subtle theme that the child is humming on the way to the session. Perhaps the child selects a favorite song of the parent's, or is cued by a parent to sing a song of preference. The therapist responds to such cues and provides space to work with the theme in a playful way. Quite often a song is associated with a significant piece of information, reflective of an experience, thought, or emotion that may be worth exploring in the session. With younger children, familiar songs and nursery rhymes often linger in their consciousness. The music therapy session provides an arena for such play to be extended and pursued. The therapist opens the door for such exploration by using a variety of techniques. A common way to enhance a child's ability to extend a theme musically is to prompt—repeating a phrase of a song, perhaps without the words, but with in-the-moment created lyrics (improvisation) that may reflect what the child is doing: "Bobby is playing the cymbals softly. . . . "

STORY SONG AND MUSICAL PLAY

"Story song" is a music therapy technique (Rubin-Bosco, 2002) that combines music and story to provide children with a creative means of working with significant issues, and is illustrated in the cases of Jeremy and Scotty to follow. This technique reflects the creative construction of theme, countertheme or conflict, variation, and resolution (and/or recapitulation). The theme is an aspect or issue that is familiar or understood by the child. In the music sense, the theme is presented through a known melody, song, or tale. Embedded in the presenting theme is the core focus of what is known and safe to the child. For example, children often ask to sing and/or play "The Wheels on the Bus," a traditional song in which the theme reflects what occurs during a familiar transition—riding the bus to and from school.

Once the child requests the song, the therapist can accompany the singing and can offer the child a musical instrument such as a tambourine. One child may sing the song and then talk about school. Another child may talk about, or be encouraged to sing about, what it is like to be in the hospital and missing school. Another child may pretend to drive the bus, using the tambourine as a make-believe steering wheel. A bell may be chosen to represent the horn as the child creates a tooting sound. Such a song can affirm a familiar routine or structure that creates a feeling of safety in the child's day-to-day life, while at the same time it can lead into the expression of feelings related to school, both inside and outside the musical context.

When song is used improvisatorily, which often occurs after the familiar verses are sung, there are opportunities for a host of issues related to the broader theme to unravel. In "The Wheels on the Bus," for instance, the therapist may create a verse about where the child is going on the bus. This could lead to an open inquiry about where the child desires to go, about whom he or she is often visiting, or about an unfamiliar fantasized place that could represent a significant need.

In story song, the therapist may find it useful to start with a structured theme, playing it as the child knows it before moving into the child's issue by opening the theme for play. It is not uncommon for traumatized children to request themes that relate to broken and fixed, such as "Humpty Dumpty" or "Ring around the Rosie." Another well-known tune commonly selected by children in the hospital is "London Bridge." "Humpty Dumpty" is a theme that (historically) reflects human mortality; "London Bridge" deals with falling down and building up. When used playfully, such songs provide a means for the child to experience the "great fall" (as in "Humpty Dumpty") or "falling down" (in "London Bridge"), which could resonate with a child's powerlessness, vulnerability, or out-of-control feelings.

Through musical support and collaborative play, the therapist can carefully support a child's reenactment of a trauma via the simple structure of music. The therapist may play chords on the guitar or piano to a child's selected song. Perhaps the supportive accompaniment may shift as the therapist follows the development of a musical theme; the therapist may use a drum to encourage a "building up again" (gaining strength and power) for a child who is feeling vulnerable (as in "The Three Little Pigs" after the wolf has blown each little pig's house down). A drum and solid repetitive rhythm may provide a means of control and an experience of containment for an emotionally difficult time. When a child uses a musical instrument of his or her choice to reflect inner feelings of trauma playfully and musically, the therapist can provide in-the-moment support as the musical relationship is ventured together. This unique aspect of music therapy is not experienced in verbal processing.

The conflict that is reflected in the therapeutic experience should be child-directed. It may or may not come from the basic story song theme, though most stories and songs have a beginning, a conflict, and an ending. When a precomposed song or story moves from the beginning and into the conflict section, the therapist may make musical possibilities for the child to create his or her own unique ending/resolution. In the music, the conflict often presents itself as a countertheme. For instance, in "The Wheels on the Bus," it is not uncommon for the bus to break down or need gas. In this situation, the child may experience resolution by creating new words to the familiar song, thus directing the music toward a spontaneously transforming conclusion.

For a child who is critically ill, bus breakdowns may reflect the frustrations of everyday life with the illness. In the case of the bus that requires gas, perhaps the child needs to be nurtured; in a parent–child session, the therapist may choose to encourage a parent to "fill it up" with different selections of instruments that the child selects for the parent to play. The therapist follows the child's cue and may move the theme into a minor musical key, or the dynamic of the music may become louder or more intense. Perhaps a complicated rhythm may unfold, and the child will select a drum that represents the bus rolling down a bumpy hill. The child is encouraged to develop the musical plot in any way he or she desires.

In the conflict presentation, it is essential for the therapist to provide musical support, and to offer resource options at critical junctures for a child who is demoralized, defeated, or in crisis. Such was the case for Jeremy, a 7-year-old boy who was hospitalized for asthma and had lost his mother 6 months prior as the result of asthma exacerbation. He created a myth about the stars in the sky being unable to shine, to the third verse of "Twinkle, Twinkle Little Star." He used the wind chimes to put the stars to sleep. It seemed as though he was mourning, and that this metaphoric experience provided opportunities for musical grief expression:

JEREMY: (*Cueing the therapist to stop playing the chimes, and singing to the tune of "Twinkle"*) The stars all slept, they had had their time, the darkness came again and let them lie. (*Whispering*) They were done, but they did not know it—they never knew it, they just stopped shining.

THERAPIST: (*Singing*) They just stopped.

JEREMY: (*Whispering*) They were sleeping, these chimes were the wind, and they made them go to sleep, for a long, long time.

THERAPIST: (*Whispering*) For a long, long time . . . but we still know they are there in the sky. I wonder if we can take some time or use some music to say goodbye to the stars. Maybe we can use our own wind, to create a goodbye song for the stars on the flute.

JEREMY: Let's sing the real "Twinkle" song again, and then each chime will kiss each star, and then I will sing and blow to the stars. Can we use a blanket and make them go to sleep? You play the guitar again?

THERAPIST: OK, sounds like a plan.

At this point in Jeremy's treatment, his asthma was under better control, and the last session prior to discharge was approaching. The therapist called upon Jeremy's own physical strength, which had emerged over previous sessions during the hospitalization (flute work), to empower his ability to say goodbye. The music (both the original "Twinkle" theme and the expanded play involving the flute that the therapist suggested) provided a means for Jeremy to reach closure. Saying goodbye to the stars may have been related to the loss of his mother and his need to say goodbye to her. At the same time, his ability to go on living (his physical strength in singing and blowing the flute) with a chronic illness that had taken his mother's life was imperative. The therapist and Jeremy were able to work within the musical play and address these multiple issues through our improvisatory story song.

Using variations on a theme, a multitude of options can be explored through musical play. The child leads the music and the story, as the therapist frames the development of coping strategies wherein the musical options can be explored and applied to the conflict within the context of the musical relationship.

CHILD TRAUMA: THE CASE OF SCOTTY, AGE 7

Scotty was an only child who benefited from music therapy in helping to manage his pain, which was the result of a chronic illness. Music therapy was an integral part of Scotty's treatment plan, with music therapy interventions taking place throughout his frequent hospitalizations. Within the past 2 years preceding 9/11, these hospitalizations occurred three to four times per year, and more often in prior years. Scotty also attended music therapy groups sporadically on an outpatient basis. The music therapist in Scotty's case (the "I" in the description that follows) was Joanne Loewy.

Scotty's family history was complicated. He was separated from his family for 2 years when he was 4 years old. He never had contact with his birth father and could not remember ever knowing him. There were reports that his father was at home until Scotty was 1½ years old, but his whereabouts as of 9/11 remained unknown.

From the ages of 4 through 5, Scotty's hospitalizations related to his pain crises increased, and music therapy was an integral part of his treatment. Through individual music therapy sessions, Scotty's pervading themes included fear, loss, detachment, and abandonment. The therapeutic goals were to increase his trust of self and others, to expand his range of affect, and to ease his acceptance of and ability to tolerate temporary separations from significant others. The staff noted that sleep was difficult for him, and he was unwilling to allow his caretakers to go home at night or leave during the day. He created several story songs, which were audiotaped to allow him to reflect and expand upon his created characters.

Scotty's Music Therapy History

When Scotty was 5 and 6 years old, music therapy sessions addressed his feelings regarding his lack of control. These feelings related to his body, because he would often have extreme pain in his joints, affecting his ability to walk. At the same time, out-of-control feelings seemed to pervade his inner fantasy life. In particular, he would create the soliloquy of a young boy at home in his bed, with no one else in sight. This little boy would not want to go to sleep, as there were monsters outside the window and in the closet. These monsters would come in and tantalize the frightened boy. During prior admissions, the music therapy sessions were focused on atmosphere building and the development of spooky characters. The teachers at his school had noted his obsession with monsters.

I built a rapport with Scotty in seeking to learn about his demons. I felt that he needed to know that I did not judge his monsters, nor did I think it was healthy simply to make them go away. My understanding, from the way that he portrayed these demons and from case conferences with the staff, was that teachers and other adults in his life did not accept or want to deal with the monsters' presence.

Our sessions were structured around play involving the monsters, in which Scotty was encouraged to create improvisatory themes about the characters. At times we would audiotape the story songs, and Scotty was eager to assign me the most gruesome characters. At one point, the cinema character Chucky (the killer doll from the movie *Child's Play*) joined the monster team. Scotty made some statement of pride about being able to watch Chucky, which reflected an awareness that this kind of character was probably not what he should have been allowed to watch; this was addressed with his social worker. However, his mind was working with the "evil," and this needed attention. We used musical instruments, particularly the drum and guiro (which can make a sustained creaky noise), to create a scary atmosphere of terror and unknowns, which we could address interactively within a safe therapeutic context.

I used minor keys on the piano and chromatic-sounding idioms to reflect the kind of setting that Scotty's mind was experiencing. After creating a "Once upon a time . . . " recitative that opened the door for character introduction, Scotty would use the theme as a frame to sing and introduce many monsters, one by one. His apparent goal in the musical play seemed to be that each monster would terrorize the boy. Most often, he would play the role of the boy. The scariness would escalate in the music play to the point where he (the boy) needed to figure out what he could do in order not to be so afraid and spooked at night.

At times, especially when listening to our story songs on tape, Scotty would take the music and spooking out of the story song context and into our live interactions. This made our exchanges full and alive. I could sense that the demons were about Scotty's sense of aloneness in his home environment, which was one of many sudden and unexpected changes. The following session excerpts illustrate Scotty's creation of a story song. He then reflects upon listening to the audiotape of the song.

(*The tape player is recording.*)

SCOTTY (*Chanting*) And the killer Chucky got together his team, they hid, one under the bed and one outside the window . . .

THERAPIST: No one will find me here. (*Playing spring drum*)

SCOTTY: (*Cueing*) . . . Now the boy went to sleep. Play sleep sounds.

THERAPIST: (*Playing metallaphone*) All was still.

SCOTTY: (*Playing C#, D, C#, D, and the A cymbal sound*) It is night—ya ha . . .

THERAPIST: (*Singing*) Here I come . . . (*To Scotty*) What do I do?

SCOTTY: Take me out of my bed, and hide me in the closet, but then you'll see bones in the closet and scream . . .

THERAPIST: (*Creating new theme on piano and singing*) I'm hiding you in the closet, I'm going to open the door, I'm hiding you in the closet, and then I'll be back for more . . . ya ha, ya ha!! (*Scotty goes to drum and plays a basic, steady beat to this tune. The therapist and Scotty improvise together for approximately 3 minutes.*)

SCOTTY: (*Singing to the theme*) Ya ha, ya ha, there's bones in there . . . but we are not afraid.

THERAPIST: No, we are not afraid . . . no, no . . .

SCOTTY: No, no . . .

THERAPIST: No, no . . .

SCOTTY: (*To therapist, whispering*) Can we listen to this?

After Scotty and I listened to the tape, we had this exchange:

SCOTTY: That was pretty good . . . maybe the skeleton could be the bones of a good guy that died. Maybe he could be, like, a relative that stayed in the closet to protect him or something.

THERAPIST: Then he would be less afraid?

SCOTTY: Yeah. There are the good monsters, well, they could be like real people in the kid's lives . . . maybe they were killed for doing bad stuff, like in another place or time or something. Like they would stab me, or take me out if I had a fight and yelled at the teacher or something . . .

THERAPIST: Do you do that? Do you yell in school?

SCOTTY: Well, I was suspended last year for mouthing off and pushing . . . but not right now . . . I get mad, but I am in control.

THERAPIST: Do you think demons punish bad children?

SCOTTY: Well, maybe not really . . . sometimes I think about it, but I don't think ghosts and stuff are really real. . . .

Though the resolution of these themes was never entirely full or complete, Scotty and I constructed a variety of scenarios through recurring music therapy session play. A few times, we were able to give a new identity to and soothe his inner beastly desires by playing music and offering the head demon, Chucky, a bed.

There were also times when some of the monsters would try to kill, but Scotty always used a very loud tom-tom drum with 16th-note rhythms to bring them back to life. Projectively, I saw this as a healthy statement about his belief in healing and medical treatment. (I also worked with Scotty's social worker to ensure that appropriate videos and television shows were watched at home.)

As the therapy progressed, we developed episodes where the music was used to tame and resolve Scotty's fears, to the point of safety and sleep. One episode led to the creation of assurances to the point of jointly composed lullabies, which we used in Scotty's routine prior to going to sleep. He chose the rainstick and asked me to play the violin. He requested that we play "Silent Night." He constructed new lyrics:

SCOTTY: (*Singing*) Silent night, not so much fright . . .

THERAPIST: Sleep, don't fear, no monsters here . . . safe and sound in my snuggly bed . . .

SCOTTY: No more screaming, just dreaming instead . . .

THERAPIST: La, la, la . . .

SCOTTY: Sleep in heavenly peace. (*Spoken*) I miss my mom . . . I hope I can go home soon.

September 11th

Scotty was admitted for a pain crisis related to his chronic illness on September 7th. He received music therapy that same day, as his pain reports were high. We used vibration—namely, the gong—to decrease his extremely painful episodes in his joints. His earlier music therapy had included vibrational work that addressed the joint pain. These sessions assisted Scotty in his ability to relax. He was encouraged to breathe and to imagine a favorite place as the gong was played above his body, assisting and easing his extreme pain. He was in too much pain to walk, so the September 7th session was conducted at his bedside. Through the use of the gong and imagery, Scotty was able to fall asleep.

By the 11th, Scotty was medically cleared and ready to go home, as his pain had diminished (to a level of 2 on a scale from 0 to 10) and he was sufficiently rehydrated. Consequent to the 9/11 terrorist attacks, however, streets were blocked and public transportation was inaccessible. Scotty and the aunt who had come to pick him up could not leave the hospital, as they were unable to find a mode of transportation or a route that would enable them to travel home. By the time he was approached for music therapy, he was clearly fearful and anxious because of the destruction. His fear remained apparent during his 40-minute music therapy session, which took place at approximately 1 P.M.

At the time of this session, most of the medical center's staff members were in a temporary "holding" mode; we were expecting to be paged to facilitate the treatment of hundreds of new patients. We had bought food and clothing for the initial handfuls of World Trade Center workers we had treated, but had expected many more patients to be admitted. We had opened new units and made beds. In the interim, we went to our assigned floors to take care of patients already in house.

Entering Scotty's hospital room, I noticed his aunt lying on his bed, seemingly asleep. Scotty was sitting in the chair watching the news on television. It was showing repeated images of the World Trade Center towers falling over and over again. It was the first glimpse that I had seen of their falling, even though I had spent the morning assisting patients who made it out of the towers to the hospital for care. I was quite concerned about Scotty's viewing the images of the buildings falling and the people running. I would not previously have predicted that any of the patients on the pediatric unit would have internalized the unfolding events of 9/11 to the extent that I soon learned Scotty had. The session I had with Scotty on that afternoon was unlike other sessions, and this surprised me.

I awoke Scotty's aunt once Scotty had agreed to come to the music therapy studio. I turned off the television in Scotty's room and informed the aunt that we would return in 40 minutes. After our warm-up/greeting song, Scotty pointed to my animal puppet box, which was a new request for him. We created a theme about each animal. He gave the animals names and then provided them each with a musical introduction before using the music to create different kinds of food for them.

He was first most interested in using the music to cook a variety of dishes for each animal. And then, to my surprise, he shifted the cooking into pretend feeding:

SCOTTY: Now let me feed you, Mrs. Cow. Here's the oatmeal. (*He takes the woodblock and, using a seven-note theme and a corresponding rhythm, sings.*) The cow will eat the oatmeal. (*Speaks*) Come here, you little cow . . . (*He pretends to feed the therapist.*)

THERAPIST: (*Singing*) That was yummy, thank you.

SCOTTY: And now the butterfly. (*He takes a bell and flies it in the sky, singing.*) Butterfly will have some butter that I churned. . . . (*Again, he pretends to feed the therapist.*)

THERAPIST: (*Singing*) That was just delightful, thank you . . .

SCOTTY: Sing it like this: Ahhh, it is so yummy . . .

THERAPIST: (*Moving to the piano*) Oh this is so, oh this is so, oh this is so yummy. I'm so grateful, I'm so pleased, Scotty's cooking—thank you, please!

It was significant how each animal ate and then said "yummy," which seemed indicative of the thankfulness of how they each received the food. Scotty was clearly enjoying eating and caretaking. He seemed to be expressing a need to feed, and perhaps at the same time to be fulfilled.

As we distanced ourselves from the play and moved into some musical improvisation, Scotty talked about being ready to go home, but there being "no way to get out." He spoke about his perception of the falling buildings, which for him translated into there being no cabs and "Auntie's getting tired of waiting":

SCOTTY: We had macaroni and cheese for lunch yesterday . . . looks like we may have lunch and then dinner here too. We can't get out, there's no cabs. The buildings fell down because of the plane accident, and there isn't even a bus. Auntie's getting tired of waiting.

THERAPIST: She's tired of waiting . . .

SCOTTY: We have to take care of the rest of the animals, so they can go to sleep too . . . but they are still really hungry. This time you cook, and I will be the animals. (*Goes to bells and sings.*) The little frogs are hungry, they've been hopping in the mud all day . . .

THERAPIST: (*Singing and playing guitar*) I'll give them some spaghetti, so they can eat and then sleep until they want to play . . .

When the session was over, we took a favorite bird puppet back to his room. I turned off the TV (which had been turned on in our absence), and we told his aunt about the animals and how good it had felt for Scotty to have had the opportunity to feed them. At this point, Scotty and his aunt were ready for lunch, and we ordered a food tray. While Scotty ate, I quietly and respectfully discussed with his aunt the negative impact television and the images of the falling towers might have on Scotty. She seemed to understand and said she would monitor his television watching more carefully.

I saw this unique session as an important one. It was a shift to see Scotty wanting to take care of things. I interpreted this as a reaction to his perception of things falling around him, which directed him to call upon his inner resources to nurture, to soothe, and to comfort. I saw the value in the way he was able to enact this through play that was focused on feeding and eating. It seemed to provide Scotty with some internal comfort on a day where there were shifts, chaos, and fear occurring all around him, and only a television set with images for him to try to piece together.

CARING FOR THE CAREGIVER: A PROGRAM APPROACH

The development of a new, integrative group therapy model for working with traumatized individuals began with the desire to help meet the expressed needs of a group of adult caregivers who were striving to cope, both personally and professionally, with the traumatic effects of 9/11. The therapeutic model that became the Caring for the Caregiver program was based upon the combination of current findings from trauma research with the use of music and music therapy techniques to facilitate this work.

The Caring for the Caregiver concept was created by Joanne Loewy and coordinated by Kristen Stewart in direct response to the events of 9/11. The project was developed as part of the American Music Therapy Association's NYC Relief Project, with underwritten support from the National Academy of Recording Arts and Sciences (the Grammy Foundation). It was presented through the Armstrong Music Therapy Program at Beth Israel Medical Center in NYC, and was targeted to serve a diverse cross-section of residents and professionals in NYC and the surrounding areas, including parents, spouses/partners, health care professionals, police officers, firefighters and clergy.

Caring for the Caregiver was presented as a 9-week training series. Each training session consisted of two 45-minute sections. The first section offered the participants an experience of a unique music therapy approach and/or technique, and was led by one of a core team of eight music therapists, each with experience in the use of music therapy with traumatized individuals from various populations. After being guided through musical experiences involving the use of instruments, voice, movement, and/or selected art materials, therapists provided opportunities for verbal processing of the music. The music therapy techniques introduced in these training segments included song sensitation; clinical improvisation; sacred songs and rounds; story song; structured song; chanting and lullabies; and music and imagery.

"Song sensitation" can be defined as the progressive exploration and experiencing of a client-chosen song through the acts of relaxation, active listening, lyric analysis, and performance. Developed by Joanne Loewy, this technique utilizes the unique qualities of song (symbolic expression, unification with others through shared experience, validation of self) with specific use of lyrics as a means to "inspire both the individual listener and the community-at-large to focus on a particular idea" (Loewy, 2002, p. 35). In this case, feelings and experiences related to 9/11 were the focus, and the song selected by the facilitator was "Fragile," by Sting.

"Clinical improvisation" is the use of instrumental and/or vocal music that is composed spontaneously in the moment. This technique was used to introduce participants to the instruments, providing an experience of group collaboration, safety, freedom of expression, tension release, unconditional acceptance, and increased awareness of self and others through the leadership of the music therapist.

"Sacred songs, and particularly "rounds," are known for their simplicity. A round utilizes simple melody, repetition, and multiple voicing in an overlapping pattern. In the Caring for the Caregiver training, the round "By the Waters" was chosen to provide a holding musical form (one that is simple in structure and repeated) within which the participants could be supported in expressing and moving through the grief and sadness associated with the traumatic events of 9/11. Working with many voices in the round and sacred singing offered participants the opportunity to care simultaneously for others and for themselves in a community.

"Story song" has been described in detail above. It was used in this context with the tale of "Humpty Dumpty." The story song was first presented using vocal and instrumental music by the core team of music therapists. Participants were then invited to join as the story song was repeated. Presenting "Humpty Dumpty" in this progressive and optional way allowed group members to choose the level of participation that best matched their individual needs, with the intention of offering the experience of safe reenactment of the traumatic event without retraumatization.

"Structured song" was used both organically and in a preplanned fashion as an opening and/or closing of a music segment. The specific use of "chanting and lullabies" served to slow the systems of the body, deepen self-awareness through internal vibration, and bring individuals to a more sensate level of being (feeling present in their bodies). Further description of the use of structured song, chanting, and lullabies is provided in the case of Sidney, below.

The "music and imagery" technique is a variation of Helen Bonny's method of "Guided Imagery and Music" (Bonny & Savary, 1973), which utilizes active listening while in a relaxed state to music specifically selected by the music therapist, with the intention of supporting a symbolic "journey" through inner experience. In this program, the music therapist, after preparing group members through the use of relaxation exercises, played slow, even beats on a gong to suggest a sense of predictability. This was followed by long tones in a simple melody on the alto flute to create a sense of depth and space through the rich and tranquil tone of the flute. Voices were added to the flute play, and the experience ended with a recapitulation of the gong as a transitional instrument. An in-depth description of this and other music therapy techniques introduced throughout the Caring for the Caregiver program can be found in *Caring for the Caregiver: The Use of Music and Music Therapy in Grief and Trauma* (Loewy & Frisch Hara, 2002).

The second portion of each training session offered an educational perspective, presented by an expert in the field of trauma, grief, and/or loss. Experts included a clinical social worker, a developmental psychologist/nurse, the members of an improvisational theatre company, a psychiatrist, a licensed counselor/trauma specialist, and a professional songwriter. As many of the music techniques presented during this training series introduced participants to new means of coping with trauma-related issues through sensation and experience, the interactive lectures that followed the music portion of each training helped to reorient participants to a cognitive understanding and awareness of traumatic experience. Thus the music was enhanced by the insight provided by each guest speaker, who in presenting his or her approach to trauma, gave a deeper perspective to the experience and emphasized the healing capacity that music therapy can bring to work related to trauma, grief, and loss.

Important elements in the format of this model included awareness and respect for each member's individual needs (Britt, 1997; Cowan, 1996; Tebb, 1995; Muldary, 1983) as well as the needs of the group as a whole, and opportunities to experientially process group members' responses to the traumatic events without retraumatization (Levine, 1997). The use of music in this model was significant for its inherent capacity to address these elements. It utilized a creative and expressive modality and forum, which facilitated self-awareness, interaction, and communication, as well as validation of self and experiences, and unconditional and simultaneous acceptance of all participants in the moment (Bruscia, 1998).

Thus, the Caring for the Caregiver program's design incorporated both the needs expressed by the caregivers participating in this program and information gleaned from the literature. The program's goal was to introduce group members to several different techniques and musically therapeutic experiences, in order to broaden their perception and experience of internal and external resources in a supportive community environment.

One innovative aspect of the model developed for the Caring for the Caregiver program was that the group included caregivers with personal as well as professional associations to the traumatic events of 9/11. This design was implemented as a way of uniting community members as individuals through common experience. van der Kolk (1987) emphasizes the importance of focusing on interdependence and community, recognizing that "sharing relationships have been the central [human] mode of coping with and adapting to the environment" (p. 155). Other noted benefits of group/social support for caregivers include decreased burnout, decreased anxiety, increased sense of hope and purposefulness in life, and increase depth of process (Shamia, 1998; Coady, Kent, & Davis, 1990; van der Kolk, 1987.

MULTIPLE LAYERS OF CARING: THE CASE OF SIDNEY, AGE 42

At the time of his participation in the Caring for the Caregiver program, Sidney had been practicing music therapy for over 20 years, and worked with children and adults coping with the effects of trauma as part of his clinical practice. Sidney, his wife, and their 2-year-old son lived on the Lower West Side of NYC, close to the site of the World Trade Center. In addition to personally coping with the effects of 9/11 as a resident of the area, and as a professional working in a neighboring community, Sidney continues to be an integral part of a 9/11 relief effort targeting outreach to members of the World Trade Center community and beyond.

This was how Sidney expressed his feelings and his desire to participate in the Caring for the Caregiver program as he struggled with stress relating to his personal and professional connections to 9/11:

> "I think, in general, my response to something traumatic is to protect myself by feeling anxious and supervigilant. What I discovered during the preparation for leadership of the [9/11 trauma] workshop was that—that supervigilance and anxiety was a protection from allowing myself to feel, to get to the grief."

> "Consciously, when I was sitting there on 9/11, I wanted to go out and do something, take some action rather than to feel helpless ... to help others and also to give myself a sense of purpose."

> "9/11 impacted me, more than any other reason, because of my worry for my son and the future ... knowing that, at any moment, something tragic could happen."

The difficulties of coping with the trauma-related stress as it surfaced in these many layers of caregiving (caring for himself and for others, both personally and professionally) were also observed by Sidney in his music making, both as a participant in the Caring for the Caregiver program and in his work as a music therapist. This became noticeable to Sidney as a lack of feeling freely expressive and as an avoidance of utilizing the upper and lower tonalities of certain harmonic instruments, such as the keyboard and piano. Sidney explained these behaviors as an expression of his fear of exploring sounds and music that might trigger memories and images of the traumatic events.

> "I was aware of the connection between my playing and my emotional process . . . avoiding my feelings of vulnerability . . . feeling a need for control . . . feeling a loss of a basic sense of security."

Specific issues relating to his self-care needs as a professional working with trauma surfaced for Sidney as well:

> [Speaking of a copresenter in the 9/11 relief project:] "I thought she did a great job, but I was so aware of how it was going, and in my feeling 'out' of what was going on, it was hard for me to relax and get into the experience itself. Also, I was playing [involved instrumentally in the presentation], so I was just . . . serving others more than, you know, being there for myself."

> "[Conversely,] I felt of all the things I was doing in response to 9/11, that was the most directly dealing with what I wanted to do about 9/11. It gave me a sense of purpose."

This polarity of experience offers perhaps one explanation for how caregivers work for prolonged periods of time while under personal duress and neglect, placing the needs of others before personal needs, to the point where burnout and secondary traumatization may occur. The literature from the health care professions of social work, music therapy, and psychology seems to indicate this as well (Hartley, 2001; Thompson, 1999; Coady et al., 1990; Muldary, 1983; Patrick, 1981). Documentation of the causes, effects, and frequency of burnout—particularly for professionals working with clients who have high-intensity needs, such as individuals coping with past or present trauma—are notably abundant. However, the literature prior to 9/11 is virtually void of documentation on self-care and coping methods for professionals.

According to Sidney, a significant occurrence in the early part of the

Caring for the Caregiver program was the moment when he was able to clearly differentiate his involvement as a participant in the program from his role as a presenter. This insight points to the multiple levels of caregiving awareness taking place in this moment for Sidney. The comments below refer to Sidney's experience during the guest speaker portion of the first Caring for the Caregiver training session. As guest speakers for this first session, members of the Playback Theatre Company used music and improvisational theatre to act out the individual stories of viewers who volunteered to share a significant occurrence or memory. Performing in hospitals, schools, prisons, and communities, as well as in theatres and clubs in NYC, this company offers the opportunity to hear and experience one's personal traumatic story in a manageable way. In this training, Sidney followed his impulse to join the improvisatory experience as a participant, choosing to musically support the sharing of another participant's story. This was a shift for Sidney in his capacity to expand his perception of his role as a cofacilitator, and to allow his intention to participate to remain strictly voluntary, without a sense of the responsibility for leadership.

> " . . . I just remember Playback allowing me to get into the experience, in a way, because I wasn't there as a facilitator of the music. I was there living in their facilitating for me, so that felt very powerful. . . . Where I was—frozen, shut down on an emotional level, this experience unlocked for me. I just took it to a very deep level, to feel that I could serve as a music maker . . . you know, not in particular as a therapist, [but] to just be there. . . . To me, this meant a lot on a personal level. It made me feel like there's a reason to be here. I think it helped me to be present. It sensitized me to other people."

As the training series progressed, Sidney continued to note his reactions to the various musical and educational segments of the training, and to recognize their impact on his ability to cope in many different ways. In week 7, the music presented included the use of a gong, hand drums, and structured song. The goal was to provide the group with an experience of "how music and sound could activate the sense of trauma resident in the body in the interest of working it through and out of the body" (Bosco, 2002, p. 74). The experience began with the use of the gong to provide a safely heightened sonic reenactment of the events of 9/11 in a controlled environment (a musical experience that Sidney recognized he had been avoiding up to now). A drumming activity was then led by the music therapist to facilitate a controlled discharge of the latent energy that had been stored in participants' nervous systems in response to the traumatic events of 9/11, and that had now been brought to the surface through the gonging. After the participants were given the opportunity to release the surfaced nervous energy through the structured drumming improvisation, the use of structured song ("Imagine," John Lennon) was chosen to enhance a feeling of safety and reconnection. The structure of precomposed music enhances a feeling of predictability and familiarity in the song form, and provides an opportunity for the body's experience to settle and reconnect with both an inner and an outer sense of order.

The music segment offered in week 8 used structured song, chanting, and lullabies as tools for expression and self-nurturance. The session began with structured song ("Sing with Me", an original composition by the presenter) as a means to engage participants and establish a musical structure to the session. With the intention of increasing awareness and openness of the physical body, the music therapist then led participants in a series of body stretches. This was followed by a combination of chants and lullabies designed to create the sense of nurturing oneself in the moment and tapping into one's innate capacity for self-healing. Both weeks 7 and 8 incorporated discussion and verbal processing to balance these experiences. Here are Sidney's comments on these sessions:

[Week 7:] "The music therapist was very helpful, in that I felt he took a risk that went to the very depths of the fears and anxieties that people may be living in, and certainly I found myself responding to the gong."

"[After the drumming,] . . . when I was there I felt that it was a safe haven. . . . the feeling right after we played was more alive. I was aware that the room felt different."

[Week 8:] "I think there really was a process of getting more deeply involved in the music. . . . Maybe that's why I had a memory of the music therapist's use of voice in one of our sessions . . . because that was already late in the process. Maybe at that point I just felt relaxed enough to get into the experience. . . . there was a certain fragility to it that was very clear, and I felt that this music therapist did it [presented] in a very genuine way, and I was moved by that."

[Of the music experiences in general:] "It helped me to feel. It helped me to have a sense of the future—hope for the future. It helped me to get angry. It helped me . . . to plead, to yearn. It helped me to have some sense of belonging . . . to feel like I fit somewhere."

CARING FOR THE CAREGIVER: A SUMMARY

The implementation of this model provided insights into the parallels between the reactions of caregivers and the reactions of traumatized individuals coping with the actual traumatic events. Such parallels have also been reported by Diane Poole Heller (1999) in her work with parents and children affected by the traumatic events at Columbine High School, particularly in the way trauma is experienced in the body through "autonomic nervous system over-activation" (p. 22). Though manifested symptoms may vary, Poole Heller recognizes the common reactions in individuals' nervous systems to a traumatic event (or to secondary traumatization, as is often the case for caregivers.)[1]

Figley (2002) defines secondary traumatic stress disorder as "nearly identical to PTSD, except that it applies to those emotionally affected by the trauma of another" (p. 3). He also points to an increased risk of experiencing secondary trauma for parents, family members, and caregiving professionals with inadequate coping skills and supportive resources.

By providing an opportunity to recognize the simultaneous experiences of trauma from a variety of caregiving perspectives, the Caring for the Caregiver program offered Sidney and other participants a unique and vital approach to working with the effects of traumatic stress. It enabled a mutuality of experience among participants by inviting them to shed their traditional professional roles of caregiving and explore a multidimensional approach to caring for the self.

The fact that this program was defined as training, rather than as therapy, allowed this opportunity for mutuality to extend also to the leaders, thus modeling personal and professional "caring for the caregiver" in the moment. Having a core team of eight music therapists, along with the project coordinator, facilitated the team's exploration of functioning in multiple roles within the singularly presented experiences.

Through the Caring for the Caregiver program, a diverse cross-section of individuals were able to explore and evaluate the use of music and music therapy in the treatment of trauma, grief, and loss. The participants acknowledged the medium of music as both viable and effective in this work. Feedback on the effectiveness of the music process and group model, received via two surveys conducted during the course of the program, confirmed Sidney's comments as shared above. The most helpful components the Caring for the Caregiver program were identified as

---

[1]Poole Heller's work with traumatized families in the Columbine community is based on the work of Peter Levine. Levine's approach, Somatic Experiencing®, is a product of his study of prey animals in the wild, in combination with an understanding of the physical body's innate ability to regulate and discharge energetic activation due to trauma, through the awareness of body sensations.

(1) being a part of a group and experiencing a sense of belonging to a community, and (2) feeling the impact of the music. As noted by one anonymous Caring for the Caregiver participant, music and music therapy can facilitate "deal[ing] with deeply embedded traumatic issues, acknowledging them and striving to cope with them in the moment."

The use of music and music therapy can touch upon many layers of trauma for those directly and indirectly traumatized. This chapter has sought to illuminate ways in which music and music therapy can serve both the givers and receivers of care in coping with traumatic experience.

REFERENCES

Bonny, H. L., & Savary, L. M. (1973). *Music and your mind*. New York: Station Hill Press.

Bosco, F. (2002). Daring, dread, discharge, and delight. In J. V. Loewy & A. Frisch Hara (Eds.), *Caring for the caregiver: The use of music and music therapy in grief and trauma* (pp. 71–82). Silver Spring, MD: American Music Therapy Association.

Britt, D. E. (1997). Psychologist self-care. *Dissertation Abstracts International, 58*(5), 1598A.

Brodsky, W. (1989). Music therapy as an intervention for children with cancer in isolation rooms. *Music Therapy, 8*(1), 17–34.

Bruscia, K. (1998). *Defining music therapy* (2nd ed.). Gilsum, NH: Barcelona.

Caine, J. (1991). The effects of music on the selected stress behaviors, weight, caloric and formula intake, and length of hospital stay of premature and low birth weight neonates in an NICU. *Journal of Music Therapy, 28*(4), 180–192.

Coady, C. A., Kent, V. D., & Davis, P. W. (1990). Burnout among social workers with patients with cystic fibrosis. *Health and Social Work, 15*(2), 116–124.

Cowan, D. S. (1996). Meeting whose needs?: The personal needs of the therapist. *Music Therapy Perspectives, 14*, 50–52.

Dossey, L. (1982). *Space, time and medicine*. Boulder, CO: Shambhala.

Edwards, J. (1999). Anxiety management in pediatric music therapy. In C. Dileo (Ed.), *Music therapy and medicine: Theoretical and clinical applications* (pp. 69–76). Silver Spring, MD: American Music Therapy Association.

Figley, C. R. (Ed.). (2002). *Treating compassion fatigue*. New York: Brunner-Routledge.

Griggs-Drane, E. (1999). The use of musical wind instruments in the treatment of chronic pulmonary diseases. In C. Dileo (Ed.), *Music therapy and medicine: Theoretical and clinical applications* (pp. 129–138). Silver Spring, MD: American Music Therapy Association.

Hartley, N. A. (2001). On a personal note: A music therapist's reflections on working with those who are living with terminal illness. *Journal of Palliative Care, 17*(3), 135–141.

Levine, P. A. (1997). *Waking the tiger, healing trauma: The innate capacity to transform overwhelming experiences*. Berkeley, CA: North Atlantic Books.

Loewy, J. V. (2000). Music psychotherapy assessment. *Music Therapy Perspectives*, *18*, 47–58.

Loewy, J. V. (2002). Song sensitation: How fragile we are. In J. V. Loewy & A. Frisch Hara (Eds.), *Caring for the caregiver: The use of music and music therapy in grief and trauma* (pp. 33–43). Silver Spring, MD: American Music Therapy Association.

Loewy, J. V., & Frisch Hara, A. (Eds.). (2002). *Caring for the caregiver: The use of music and music therapy in grief and trauma.* Silver Spring, MD: American Music Therapy Association.

Loewy, J. V., MacGregor, Richards, K., & Rodriguez, J. (1997). Music therapy and pediatric pain management: Assessing and attending to the sounds of hurt, fear and anxiety. In J. Loewy (Ed.), *Music therapy and pediatric pain* (pp. 45–56). Cherry Hill, NJ: Jeffrey Books.

Malone, A. (1996). The effects of live music on the distress of pediatric patients receiving intravenous starts, venipunctures, injections, and heel sticks. *Journal of Music Therapy, 23*, 19–33.

Muldary, T. W. (1983). *Burnout and the health care professional: Manifestations and management.* Norwalk, CT: Capistrano Press.

Patrick, P. K. S. (1981). *Health care worker burnout: What it is, what to do about it.* Chicago: Blue Cross Association.

Poole Heller, D. P. (1999). *Columbine: Surviving the trauma.* Unpublished manuscript.

Priestley, M. (1975). *Music therapy in action.* London: Constable.

Robb, S. (1996). Techniques in songwriting: Restoring emotional and physical well being in adolescents who have been traumatically injured. *Music Therapy Perspectives, 14*(1), 30–37.

Rubin-Bosco, J. (2002). Resolution versus reenactment: A story song approach to working with trauma. In J. V. Loewy & A. Frisch Hara (Eds.), *Caring for the caregiver: The use of music and music therapy in grief and trauma* (pp. 118–127). Silver Spring, MD: American Music Therapy Association.

Shamia, M. (1998). Therapist in distress: Team-supervision of social workers and family therapists who live under political uncertainty. *Family Process, 37*(2), 245–259.

Stewart, K. (2002). Models of caring for the caregiver. In J. V. Loewy & A. Frisch Hara (Eds.), *Caring for the caregiver: The use of music and music therapy in grief and trauma* (pp. 9–22). Silver Spring, MD: American Music Therapy Association.

Stewart, K., & Schneider, S. (2000). *Music therapy in the NICU.* New York: Satchnote Press.

Tebb, S. (1995). An aid to empowerment: A caregiver well-being scale. *Health and Social Work, 20*(2), 87–92.

Thaut, M., & McIntosh, G. C. (1992). Effect of auditory rhythm on temporal stride parameters and EMG patterns in normal and hemiparetic gait. *Neurology, 42*, 208–216.

Thaut, M., Rice, R., & McIntosh, G. (1997). Rhythmic facilitation of gait training in hemiparetic stroke rehabilitation. *Journal of Neurological Sciences, 151*, 7–12.

Thompson, T. L. (1999). Managed care: Views, practices, and burnout of psychologists. *Dissertation Abstracts International, 60*(3), 1318B.

Turry, A. (1997). The use of clinical improvisation to alleviate procedural distress in young children. In J. Loewy (Ed.), *Music therapy and pediatric pain* (pp. 89–96). Cherry Hill, NJ: Jeffrey Books.

van der Kolk, B. A. (1987). The role of the group in the origin and resolution of the trauma response. In B. A. van der Kolk (Ed.), *Psychological trauma* (pp. 153–172). Washington, DC: American Psychiatric Press.

Winnicott, D. W. (1965). *The maturational processes and the facilitating environment.* London: Hogarth Press.

CHAPTER 10

Sandplay, Art, and Play Therapy to Promote Anxiety Reduction

LOIS CAREY

Traumatic stress is an overwhelming response to violent acts such as those described by Nancy Boyd Webb in Chapter 1 of this book. The events of September 11, 2001—the attacks on the World Trade Center (WTC) and the Pentagon, and the downing of the plane in Pennsylvania—are prime examples. This chapter discusses creative techniques that are helpful in resolving disturbing responses to many situations of trauma.

I am a social worker in private practice in a suburban area of New York City. My office is approximately 25 miles from what is now known as "Ground Zero," and as such is somewhat removed from the epicenter of that particular tragedy. However, many families who live in this area are employed in the city, and unfortunately, a number of their members were victims. In addition, many of our local police officers and firefighters are employed in the city and were on volunteer duty for the weeks and months following "9/11." I present a case in this chapter of a child whose father was involved in the rescue efforts.

In addition to being a play therapist, I am a family therapist and have incorporated into my work some creative forms of therapy, along with more traditional verbal therapy in both individual and family treatments. My primary specialty is sandplay therapy, with art therapy as my secondary interest.

Many cases throughout my years in practice have involved children traumatized by sexual abuse, loss/bereavement, adoption, and neurological impairment. These cases cover many of the standard diagnostic categories, such as anxiety, depression, attention-deficit/hyperactivity disor-

216

der, oppositional defiant disorder, developmental delay, and Tourette's syndrome. The case presented in this chapter is that of an anxious child whose symptom of migraine headaches was exacerbated by the events of 9/11.

SANDPLAY, ART, AND PLAY THERAPY

Why does one choose play, sandplay, or art therapy? Primarily because children readily accept and understand these techniques, which immediately help to lower any resistance to being "in therapy." Play therapy has become the accepted method for most child therapy, because play is the way that children traditionally handle their problems. Garry Landreth (1991, p. 10) tells us:

> For children to "play out" their experiences and feelings is the most natural dynamic and self-healing process in which children can engage. Play is a medium of exchange and restricting children to verbal expression automatically places a barrier to a therapeutic relationship by imposing limitations that in effect say to children "You must come up to my level of communication and communicate with words."

One can readily see that any form of therapy that is essentially creative, and that can be nonverbal as well as verbal, holds a definite advantage for a child who has been traumatized (no matter what the cause). My preference, because of my training, is to utilize sandplay therapy, art therapy, and play therapy, all of which were used in the case to be discussed.

Sandplay therapy is directly related to art therapy and play therapy. Dora Kalff, a Jungian analyst in Switzerland, developed sandplay therapy about 50 years ago (see Kalff, 1980a). Kalff's work grew out of her studies with Margaret Lowenfeld in London, who developed a therapeutic technique referred to as the "world technique" (Lowenfeld, 1979) that used toys and miniatures. Kalff's analytic training had incorporated knowledge of myths and archetypes as a means for understanding and deepening the analytic process. Kalff had an allied interest in Zen Buddhism, which she integrated into her understanding of this new form of treatment with children. She believed that it was imperative to apply a child's understanding of what was produced, rather than to impose any of her own interpretations. This is associated with a Zen Buddhist guru's practice of not answering any question posed by a seeker; instead, the guru returns the question to the seeker to find his or her own answer.

Another influence on Kalff's work was the theory of Erich Neumann, a German analyst. Kalff noted that Neumann's theories of child psychological development were directly applicable to what she observed in sandplay. Neumann developed his ideas in his 1973 book *The Child*, in which he demonstrated three stages that a child goes through to separate from the mother and to become a fully functioning individual. He called these (1) the animal–vegetative stage, (2) the fighting stage, and (3) the stage of adaptation to the collective, all of which are visible in the sand pictures that a child produces. In addition to these stages, Kalff observed that her young clients often reached a time in therapy when at least one "special" picture was produced. Such a picture indicated that a child's ego and self had been reunited, thereby permitting deeper healing. This type of picture, often in a mandala form, holds indications of a child's (or adult's) deep level of spirituality. Kalff (1980b) termed these pictures "the constellation of the self," and they could be likened to an "aha" moment in verbal therapy.

Kalff was the originator and primary teacher of this technique, and spread her expertise in numerous geographical areas until her death in 1990. She had the great advantage of language fluency and could lecture in the languages of the countries where she taught. In addition, she held many seminars in her private home and office, located just outside Zurich, Switzerland. I was one of her trainees during the 1980s and made many trips to Zurich for the experience. I also attended several of her trainings in California and feel quite privileged to have had these opportunities. I use her theories in my teaching and lecturing, as well as with the children and adults I treat.

Materials for Sandplay

Sandplay therapy is optimally conducted with two sandboxes that are 19½ × 28½ × 4 inches deep. Each is half filled with sand, and the bottoms and sides are painted blue, in order to represent water or sky when the sand is pushed to one side. In addition to providing limits, this is a comfortable size for the eye to encompass in one glance. Two boxes are provided, so that one can contain wet sand, the other one dry. This presents the child with an initial choice of medium, and the choice can be diagnostically relevant. The other important component of a sandplay office is a broad assortment of miniatures from which a child can select to create a "sand picture" or scene. Miniatures include various categories: animals (domestic, wild, prehistoric); birds (many varieties, including storks, peacocks, penguins); buildings (houses, barns, churches, etc.); people (various occupations, both genders, different ages, different ethnicities); spiritual/religious figures; fantasy figures (fairy tale characters, superheroes); natural items (trees, shells, stones, rocks, etc.); transportation vehicles (cars, trucks, planes, boats); and miscellaneous items (fences, bridges, caskets, headstones). The collection of miniatures can be as broad as space and money permit; however, it is suggested that a collection hold only those items of which the therapist has some mythological or archetypal understanding. Otherwise, the value of the items would be limited by the therapist's lack of knowledge. A fuller discussion of sandplay therapy appears in my book *Sandplay Therapy with Children and Families* (Carey, 1999).

Materials for Art Therapy

Art therapy is an older and more widely recognized form of treatment than sandplay therapy, and is therefore more widely accepted and understood. The equipment required for art therapy is somewhat different from that needed for sandplay therapy. The art therapy office is equipped with various sizes and shapes of paper, different types of media (oils, crayons, markers, watercolors), fabrics, magazines (for cutouts), clay, Play-Doh, easels at varying heights, chalkboards, and the like. Again, the selection can be as broad as space and money permit. For a much fuller discussion of art therapy, see Malchiodi (1998).

Play Therapy Materials

The traditional play therapy room often includes art materials as well as puppets, dollhouses, wheeled vehicles, bop bags, and (less often), sandplay equipment. This may be because sand takes up more physical space and because most play therapists already possess art materials. In addition, training in art therapy is more readily available than that in sandplay therapy; therefore, art therapy techniques are more familiar to many play therapists. The similarity that exists between art and sand is that both can be used nonverbally as well as verbally—a definite advantage when one treats any child, and especially a traumatized child.

The physical arrangement of my own office allows for separate spaces for verbal and nonverbal sessions: The sandplay/art room is separate from the interviewing office. This affords a child an initial choice between the two when he or she comes for therapy, having seen both areas during the intake appointment. There are times when both areas are used within a given session, and at other times the child chooses one site or the other. Because the work I do is primarily child-centered, I follow the child's lead.

The sandplay therapy process begins by inviting the child to touch the sand in both boxes to see which one might "feel better." He or she is then directed to look at all the miniatures that are arranged on shelves around the room. The child then selects as many or as few toys as needed in order to construct a sand scene. I tell the child that a photograph of the scene will be taken when he or she states that it is complete. (I take two pictures: a Polaroid that the child can keep at the conclusion of therapy, and a slide that I explain is for teaching or writing purposes. The parent signs permission for this use; the child gives his or her permission as well, depending on the age and understanding of the child.)

When the child has completed his or her first (and subsequent) sand scenes, I invite the child either to say something about it, to name it, or to tell a story about it. However, if the child does not want to say anything, that is fine as well. The most important part of sandplay therapy is that any verbalization is kept within the metaphor of whatever has been depicted in the tray. For example, if there is a threatening scene with a tiger about to devour a kitten, the therapist might say something like this: "I see you have a tiger and a kitten—I wonder what the tiger and/or the kitten might be feeling." In this way, the therapist acknowledges the feeling tone in the scene without interpreting it as a real-life situation or assigning roles to the figures. This is similar to some forms of play therapy interactions: The therapist takes great care in moving slowly toward the deeper, somewhat more obvious (to adults), connections. My belief is that a child will eventually make connections when he or she is ready to do so, and that if a therapist moves too quickly, the child can become defensive and unavailable to the therapeutic process.

The healing process in sandplay therapy appears to come about through the *process* of creation, rather than through the *content* of any single picture. Sandplay moves through developmental stages, in accordance with a child's chronological and psychological age. The role of the therapist here is vitally important. The sandtray is the healing vessel, sometimes called the "temenos" (place of healing), and the therapist's function is to witness and "hold" the unconscious of the child's psyche while a transformative process takes place. My belief is that it is the person of the therapist, combined with the medium of the sand equipment, that determines success or failure with this technique. Anyone can own a sandbox and toys, but the training, care, and compassion of the sandplay therapist will determine just how healing this form of therapy will be.

CASE EXAMPLE

The following case example involves an "indirect victim" of the WTC tragedy. This was a 10-year-old boy who was brought to me by his mother in October 2001. I will call this boy Alexander. He was suffering from severe migraine headaches that had become much more frequent after the WTC attacks.

During the intake, I explored all of the relevant facts about Alexander and his family, using the tripartite crisis assessment model developed by Nancy Boyd Webb (1999; see also Chapter 2, this volume). This assessment model describes three different sets of interacting variables that should be considered for each unique crisis event: (1) the nature of the crisis situation, (2) the idiosyncratic characteristics of the individual, and (3) the strengths and weaknesses of the individual's support system.

The Nature of the Crisis Situation

The nature of this particular crisis situation was unlike any that had ever been experienced in the United States prior to September 11, 2001. The WTC in New York City was one of the targets of terrorists, who had hijacked four planes and deliberately crashed two of them into the towers. The entire U.S. way of life was immediately changed and threatened; the country had never before experienced such a horrific act. Indeed, there had never heretofore been such a major attack on the U.S. homeland. The impact of this tragedy affected people throughout the country—but especially in the New York City and Washington, D.C. areas. All four of these planes had been deployed to those two cities, but only three succeeded in their mission. The fourth one, meant for Washington, was brought down in Pennsylvania due to the incredible courage of passengers on that flight.

Other parts of the country were affected as well. However, the closer one was to any of these crisis areas, the more intensely the effects were felt (Pynoos & Nader, 1989; Nader, Pynoos, Fairbanks, & Frederick, 1990). Therapists, too, in these geographical areas were deeply shaken, having had very little (if any) prior experience with such an overwhelming event. Although there had been some earlier terrorist attacks, such as the 1993 WTC bombing and the 1995 Oklahoma City bombing, none were of the magnitude of the 9/11 atrocity. All of us in the helping professions were aware that our services would be vitally needed for quite some time because of this tragedy. We struggled to maintain our own balance in order to be of assistance to those who might need our help and expertise.

The Idiosyncratic Characteristics of the Individual

A complete psychosocial history is integral to the assessment process. Alexander, age 10, a latency-age boy, had suffered with migraines since the age of 5. Some were preceded by an aura. The migraines appeared to stem from an anxiety disorder. They had been controlled with medication (verapamil, 180 mg/day, and Aleve at the onset of a headache or an aura). Prior to 9/11, Alexander was experiencing approximately one headache per month. After that date, he began having about 10 per month. His anxiety appeared to increase his symptoms. Many of his headaches necessitated full-day absences from school; with others, he was able to attend only part of the day.

Alexander was a nice-looking, well-groomed boy who attended a religious school in his community. He was an honor student and took his schoolwork seriously. In addition, he was active in several sports, where he was one of the star players. He was a very serious-minded boy who was polite and respectful, almost to excess. For example, when I would hand a toy or art materials to him, he would always say "thank you." Sometimes there might be 10 or 12 "thank yous" within 5 minutes. I assured him that he did not need to thank me so profusely. Everything he did, from his schoolwork performance to his sports activities to parties that he attended, was accomplished with the utmost intensity and enthusiasm. His history, according to his parents, was that he had always been a tense child and appeared to internalize things deeply. He never had to be reminded to attend to his responsibilities, and he diligently did whatever was required of him.

The Strengths and Weaknesses
of the Individual's Support System

When one assesses a young child, it is important that the family dynamics be explored as well. This intact family, which I will call the Hobarts, consisted of the following:

> Client: Alexander, age 10, a fifth grader with a history of migraine headaches.
> Mother: Jeannette, age 39, a part-time sports coach.
> Father: Anthony, age 40, a New York City firefighter.
> Brother: Douglas, age 14, a ninth grader.

There was also a very large, close-knit extended family that celebrated numerous family events.

On 9/11, Mr. Hobart, along with almost all the firefighters and police officers in the New York City area, was assigned to the WTC site and spent two to three months there as part of the search and rescue team. Numerous other rescue volunteers came to assist from across the nation, and from foreign countries as well, in the frantic search for survivors and/or remains.

A significant number of Mr. and Mrs. Hobart's friends and colleagues, unfortunately, died during the rescue operations. These deaths required attendance by both parents at numerous funeral services. The children also attended one or two of the services because they were friends of the children whose parents had died. The mood in the Hobart household was one of devastation and utter depression as one funeral followed another.

Alexander, the younger child of this couple, was the one who internalized most of the family pressures. As noted earlier, he had a history of tension and anxiety, as evidenced by migraine headaches. His tension was further revealed by the fact that his nails were bitten quite far down. He had been taken to many specialists for his migraines. Up until 9/11, the medication he was taking was effective, at least most of the time. After that, it did not appear to help.

Alexander's family support system was a strong one, as indicated above. He also performed well in school and sports, had good peer relationships, and was well thought of by teachers and peers. He had many ego strengths, but his coping mechanisms did not always serve him well. His major complaint was the migraine condition, which was linked to those times when he became too anxious and intense over a test or a sport activity (or even, at times, playing too hard at family parties).

This is the information I acquired during the assessment process. During that time, I also explained my method of treatment to Alexander and his parents. I requested that Mrs. Hobart keep a log in order to see what, if anything, precipitated his headaches. The other son, Douglas, was not included in the assessment. The option was left open for him to attend some of the treatment sessions later if that was deemed necessary.

Treatment

Excerpts from Mrs. Hobart's log for the first week (and Alexander's first individual session) follow:

Gave an Aleve at 8 A.M. as Alexander had an aura. At 1:55 P.M., took him out of school as he felt nausea; he had NO headache, yet expressed great nervousness about the planned meeting with play therapist, Lois. Alexander's 3 P.M. visit with Lois was great! He said, "I want to go once a week for the rest of my life!"

[Two days later:] A #4 headache [the Hobarts rated the headaches on a scale of 1–10, 10 being the worst]. Gave Aleve at 9 P.M. Alexander had a busy day: school, followed by 4 P.M. Halloween dance/party at school. At 5:30 P.M. he had soccer practice. He was not himself at practice . . . a "bad" performance, he said.

[Two days later:] He woke up with #4 headache. Gave verapamil (as I do every morning, 180 mg/day) and Aleve. We went to 9:15 Mass, and Alexander took note that I moved during Mass closer to his father (who was getting upset at Mass). After church, Alexander asked me about the move, and I told him that I wanted to be near Daddy because I loved him and he needed to have me near him at that time. Alexander had an 11:30 A.M. soccer game and mentioned he was nervous. The game went well, and he was fantastic! We went to ShopRite after dinner, where Alexander's ears turned bright red and he was hot. He said he felt weird and wasn't sure if it was an aura or what. I gave him an Aleve, and he was asleep by 9 P.M. [One of the symptoms of a migraine was that his ears turned bright red.]

[Next day:] He said he woke up "dizzy." He still had that "hot" feeling as well (but no temperature). Gave him an Aleve around 8 A.M. and we all went to school (I work where Alexander attends school). Alexander was in the RN's office at 9:30 A.M. with a #3 headache. His grandfather took him home. His eyes were black and appeared swollen, and his body looked hot. He slept for an hour and felt much better.

I will not report Mrs. Hobart's notes for the following weeks verbatim, but they revealed that he had numerous headaches during the first month to 6 weeks of treatment. There were several reports of his being "nervous" prior to sessions, but he always wanted to attend. Most of the reported headaches occurred in relation to overexertion, to being overtired, and/or to being overexcited. A record was kept of the numbers of headaches he had during the first 6 or 7 months of therapy: 10 in October, 8 in November, 6 in December, 7 in January, none in February, 2 in March, 2 in April, and 2 in May.

As part of my evaluation of a child, I frequently use the House–Tree–Person test because it is a good indicator of some of a child's personality features and/or can provide the trained therapist with clues to the child's needs. I asked Alexander to complete these drawings during our first individual session (Figure 10.1). The instructions are to draw a house on one page, a tree on another page, and a person on a third page. In order to save space, I have placed all of the drawings on one sheet. They are reproduced here in their actual size, but each was drawn on a separate page measuring 8½ × 11 inches.

Each drawing was executed quickly, suggesting that this was an anxiety-ridden task. Several things are notable about these drawings. First is the very small size of each image. This usually indicates how

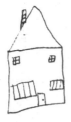 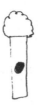

FIGURE 10.1. Alexander's House–Tree–Person test drawings.

small and helpless a child sees him- or herself as being. I assumed, therefore, that Alexander needed some boosting of his self-esteem and his ego, as well as a significant amount of anxiety reduction. The house has windows on the lower floor that almost look like teeth, suggesting some oral rage. This might indicate that he was internalizing much of his anger, which could be a factor contributing to his numerous migraine headaches. It is a two-dimensional house, which is unusual for a child of this age; there is also no ground line, suggesting that he did not feel that he had a solid base. In other words, Alexander's feelings of security had been badly undermined.

Like the house, Alexander's tree has no ground line, and there is a hole halfway up. When one looks at a tree with a hole in it, one considers that the height of the tree represents the age of the child, and that the relative placement of the hole indicates the age of a past wound or trauma. If we consider that Alexander was now age 10 and the hole is halfway up, this might suggest that the trauma occurred at about age 5, the age when his migraines began. There were no significant family events that anyone could recall during his fifth year.

The person that Alexander drew is of a nondescript nature, with the arms raised, almost like a baby reaching up for its mother. This drawing is typical of a younger child. Also of note is (once again) the lack of a ground line, as well as the fact that the feet point backward. The placement of the feet suggests that he felt safer in the past than presently.

Alexander did his first sand picture (Figure 10.2) during that session, and it revealed some amount of inner chaos—many figures were used, with no logical theme. This is typical of many first pictures, especially of those by children with an anxiety disorder.

As discussed earlier, sandplay therapy reveals developmental stages. Chaos can often be the first stage, followed by the animal–vegetative stage, the fighting stage (with the theme of good–evil), and finally an indication that a state of positive ego development has been reached and there is movement toward an increased ability to deal with problems. Dora Kalff (1980b) found in some of her cases that a spiritual connection was revealed, and she termed this "the constellation of the self," as noted earlier. She believed that it signaled a turning point in therapy, and it was a positive indication to her that the ego and the self, formerly separated by trauma, had been reconnected.

Space does not permit the illustration of all these elements. However, I would like to focus on a few examples. Figure 10.3 is a typical fighting-stage sand picture, with teams facing off against each other. This was made about 3 weeks after the first picture. Figure 10.4 was made about 6 weeks into therapy and is Alexander's version of the rescue scene at the WTC twin towers. He asked me what I might have that could represent

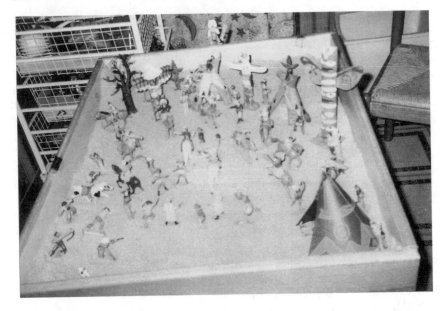

FIGURE 10.2. Alexander's first sand picture, revealing inner chaos.

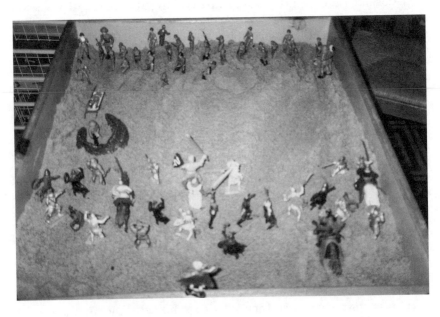

FIGURE 10.3. Alexander's fighting-stage sand picture.

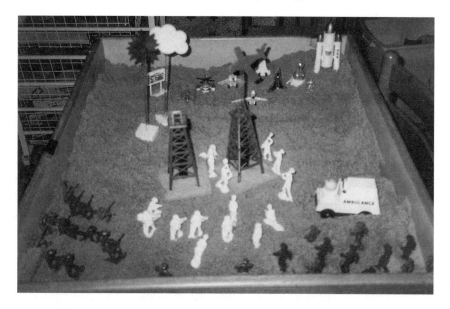

FIGURE 10.4. Alexander's sand picture of the WTC rescue scene.

the towers, and I gave him two miniature oil wells in my collection. He added an airplane soaring nearby. Then he placed numerous firefighters and rescue vehicles in attendance. Alexander and I both felt a sense of loss and devastation as we looked at this scene.

Some 3 or 4 months after therapy began, Alexander asked whether he could draw rather than use sand, and he produced Figure 10.5. This is a picture of the firefighters attempting to rescue those falling from the two WTC buildings. One building is red and signifies the fire. The number "18" on the fire truck is, I believe, the number of his father's detail. This same type of drawing was made by numerous children after 9/11. I saw many during my crisis work in New York City.

Figure 10.6 was made about 5 months after Alexander began therapy and was his depiction of people visiting the Statue of Liberty. They appear to be paying homage to what the statue represents. I commented to him that it looked as if the people (who form a cross) are placing their hope for the future with God. He was quite moved by my observation and agreed. I intuitively believed that his religious upbringing and innate spirituality were being revealed unconsciously in this picture. This is an example of the spiritual component in a sand picture.

The resolution, or turning point, of sandplay therapy is often illustrated by a sand picture, sometimes in a mandala form such as that seen in Figure 10.7; again, Kalff would refer to such a picture as "the constella-

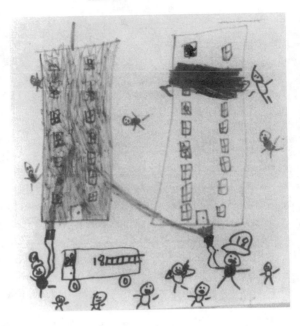

FIGURE 10.5. Alexander's drawing of the WTC rescue scene.

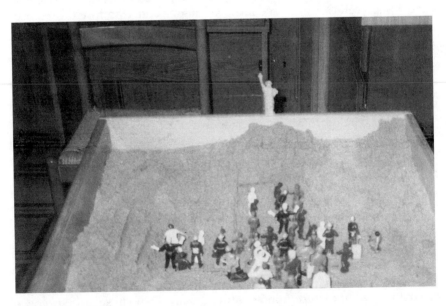

FIGURE 10.6. Alexander's sand picture of people visiting the Statue of Liberty.

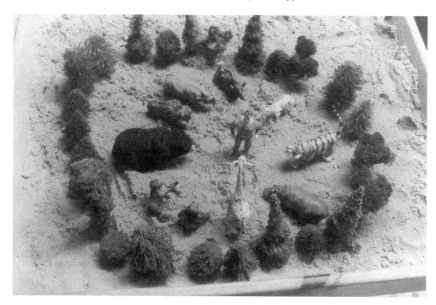

FIGURE 10.7. Alexander's mandala-like sand picture ("the constellation of the self," in Kalff's words).

tion of the self." This scene shows Superman in the center of a circle of wild animals, which in turn are surrounded by a circle of trees. Alexander had progressed from the very tiny self-portrait illustrated in Figure 10.1 to Superman (possibly his new self-figure) taking on the wild animals. One can only hope that Superman (Alexander) will be the victor!

This series of sandplay pictures and artwork illustrates the power that can exist in a nonverbal milieu. A child is able to verbalize his or her deep concerns in a way that is nonthreatening, nonverbal, and nonconfrontative.

The drawings and sand pictures, however, do not cover all that transpired during Alexander's therapy. Several sessions were held with one or both parents, some without Alexander and some when he was present. Mrs. Hobart, in particular, carried a tremendous burden. She was concerned not only about Alexander, but also about her husband. Mr. Hobart developed a lung condition as a result of his duties at the WTC and was on medical leave for a lengthy period of time. He was also extremely depressed about the loss of so many of his friends and colleagues. Mrs. Hobart needed to be the "glue in the infield," and she performed that role admirably. Alexander was not told about his father's mental or physical condition, in order to prevent any exacerbation of his own struggle. (However, he undoubtedly sensed the tension in the family.)

Mr. Hobart wrote an impassioned article that was printed in a trade magazine, in which he exhorted the need for firefighters and engineers to be aware of each other's needs. He described the problems there had been in the WTC with communications, egress, hidden stairwells, and so forth, all of which contributed to the huge loss of firefighters' lives. (I am not listing this publication in the references, in order to maintain the confidentiality of this case, but Mrs. Hobart believed that writing the article helped her husband achieve some resolution of his emotional distress.)

Alexander began to exhibit major separation anxiety when his mother had to go out of town on her coaching assignments. This disorder developed shortly after the WTC incident. Many of her travel dates could be directly identified as factors contributing to his headaches. He was able to verbalize that he was terrified that she would have an auto accident and thus be taken from him. He could not or would not go to sleep until she arrived home—often at midnight or later. Once or twice, she had to remain away overnight, and he stayed with an aunt. He was quite anxious on those occasions.

Alexander became somewhat resistant to therapy after about 6 months. He would tell his mother before a session that he didn't want to come any more, but he did not tell me. I explored these feelings of resistance with him, but he could never verbalize his thoughts about this. His answers to my questions were either "I don't know," or "Just because." My inner interpretation of the resistance was that he was being confronted with separation issues at this time and was terrified of any change that might ensue. He continued to be in need of the security of his mother's presence, and feared anything that was a threat to his relationship with his mother.

Another factor intervened: Alexander and his mother had to see the neurologist for a medication review. At that appointment, Mrs. Hobart brought up Alexander's resistance to therapy. The doctor suggested that therapy should definitely be continued, but thought perhaps play therapy was "too babyish" for 10-year-old Alexander. My own opinion was different. I believed that Alexander was stuck in the separation–individuation phase that is usually mastered by children by the age of 2 or 3. In addition, his nail biting and overall tension continued, and I sincerely believed that play therapy was the treatment of choice. However, given this family's cultural background where "the doctor knows best," there was nothing I could do but switch to a more verbal form of therapy. I also reduced the sessions to two per month at that time, to lower his resistance further. The doctor had suggested that Alexander and Mrs. Hobart discuss the separation issues together at a therapy session, which we did. I was able to interweave those verbal sessions with others where a more nonverbal modality was used. The picture with Superman as Alexander's apparent self-image (Figure 10.7) was constructed during that time. This indicates a more age-appropriate stance with regard to the separation issue—Superman does not need a dependent relationship—and it was hoped that Alexander no longer needed to cling to it either.

In the aftermath of 9/11, many rescue personnel from other countries offered help. One firefighter in Germany collected a large sum of money from his colleagues. He made several phone calls to various places in New York and found no satisfactory answer as to how these funds could be dispersed. Because he felt so strongly about this, he came to New York in person to ascertain the best way to distribute these funds.One of his first stops was the firehouse where Mr. Hobart was on duty. This was the first of several such meetings between Mr. Hobart and this "good Samaritan." The outcome was a plan to provide many survivors of the families of firefighters and Pentagon workers with an all-expense paid trip to Germany in the summer of 2002. The Hobart family was one of those included. There were over 70 persons in the Hobarts' group; three other equally large groups made a similar trip. Mr. and Mrs. Hobart were interviewed for a documentary that was being produced, and they hoped eventually to receive a copy of the film. It was truly gratifying to me to know that there was such an outpouring of love, care, and concern for the many victims of this unbelievable tragedy. The human spirit cannot be deterred when such a need exists. I would only pray that this type of humanitarian aid could spread to other parts of our troubled world without such a tremendous, senseless loss of life.

After the Hobart family returned to the United States, I met again with Alexander and his parents for a reevaluation of his condition. He had seen his neurologist on the day previous to our session, and Mrs. Hobart reported the doctor's observations. Mrs. Hobart told him what had transpired during the trip—primarily, that Alexander had not had a single migraine. She had given him approximately five Aleves during the trip, because she thought she could anticipate those situations that might lead to a migraine and thus head them off with the medication. Alexander was also taking the usual daily dose of verapamil. The doctor expressed concern about the frequent use of Aleve, and it subsequently was agreed that Alexander would ask for one when he felt it to be necessary—either when a migraine had developed or when he noticed an aura. In other words, Alexander was being encouraged to take control of his own condition, instead of Mrs. Hobart's being the monitor. The neurologist asked to see him again in 6 months, and it was (and is) hoped that eventually Alexander may not need much medication.

During the reevaluation session with Alexander, we agreed that treatment should be continued for the following several months on a bimonthly basis, and that we would focus on more expressive, nonverbal activities. This decision was based on my knowledge of Alexander—particularly his underlying anxiety state combined with his resistance to verbalizing any of his concerns. It appeared to me that a nonverbal modality was a far better approach to reducing his continuing anxieties than a verbal one.

Alexander was due to begin school again (this reevaluation occurred in the late summer of 2002), and this would undoubtedly contribute to an increase in his stress level. I explained to the parents and the child my difference of opinion from the neurologist by saying that I truly felt the best way to treat him was to focus on his underlying anxiety rather than on the number of migraines that he experiences. This new treatment plan was based on his stated wish to overcome some of the separation anxiety that continued to persist when his mother needed to travel. I explained the positive sign represented by Superman in Figure 10.7, but I also noted that Superman needed now to meet and confront some of those other things that continued to keep him from achieving true ease and comfort with his situation.

SUMMARY

This chapter has focused on one anxious child's reaction to the events at the WTC on 9/11. He was at risk because of several factors: (1) his history of migraine headaches; (2) his father's role in the WTC search and rescue operations; (3) the exacerbation of a separation anxiety disorder.

Art therapy, sandplay therapy, and family therapy were all employed in this child's treatment. Improvement was noted after the first few months, signified by the lessened frequency of his migraines and confirmed by what was revealed in the sand pictures. Alexander's resistance to attending therapy was ameliorated by decreasing the frequency of the sessions and by his recognition that his symptoms, though not fully resolved, were abating.

Several pictorial examples of Alexander's journey toward healing have been included. These demonstrate how, through the use of these creative milieus, he did indeed accomplish some resolution of his fears. In so doing, he was able to reduce some of his symptoms. Alexander agreed to continue therapy with the objective of addressing his remaining anxieties.

I would add that although the case example described is one of an existing condition that was exacerbated by a national crisis, the techniques used are applicable to other children who suffer from anxiety, depression, family issues, or overall limited emotional and/or developmental functioning. Sandplay therapy and art therapy are valuable avenues to explore when children have limited verbal skills or lack the maturity necessary to help them express their innermost fears.

The immediate post-9/11 time was one of major significance for all of us in the helping professions. We struggled to keep our own equilibrium and not to allow our personal issues to infect the work that we were doing, in order to serve the children and families that came to us. My own situation included the fact that my husband, who had suffered a stroke about 3 weeks prior to 9/11, was in a rehabilitation hospital when the attacks occurred. My son developed posttraumatic stress disorder after the crisis. He worked in the financial district, and had to walk home on the day of the attack with the black cloud following him. With all of these personal and professional stresses that were plaguing me, I considered retiring. However, with the help of colleagues, friends, and church, I have continued to perform what I believe to be the prime mission in my professional life—to serve children and families to the best of my ability, using my knowledge, my creativity, and my past experience in this career that I have chosen.

REFERENCES

Carey, L. (1999). *Sandplay therapy with children and families.* Northvale, NJ: Aronson.

Kalff, D. (1980a). *Sandplay: A psychotherapeutic approach to the psyche.* Santa Monica, CA: Sigo Press.

Kalff, D. (1980b). *Jungian sandplay.* Lecture presented at Jung Institute, Zurich, Switzerland.

Landreth, G. (1991). *Play therapy: The art of the relationship.* Muncie, IN: Accelerated Development Press.

Lowenfeld, M. (1979). *The world technique.* London: George Allen & Unwin.

Malchiodi, C. (1998). *Understanding children's drawings.* New York: Guilford Press.

Neumann, E. (1973). *The child.* New York: Putnam.

Nader, K., Pynoos, R. S., Fairbanks, L., & Frederick, C. (1990). Children's PTSD reactions one year after a sniper attack at their school. *American Journal of Psychiatry, 147,* 1526–1530.

Pynoos, R. S., & Nader, K. (1989). Children's memory and proximity to violence. *Journal of the American Academy of Child and Adolescent Psychiatry, 28,* 236–241.

Webb, N. B. (Ed.). (1999). *Play therapy with children in crisis* (2nd ed.): *Individual, group, and family treatment.* New York: Guilford Press.

Community Outreach and Education to Deal with Cultural Resistance to Mental Health Services

LIN FANG
TEDDY CHEN

The Bridge Program, an innovative model that integrates mental health services and primary care, was established in 1998 to provide mental health care for the Chinese American community in the New York City metropolitan area. Through understanding the cultural attitudes and service utilization pattern of the community, the program aims to increase access to mental health care, promote the skills of primary care providers, and raise community awareness of mental health issues. This is accomplished by offering integrated clinical services, provider education, and public education and outreach. This chapter illustrates how this program breaks through cultural resistance to mental health in order to respond to the mental health needs of children and families in the Chinese community through comprehensive and innovative approaches. Because we know that many other cultures in addition to Chinese Americans avoid seeking mental health services (Webb, 2001), we hope that the approaches presented here can be broadly applied.

MENTAL HEALTH SERVICES UTILIZATION AND THE CHINESE AMERICAN COMMUNITY: DISPARITY BETWEEN NEEDS AND SERVICES

As the fastest-growing racial group in the United States, the Asian American population has increased at least 172% (from 6,908,638 to 11,898,828) from 1990 to 2000 (U.S. Bureau of the Census, 2000). In New

York City, Asians constitute 10% of the city population, and 45.9% of these Asians are Chinese (U.S. Bureau of the Census, 2000). The need for mental health services is increasing as this population—largely foreign-born and linguistically isolated—rapidly grows. However, significant disparities between mental health needs and services for racial and ethnic minorities exist, as indicated in a report of the Surgeon General (U.S. Department of Health and Human Services, 2001).

Among all ethnic groups, Asian Americans have the lowest mental health service utilization rate (Cheung & Snowden, 1990; Snowden & Cheung, 1990; Sue, Fujino, Hu, Takeuchi, & Zane, 1991; Uba, 1994; Durvasula & Sue, 1996; Matsuoka, Breaux, & Ryujin, 1997; Snowden & Hu, 1997). As a result, when they finally reach mental health professionals, Asian Americans are often more severely ill or in crisis (Snowden & Cheung, 1990)—conditions that are costly to treat and may require lengthy inpatient services.

Three important sets of contextual factors explain the low utilization of mental health services by Asian Americans in general and Chinese Americans in particular:

- Limited availability and accessibility of services
- Cultural factors (such as shame and stigma, cultural beliefs about mental health, and symptom presentation)
- Underrecognition of needs by primary care providers

Limited Availability and Accessibility

Availability

The low availability of bilingual and bicultural mental health services in Asian American communities is a significant factor. A severe shortage of bilingual and bicultural professionals has been a long-standing obstacle for service delivery among most human service organizations in Asian American communities, and there is no exception in the mental health field. Furthermore, due to the constraints of personnel and financial resources, only a few mental health programs are offered; the results are often long waiting lists and long delays for potential clients (Chung, 2002).

Accessibility

The obstacles to accessing the health care system also explain the lower mental health service utilization rate among Chinese Americans. Financial constraints limit the access of Chinese Americans to the overall health care system. According to the Surgeon General's report, 20% of Chinese Americans have no health insurance. The rate of Medicaid coverage for

Asian Americans and Pacific Islanders is also far below that of European Americans. Only 13% of Chinese Americans who have family incomes below 200% of the federal poverty level are covered by Medicaid, compared to 24% of European Americans at the same income level (U.S. Department of Health and Human Services, 2001).

Cultural Factors

Shame and Stigma

The cultural inhibition surrounding mental health issues has a powerful negative impact on service utilization among Chinese Americans. The shame and stigma attached to mental disorders deter people in the Asian American communities from seeking mental health services. There are two major bases for this stigmatization. In the first place, individuals who fail to resolve difficulties themselves and who admit to having mental health problems are believed to be immature, weak, and low in self-discipline. Second, mental disorders are regarded as hereditary flaws of the patient's family. Therefore, the mental disability of an individual brings shame on the entire family. Such a belief places great pressure on patients and their families, and as a result, many choose to deny having any form of mental disorder to protect the family name (Uba, 1994).

Cultural Beliefs about Mental Health

Great differences in conceptions of mental health and treatment exist between Asian and Western cultures. These cultural variations affect definitions of mental health and mental illness, expressions of psychopathology, and coping mechanisms (Marsella, 1982; Wu, 2001). Preferences for alternative therapies, such as traditional herbalists, home remedies, and dietary measures, are documented in the literature (Pearl, Leo, & Tsang, 1995; Ma, 1999). The unfamiliarity with mental health services is also reflected in differences in conceptions of a problem and its treatment, and differences in choices of problem-solving strategies.

Symptom Presentation

Many Asian Americans do not seek mental health services because of the way in which their symptoms are manifested (Uba, 1994). Research findings reveal that Asian Americans are more likely to express somatic complaints than European Americans (Kleinman & Good, 1985). Several factors can explain the higher rate of somatization among Asian American groups. First, the somatic process indicates a holistic view of mind and body, which is commonly accepted in Asian culture. Moreover, expression of emotional distress through physical symptoms is appropriate or more acceptable to others from the same culture. Finally, reporting somatic symptoms to physicians or nurses is a legitimate way to gain access to mental health services at medical facilities without having to face stigma or shame (Akutsu, 1997).

Underrecognition of Needs by Primary Care Providers

Somatization or focusing on somatic symptoms of psychological distress naturally leads Asian patients to seek treatment from medical providers, rather than from mental health professionals. However, Chung (2002) has indicated that primary care practitioners, including Asian physicians who speak the language and share the culture of Asian patients, often fail to address mental health issues with patients during their consultations due to fear of embarrassing the patients, their own negative feelings and inaccurate myths about mental illness and its treatment, and lack of sufficient training to provide adequate assessment.

THE BRIDGE PROGRAM: A MENTAL HEALTH PROGRAM INTEGRATED WITH PRIMARY CARE

The Charles B. Wang Community Health Center (CBWCHC), formerly known as Chinatown Health Clinic, has had a long-standing relationship with the Chinese community in metropolitan New York since it was established in 1971 to provide bilingual and bicultural health care. The Bridge Program was established in 1998 as an innovation to address the disparities between mental health needs and services of the Chinese community as described above. The purposes of the Bridge Program are to connect appropriate mental health services for patients with identified needs, to empower physicians and other service providers, and to counter the misconceptions of mental health issues in the community. The program has three distinct aims:

- Clinical services
- Provider education
- Public education and outreach

Clinical Services

On-site mental health clinicians, including psychiatrists and psychiatric social workers, receive referrals from the primary care physicians at the health center and provide timely consultations, mental health evaluation, and treatment in the primary care setting. The integration of mental health services into the primary care setting decreases the mental health taboo, addresses the somatization issue, breaches the gap between primary and specialized care, and increases patients' access to the mental health care system.

Provider Education

In order to enhance the capacity of primary care providers (as well as other care providers from social service agencies) to ensure early detection of patients with psychiatric disorders, ongoing training is organized to improve the providers' skills and knowledge base in the identification and treatment of mental health disorders commonly seen in their work settings.

Public Education and Outreach

In order to raise the awareness of mental health issues and overcome the stereotypes of mental health problems and their treatment, ongoing community education as well as outreach activities are provided through a variety of means. These include the development and dissemination of bilingual literature, community workshops, health fairs, community mental health screenings, and radio/TV programs through the local Chinese-language media.

As a community health center that attempts to address the primary health care concerns of the local residents, CBWCHC provides a wide range of health-care-related services through its Health Education Department, its Social Service Department, and the federal Women, Infants, and Children program, in addition to medical care. Such a multidisciplinary setting allows the Bridge Program to serve the mental health needs of the Chinese community through a comprehensive and holistic approach.

TRAUMA, STRESS, AND LOSS EXPERIENCED BY CHILDREN AND FAMILIES IN NEW YORK CITY'S CHINESE COMMUNITY

Mental Health Needs of Chinese American Children and Families

Because Chinese Americans and other Asian Americans are usually regarded as "model minorities," the mental health needs of Chinese American children and adolescents have been often overlooked (Crystal, 1989; Lee, 1995; Tang, 1997). Not surprisingly, little has been learned about the mental health needs of Asian children and adolescents, due to the lack of studies (Lee, 1995; U.S. Department of Health and Human Services, 2001). Although in recent years a growing number of empirical and conceptual reports have discussed the psychological reactions of children to traumas, most of these reports are based on European American populations (Rabalais, Ruggiero, & Scotti, 2002), and very limited efforts have been focused on the needs of Asian children. However, despite the paucity of research on trauma and stress in Chinese American children, some findings indicate that mental health problems do exist among Chinese Americans (Crystal, 1989; Lee, 1995; Tang, 1997; Wang, 2001). For example, Sue and Zane (1985) found that Chinese immigrant university students have higher levels of anxiety than other university students. A study investigating suicide among Asian American youth aged 15–24 indicated that suicide was the third major cause of death in 1992 for Chinese Americans of this age group (Coalition for Asian American Children and Families, 1999). Based on the available literature and our practice experience, two distinctive risk factors encountered by the Chinese children and families of New York City are low socioeconomic status and immigration.

Socioeconomic Status

In New York City, more than half of the Asian American children born in 1999 (51.8%) were born into poor or low-income families that were Medicaid recipients (New York City Department of Health, 1999). The clientele analysis of CBWCHC also shows that 17% of its patients were uninsured in 2001. Such evidence suggests that New York's Chinese American community is an impoverished one. The poor socioeconomic status resulting from parental unemployment, poverty, and poor environmental conditions can contribute to a number of behavioral problems in children, especially among those from specific ethnic minority groups (Rabalais et al., 2002), such as Chinese Americans.

Immigration

Whether they leave their home countries voluntarily or involuntarily, immigrants always face the disruption of their connections with their significant contexts, which include the land, language, customs, families, social networks, culture, sense of community, and lifestyles (Marsella, 1994). These are compounded by the adjustment issues of education and language, as well as economic, social, and psychological well-being (Haines, 1989; Webb, 2001). Although immigration serves as a common risk factor for mental health problems in the local Asian communities, which largely consist of newcomers, the Chinese families are challenged by an additional unique phenomenon: It has been noted that during the past decade, Chinese newborns have often been sent back to China for child care soon after birth and return to the United States at about school age, due to family financial considerations (Zheng, 1999). The literature indicates that children and adolescents who are reunited with their parents after such a separation commonly experience multiple adjustment problems resulting from disruptions of their significant relationships with grandparents, extended family, peers, language, and culture in the home country, and are confronted with harsh environmental changes that include the different educational system, racism, gang violence, and discrimination against ethnic minorities in the United States (Alvarez, 1995; Crawford-Brown & Rattray, 2001). Given the long-standing stigmatization of mental health issues in the Chinese culture, these adjustment issues as well as children's manifestations of depression, sadness, anxiety, and anger are often overlooked; the results are higher risks of developing emotional disorders.

IMPACT OF THE WORLD TRADE CENTER DISASTER

Because Chinatown is the ethnic minority community in closest proximity to the site of the World Trade Center (WTC) in lower Manhattan, the terrorist attacks of September 11, 2001 on the WTC made a tremendous psychological and economic impact on Chinatown residents. A community survey done 5 months after "9/11" interviewed 555 Chinese residents; the survey showed that 88% had one or more major psychiatric symptoms during the first 2 weeks after the disaster, and that over half (53%) still reported one or more symptoms 5 months after the disaster (Chen, Chung, Chen, Fang, & Chen, 2003). A study conducted among 8,266 New York City public school students in grades 4–12 revealed that one-fourth of the Asian students met the criteria for one or more psychiatric disorders and also reported problems in their day-to-day functioning after 9/11. Among the problems reported were agoraphobia (13%), separation anxiety disorder (10%), posttraumatic stress disorder (PTSD) (9%), generalized anxiety disorder (9%), major depressive disorder (9%), conduct disorder (6%), and panic disorder (5%) (Applied Research and Consulting, L.L.C., Columbia University Mailman School of Public Health, & New York State Psychiatric Institute, 2002).

A COMPREHENSIVE APPROACH TO ADDRESS NEEDS FOR CHILDREN AND FAMILIES OF THE COMMUNITY

Public Education and Outreach Activities

In conjunction with the Health Education Department of CBWCHC, the Bridge Program has conducted a series of community outreach programs, including community workshops, writing contests, bilingual literature development, and broadcasting. This has been accomplished through working with schools, community social service, health agencies, local Chinese newspapers, and radio networks. The aim of these efforts is not only to reach a greater number of individuals, but also to target the larger community through establishing community partnerships.

Parent Workshops

Since 2000, CBWCHC has collaborated with New York City Community School District 2 on Project Excellence in Social and Emotional Literacy (EXSEL) to promote students' social-emotional development and academic learning. Serving in an advisory role, a the health educator from the Health Education Department and a clinical social worker from the Bridge Program are involved in a curriculum design for Project EXSEL that includes counselor training on the topic of how to work with Chinese parents while respecting the cultural norms of Chinese family values; such training is intended to promote counselors' awareness, sensitivity, and competence. In addition, the staff members work with local school guidance counselors and Chinese parents to identify the needs of the parents and to design the curricula for a series of workshops. In an interactive format, parents are encouraged to raise their concerns and to exchange ideas with the clinical social worker and health educator in discussions of their children's social and emotional needs, appropriate discipline methods, communication skills, and available community resources. After the 9/11 WTC disaster, the focus of the workshops was adjusted to include content about stress, anxiety, and depression. The following list presents the discussion topics from a workshop conducted at P.S. 130 in Chinatown in December 2001, and attended by approximately 30 parents:

- Triggers of stress, anxiety, and depression that can affect parents
- Signs and symptoms commonly seen in Chinese children when they suffer from anxiety or depression
- Ways in which feelings of stress, anxiety, and depression can affect parents' relationship with their children and families
- Recommendations for parents to alleviate their own feelings of stress, anxiety, and depression
- Available community resources to assist parents stressed and overwhelmed by the events of 9/11

The following aims were achieved: Guidance counselors and parents were empowered with knowledge and skills to identify, and become sensitive to children's emotional needs, to take timely and appropriate actions, and to provide a platform among themselves to share information and support each other.

Teens' Stress Reduction Workshops

In addition to conducting parent workshops, CBWCHC reaches out to members of the teenage population who are experiencing a high level of stress. Stress reduction workshops have been offered to several neighborhood high schools whose student bodies primarily consist of new immigrants. The following themes are covered in these workshops:

- What is stress?
- What can stress do to me?
- What is it like when a person is stressed out?
- What should I do when I or someone I care about has too much stress?

The workshops are conducted in the Chinese language and in an interactive way. Teens are encouraged to share their feelings and exchange ideas with one another. Specific individual concerns are addressed after the session by the presenters and followed up by school counselors or teachers.

Writing Contest

In order to increase awareness among Chinese teenagers about common emotional psychological issues such as stress, depression, peer pressure, and social skills, CBWCHC sponsored a student essay-writing contest in 2000 to promote emotional well-being among teenagers. The contest was open to students from grades 7 to 12 and was divided into Chinese and English subgroups. Participants were asked to write personal stories based on the following suggested topics:

- What are the obstacles/difficulties you have experienced in your life? How are you dealing with them? What have you learned?
- What can I do to help a friend when he or she seems unhappy or depressed?

Out of 180 submissions, 6 winners were selected by a panel of judges invited from local newspapers, social service agencies, and high schools. A formal press conference and ceremony were held to honor the winners, as well as to convey the messages to both parents and children that teens do have emotional needs and that discussions on such areas are important and appropriate.

Utilization of the Mass Media

The significant influence of mass media has been well recognized in the Chinese community. The local Chinese-language media are the major means for their audiences or readers, mostly immigrants, to receive updated information and knowledge. The CBWCHC has had a long-term working relationship with these local media. The Health Education Department has worked with several radio stations, newspapers, and TV stations, and has established regular programs such as "Health Mailbox" to provide community residents with a variety of health-related information.

The clinicians of the Bridge Program have also frequently served as guests on either taped programs or call-in programs to discuss with the audience such topics as stress reduction, ways parents can communicate with children, depression, and anxiety. Furthermore, staff members are frequently interviewed by reporters from local newspapers, radio stations, or television stations when incidents take place in the community, such as a teenage suicide, or teenage violence; after 9/11, several such interviews focused on methods to maintain emotional well-being. Frequently, articles produced as joint efforts of health educators and clinicians on various mental health issues are published in the five major Chinese-language newspapers that reach approximately 200,000 readers across North America.

Regardless of the medium utilized, the Bridge Program staff always presents the topics and content in a culturally appropriate way. Instead of sterile/medical terms such as "anxiety," "depression," or "children's emotional needs," clinicians are creative and sensitive in using more generic and acceptable phrases, such as "stress," "how to live a healthier and happier life," or "how to communicate effectively with your children." Doing this attracts broader attention, avoids possible resistance, and produces greater effects.

Literature Development and Distribution

Literature is considered an important public education tool. However, bilingual literature targeted to the Chinese American population is scarce. With this understanding, several fact sheets, brochures, and pamphlets have been developed or translated into bilingual format through the efforts of the Bridge Program, the Health Education Department, and pediatricians. Provided in both English and Chinese, these publications include the following:

- *How to Promote Children's Social and Emotional Needs*
- *Children and Teens' Reactions to Crisis and Death: Guidelines for Mental Health Staff, Teachers, and Parents*
- *Learn to Cope with Stress and Trauma*
- *Teens: Coping with Stress*
- *Attention-Deficit/Hyperactivity Disorder in Children*
- *Quick Tips for Parents–On Listening–Cooperation–Punishment*

These materials not only are available at CBWCHC, but are also distributed to schools, various social service and health agencies, and health fairs for wide dissemination. These titles are often mentioned during various public education programs, such as workshops and radio programs, to encourage the public to obtain them.

Community Screening

One of the innovative approaches of the Bridge Program is providing screenings through different settings in order to identify individuals who are in need of services, as well as to collect community epidemiological data. Since 1999, the Bridge Program has sponsored several health fairs and provided depression screenings. Individuals whose screenings are positive are referred to on-site clinicians for immediate consultation and provided with further mental health services or referral resources when needed.

After the WTC disaster, the Bridge Program designed a standardized questionnaire and interviewed 555 residents, from 8 to 86 years old, who came to CBWCHC and the Chinese American Planning Council (a major social service agency in Chinatown); the aims were to examine the psychological impact of the 9/11 disaster and to identify patients at risk (Chen et al., 2003). The comprehensive screening/referral plan developed for this effort is illustrated in Figure 11.1.

Recognizing the prevalence of teenage depression, CBWCHC plans to conduct another survey in 2003 targeting CBWCHC patients aged 12–18, to further explore the emotional needs of teenagers. A range of standardized surveys has been collected, and a working group that consists of teenagers, physicians, mental health clinicians, and health educators will select the survey tool that is most culture- and age-appropriate.

Provider Training

Because primary care providers as well as social service providers are on the front line in treating clients with emotional or behavioral problems, the Bridge Program has consistently offered continuing education to these providers both within and outside the CBWCHC. For example, several in-service training sessions on the topics of PTSD and attention-deficits/hyperactivity disorder (ADHD) have been given to an audience of pediatricians, nurses, medical assistants, social workers, caseworkers, and family health workers. These sessions have been conducted by the Bridge Program staff or outside experts. Three weeks after 9/11, a special training session on PTSD was provided by the psychiatrist and clinical social workers of the Bridge Program to the entire staff of CBWCHC, addressing the following areas:

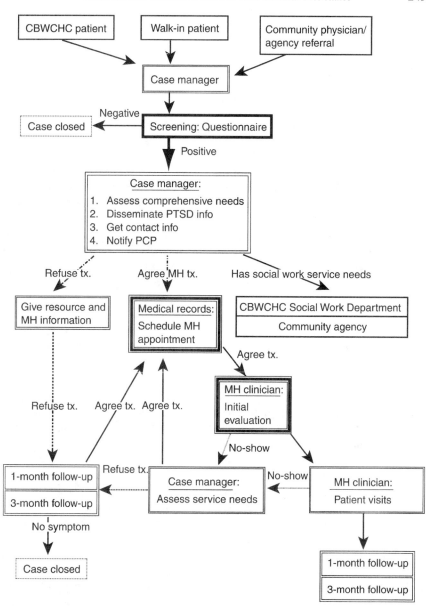

FIGURE 11.1. CBWCHC 9/11 community and clinic screening procedure. PCP, primary care provider; tx., treatment; MH, mental health. For other abbreviations, see text.

- Common signs and symptoms of PTSD among adults and children, with a focus on the symptoms commonly seen in the Chinese population
- Ways to evaluate the risks
- Available pharmacological and psychological treatments
- Case illustrations
- Tips to refer patients for further evaluation when needed
- Self-care for staff and providers

In addition, the Bridge Program has worked closely with different community agencies or coalitions. Program staff members have given presentations on such topics as recognition and treatment of depression and anxiety disorders and recognition of PTSD for providers of various programs. For example, in November 2001 the training program on recognition of PTSD was provided in collaboration with the Chinese Social Service and Health Council, an umbrella agency consisting of more than 30 agencies that serve the Chinese community in metropolitan New York. Participants in the program were case managers, nurses, social workers, physicians, and program administrators; the training focused primarily on signs and symptoms of PTSD that may be observed in the social service setting, ways to make referrals, and available community resources.

Clinical Services

Since its establishment, the Bridge Program has been one of the consultation resources for schools and social service agencies that serve children and families. Common reasons for referral include inattention, impulse control problems, truancy, unexplainable somatic complaints, anxiety, depression, adjustment issues, and parent–child relationship problems. As illustrated in Figure 11.2, children who are CBWCHC-registered patients, or those who use CBWCHC physicians as their primary care providers, will be assessed by mental health clinicians after the completion of a physical examination to rule out any physical problems.

From the initiation of the Bridge Program in 1998 through October 2002, a total of 634 patients were identified as having mental health needs and were evaluated by staff clinicians. Approximately one-fifth ($n = 134$; 21%) of those patients were aged 18 or under. Seventy-eight percent ($n = 105$) of these young patients were diagnosed with at least one mental health disorder, according to the *Diagnostic and Statistical Manual of Mental Disorders*, fourth edition, text revision (DSM-IV-TR; American Psychiatric Association, 2000). As presented in Figure 11.3, the primary DSM-IV-TR diagnostic categories were ADHD (23%), mood disorders (23%), adjustment disorders (22%), and anxiety disorders (10%). The number of

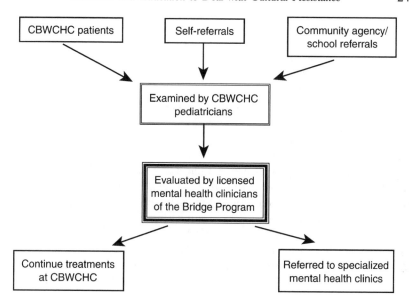

FIGURE 11.2. Mental health service procedure for CBWCHC patients.

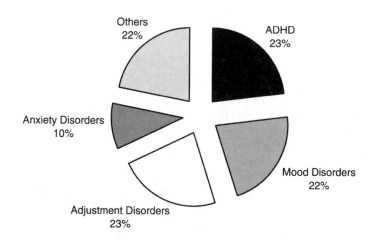

FIGURE 11.3. Bridge Program: Diagnosis distribution of patients aged 18 or under.

patients and visits has increased steadily over the years. Figure 11.4 summarizes the patient numbers and visits of the Bridge Program from July 1997 to December 2001.

CASE ILLUSTRATION

Mary, a 9-year-old Chinese American and the only child of a single-parent family, was referred by her pediatrician for a mental health evaluation in December 2002. She was a third grader at a local elementary school. This was the second referral, the first having been made in December 2001, when Mary had complained about headaches and nightmares during her physical examination. Mary reported that she started to have these problems after 9/11. In addition, she stated that she had been feeling scared most of time because of "those terrorists." No physical cause for these symptoms was identified in her doctor's visits. The pediatrician wondered whether Mary's physical condition was related to the WTC disaster, and therefore made the referral. However, her mother did not keep the initial appointment.

During the December 2002 evaluation, Mary said that she had been feeling scared since the WTC disaster. Although she did not directly witness the event, she knew about it through the extensive TV coverage during the period. She started to develop nightmares. At first her terrifying dreams were related to the WTC disaster, but recently her dreams had changed to scenes of earthquakes, after she studied earthquakes in her science class and realized that they could have devastating impacts. She knew that some distant relatives in Taiwan had had their home destroyed in an

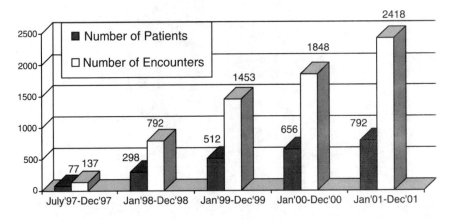

FIGURE 11.4. Bridge Program: Number of patients and number of visits.

earthquake a few years ago. She was afraid that an earthquake might take place in New York. Mary kept raising various questions related to earthquakes during the session: "Can an earthquake kill a lot of people?", "Did that ever happen in New York?", "Could it happen in New York?", "What do people do when there is an earthquake?", and "Are you afraid of earthquakes?" Mary also reported that she had started worrying a lot since the WTC disaster. She used to worry a lot about the terrorists; now she had a lot of fears about earthquakes as well. She constantly wondered whether an event similar to 9/11 or an earthquake could take place in New York. Whenever she thought about it, her heart pounded and her hands started to sweat. She could not get rid of the fearful thoughts and often could not concentrate well in school. She also avoided watching any scary movies and always needed to be accompanied by someone when she went to the bathroom.

Mary's mother was a garment factory worker. She confirmed Mary's story, and added that Mary had been a cheerful girl and had been doing well in general prior to the WTC disaster. She did not bring Mary to the scheduled appointment in December 2001, because she was hesitant to do so and was hoping that Mary would improve on her own. However, a year had passed and Mary had not improved; indeed, she was even worse. Therefore, she consulted with Mary's pediatrician again and kept this appointment, since the doctor strongly suggested that Mary should be evaluated by a mental health care provider as soon as possible.

The mother reported that Mary had changed a lot since the WTC disaster. For one thing, she had become a "worrier." Mary often called the mother at work several times a day to make sure she was safe and would be home later. The child was anxious and hypervigilant all the time. She also refused to sleep on her own any more, because she was afraid of the dark. Minor incidents could trigger Mary's strong emotional reactions. One recent example was that she cried out for her mother and burst into tears when she heard sirens outside their apartment. Moreover, Mary's grades were dropping, and she often complained of headaches and stomachaches.

The clinician approached this case on individual, family, and school levels. On the individual level, the clinician primarily focused on safety assurance and relaxation skills training. Each of Mary's worries was carefully addressed, while she was assured that people took her concerns seriously and were doing their best to protect her, her mother, her school, New York, and the entire nation. Moreover, the relaxation skills training effectively ameliorated Mary's physical discomfort. The clinician asked Mary to "play the air" (inhale and exhale) and demonstrated a breathing exercise. Several times when Mary complained of having acute stomach pain during the sessions, the clinician asked her to "play the air" right away, and the pain was gone in a minute. Mary was told that she could use the relaxation as a "medicine" whenever she could not fall asleep, felt worried, or had "heart attacks" (palpitations).

On the family level, family psychoeducation and parenting skills were the foci. The mother was provided with information related to anxiety and the ways in which it can affect a person's social and health functioning. Moreover, through several discussions with the clinician, the mother started to learn how to respond appropriately to Mary's behaviors, such as her questions related to her fearful thoughts and her frequent telephone calls. These discussions were particularly important, since this mother did not have much access to information about children's anxieties (she did not read English, and there were relatively few educational materials written in Chinese). In addition, she worked long hours in the factory and spent little time with Mary. Even when she did, she tended to rush through things without paying much attention to Mary's emotional needs. After the mother worked with the clinician and figured out several ways to handle Mary's situation more appropriately, several family sessions were facilitated by the clinician to reinforce the skills discussed during these meetings. The mother stopped saying, "It is nonsense," or "Do not think about it," when Mary asked her questions or told her that she was worried. Instead, she was gradually able to encourage Mary to express her feelings, to sympathize with Mary, and to provide her with assurance.

The school counselor and teacher were approached after receiving consent from the mother. They were surprised to learn about Mary's level of distress, because she had been always quiet and well behaved in class. After a conference among the school, the mother, and the clinic, Mary was given more attention and encouraged to ask questions in class. The school counselor also monitored Mary closely and maintained the contact with the clinician.

With the interventions, Mary's physical discomfort and symptoms of anxiety gradually decreased over the course of 2 months. She had far fewer nightmares and stomachaches. The palpitations were also less of a problem for Mary, and she was not as worried. She concentrated better in class, and her grades were improving. Moreover, she did not call her mother at work as often, because she knew "Mom would be home later." Finally, Mary seemed to enjoy her life more in general and became more engaged in school and social activities.

This case illustrates how each system—individual, family, school, and the community health center—can work together for the client's benefit. The Bridge Program plays a key role in terms of providing access to mental health care and organizing the treatment "team" consisting of different systems. Within this holistic framework, patients are provided with extensive and effective care.

CONCLUSION

In this chapter, we have first discussed the disparity between needs for and usage of mental health services in the Asian and Chinese American communities, and factors related to the low usage rate. We have then provided an example of an innovative program that increases service accessibility, destigmatizes mental health issues, and promotes the awareness of such issues in the Chinese American community. We have discussed a spectrum of culturally sensitive and creative activities, ranging from clinical practice to community action. We are pleased to share what we have learned, in the hope that our experiences can benefit other immigrant groups.

The lower utilization rate of mental health services among Asian Americans in general and Chinese Americans in particular actually reflects differences in the conceptualization of life problems between Americans of European and Asian origins. It may also reflect that the mental health system may not appear "user-friendly" to people in the Chinese community. It is necessary to address these issues in program design. In the Chinese American community, cultural factors related to mental health include people's way of conceptualizing their conditions, their cultural beliefs regarding mental health and mental disorders, their symptom presentation, and their actual help-seeking behavioral patterns. These factors were considered in the design of the Bridge Program and its services and activities.

Education is a major component of the Bridge Program. Creatively designed community education activities have attempted to normalize the concepts of mental health by making connections between behavioral health and daily life. Furthermore, education helps to increase awareness of mental health issues and minimizes the stigma attached to mental illnesses. Educational activities must also target the health care providers. The attitudes of many health care providers in the Chinese American community toward mental disorders are similar to those of the rest of the community. Through educational training that aims to enhance practice competency and sensitivity, service providers are encouraged and empowered to adopt new concepts, and thereby to become the first-line personnel in fighting mental disorders in their community.

Changes in the health care delivery system over the past decade have increased the public visibility as well as the number of patients of primary care physicians. Across different countries and payment mechanisms, the distinct features of primary care include (1) primary contact, (2) ongoing contact, (3) comprehensiveness, and (4) coordination. These components have facilitated the interface between the primary care and mental health fields (Starfield, 1998). Primary care physicians in family medicine, pediatrics, internal medicine, and gynecology confront a wide range of physical as well as mental health problems in their daily practice. In the Chinese American community, cultural factors make primary care an even more appropriate setting to provide mental health services. The generic nature of primary care lessens the intimidation and stigma associated with mental health. Taking into account the cultural factors and the practical reality of the intense schedules of health care providers, the Bridge Program facilitates systematic change by providing on-the-spot consultation by mental health clinicians. Such infrastructural design provides easy access to care for a community known for mental health service underutilization, and decreases the burden created by a tedious referral procedure. Ultimately, these interventions at the agency and community levels should prevent delays in treatment and promote the well-being of the community.

Several challenges remain. First, practice evaluation and program evaluation are needed for clinical practice and the educational activities. The Bridge Program has designed several measurements to assess the effectiveness of the clinical practice and has begun to implement these. Such analysis will help the clinicians as well as the program administrators to evaluate practice outcomes and determine areas for improvement. Another area to address relates to how best to elicit and formalize practice knowledge gained from clinical experience, and to enhance the knowledge base of social workers and health care practitioners in their work with Chinese Americans.

Second, the current community partnership consisting of health care organizations, schools, other social service agencies, and local media must be not only maintained but further expanded. In order to achieve long-term and broad effects, activities with successful outcomes, such as writing contests and workshops, should be held more regularly and involve more sponsors. In the meantime, more new activities should be explored via collective brainstorming. For example, the Bridge Program is currently attempting to engage some youth who have received mental health services, and to enlist them in working on an antidepression project. We believe that this can both empower the clients and educate the community through the consumer's perspective.

Lastly, the program's sustainability is a practical and central issue. The establishment of the Bridge Program was made possible by several grants from private foundations, including the Robert Wood Johnson Foundation, the Van Ameringen Foundation, the Pfizer Foundation, the New York Community Trust, and the Sergei S. Zlinkoff Fund. Now that the program has been developed with this seed funding, sustaining it has become a crucial task—one that directly affects the program's future direction. The continuation of educational activities inevitably depends on the grant support. Securing external funding for community services and promoting the internal productivity of clinical services are critical issues.

The Bridge Program is an interdisciplinary and multidimensional model to serve a lower-income ethnic community with great mental health needs. Despite the challenges ahead, we must continue our efforts and passion to work with our community through learning from our clients and our colleagues in daily practice. Enhancing clinical practice and continuing provider and public education are equally important for the quality of mental health services of the community. Notwithstanding some successful experiences, the learning process is ongoing; we plan to remain flexible and open to new concepts and to prepare for future challenges.

REFERENCES

Akutsu, P. D. (1997). Mental health care delivery to Asian Americans: Review of literature. In E. Lee (Ed.), *Working with Asian Americans: A guide for clinicians* (pp. 467–476). New York: Guilford Press.

Alvarez, M. (1999). The experience of migration: A rational approach in therapy. *Journal of Feminist Family Therapy, 11*(1), 1–29.

American Psychiatric Association. (2000). *Diagnostic and statistical manual of mental disorders* (4th ed., text rev.). Washington, DC: Author.

Applied Research and Consulting, L.L.C., Columbia University Mailman School of Public Health, & New York State Psychiatric Institute. (2002). *Effects of the World Trade Center attack on NYC public school students: Initial report to the New York City Board of Education.* New York: New York City Board of Education.

Chen, H., Chung, H., Chen, T., Fang, L., & Chen, J.-P. (2003). The emotional distress in a community after the terrorist attack on the World Trade Center. *Community Mental Health Journal, 39*(2), 157–165.

Cheung, F. K., & Snowden, L. R. (1990). Community mental health and ethnic minority populations. *Community Mental Health Journal, 26,* 277–291.

Chung, H. (2002). The challenges of providing behavioral treatment to Asian Americans. *Western Journal of Medicine, 176,* 222–223.

Coalition for Asian American Children and Families. (1999). *Half-full or half-empty?: Health care, child care and youth programs for Asian American children in New York City.* New York: Author.

Crawford-Brown, C., & Rattray, M. (2001). Parent–child relationships in Caribbean families. In N. B. Webb (Ed.), *Culturally diverse parent–child and family relationships* (pp. 107–130). New York: Columbia University Press.

Crystal, D. (1989). Asian Americans and the myth of the model minority. *Social Casework, 9,* 405–413.

Durvasula, R. S., & Sue, S. (1996). Severity of disturbance among Asian American outpatients. *Cultural Diversity and Mental Health, 2,* 43–52.

Haines, D. W. (1989). Introduction. In D. W. Haines (Ed.), *Refugees as immigrants: Cambodians, Laotians, and Vietnamese in America* (pp. 1–23). Totowa, NJ: Rowman & Littlefield.

Kleinman, A., & Good, B. (1985). *Culture and depression*. Berkeley: University of California Press.

Lee, P. C.-Y. (1995). Understanding death, dying, and religion: A Chinese perspective. In J. K. Parry & A. S. Ryan (Eds.), *A cross-cultural look at death, dying, and religion* (pp. 172–182). Chicago: Nelson-Hall.

Ma, G. X. (1999). Between two worlds: The use of traditional and Western health services by Chinese immigrants. *Journal of Community Health, 24*, 421–443.

Marsella, A. J. (1982). Culture and mental health: An overview. In A. J. Marsella & G. M. White (Eds.), *Cultural conceptions of mental health and therapy* (pp. 359–388). Boston: Reidel.

Marsella, A. J. (1994). Ethnocultural diversity and international refugees: Challenges for the global community. In A. J. Marsella, T. Bornemann, S. Ekblad, & J. Orley (Eds.), *Amidst peril and pain: The mental health and well-being of the world's refugees* (pp. 341–364). Washington, DC: American Psychological Association.

Matsuoka, J. K., Breaux, C., & Ryujin, D. H. (1997). National utilization of mental health services by Asian Americans/Pacific Islanders. *Journal of Community Psychology, 25*(2), 141–146.

New York City Department of Health, Office of Vital Statistics. (1999). *Summary of vital statistics*. New York: Author.

Pearl, W. S., Leo, P., & Tsang, W. O. (1995). Use of Chinese therapies among Chinese patients seeking emergency department care. *Annals of Emergency Medicine, 26*, 735–738.

Rabalais, A. E., Ruggiero, K. J., & Scotti, J. R. (2002). Multicultural issues in the response of children to disasters. In A. M. La Greca & W. K. Silverman (Eds.), *Helping children cope with disasters and terrorism* (pp. 73–99). Washington, DC: American Psychological Association.

Snowden, L. R., & Cheung, F. K. (1990). Use of inpatient mental health services by members of ethnic minority groups. *American Psychologist, 45*, 347–355.

Snowden, L. R., & Hu, T. W. (1997). Ethnic differences in mental health services use among the severely mentally ill. *Journal of Community Psychology, 25*(2), 141–146.

Starfield, B. (1998). *Primary care: Balancing health needs, services, and technology*. New York: Oxford University Press.

Sue, S., Fujino, D., Hu, L. T., Takeuchi, D. T., & Zane, N. W. (1991). Community mental health services for ethnic minority groups: A test of the cultural responsiveness hypothesis. *Journal of Consulting and Clinical Psychology, 59*(4), 533–540.

Sue, S., & Zane, N. W. S. (1985). Academic achievement and socioemotional adjustment among Chinese university students. *Journal of Community Psychology, 32*, 570–579.

Tang, N. M. (1997). Psychoanalytic psychotherapy with Chinese Americans. In E. Lee (Ed.), *Working with Asian Americans: A guide for clinicians* (pp. 323–341). New York: Guilford Press.

Uba, L. (1994). *Asian Americans: Personality patterns, identity, and mental health*. New York: Guilford Press.

U.S. Bureau of the Census. (2000). *Census 2000*. Washington, DC: U.S. Government Printing Office.

U.S. Department of Health and Human Services. (2001). *Mental health: Culture, race, and ethnicity* (A supplement to mental health: A report of the Surgeon General). Rockville, MD: Author.

Wang, J. Z. (2001). Illegal Chinese immigration into the United States: A preliminary factor analysis. *International Journal of Offender Therapy and Comparative Criminology, 45*(3), 345–355.

Webb, N. B. (Ed.). (2001). *Culturally diverse parent–child and family relationships.* New York: Columbia University Press.

Wu, S.-J. (2001). Parenting in Chinese American families. In N. B. Webb (Ed.), *Culturally diverse parent–child and family relationships* (pp. 235–260). New York: Columbia University Press.

Zheng, Y. W. (1999). *Voice of America report:Chinese immigrants send babies home* [Online]. Available: http://www.voa.gov/chinese/archive/worldfocus/sep1999/tue/092899chineseimmigrants.htm [in Chinese]

❦ PART III

Living with Traumatic Memories and Ongoing Fears

🎐 CHAPTER 12

Treatment of Psychological Trauma in Children of Military Families

THOMAS HARDAWAY

Approximately 1.8 million children in the United States live in military families. Although this number may seem numerically small when compared with the overall U.S. population of 72 million children, it represents a significant proportion of the population in geographical areas surrounding military bases, and in urban areas like Washington, DC. In addition, by virtue of available medical and mental health benefits, military children are likely to appear in the practices of civilian mental health practitioners for evaluation and treatment of mental health problems and stress. The stresses experienced by these children and by their families run the gamut from recurring and persistent chronic stresses (such as frequent moves and separations), to the moderate to severe stressor of having a parent deploy to war, to the devastating loss of a parent as a wartime casualty.

Evaluating and treating these families requires knowledge of the unique culture and military command systems in which they are embedded and in which they function. Therapists must understand the military-related issues in order to make recommendations that are realistic and relevant to such families. Similarly, therapists must understand the nature of the various stressors in the lives of military children in order to perform meaningful and helpful assessments, and to formulate effective treatment plans. The nature and severity of stressors can be divided into the following categories:

1. *Routine stressors*: frequent moves; changes in school and social milieus; and routine separations from military parents, who often must go into the field or to sea to train for up to months at a time.
2. *Acute, severe stressors*: wartime deployment of military parents; negative reactions from the surrounding civilian social structure regarding the work that a military child's parent is doing; and possible or actual injury to or death of the military parent.
3. *Chronic, recurring, and severe stressors*: living in remote, sometimes hostile foreign areas; accompanying threats or occurrences of terrorism.
4. *Complicating factors*: effects of mental health problems such as attention-deficit/hyperactivity disorder (ADHD), oppositional defiant disorder, and depression, as well as developmental delays and physical abnormalities, upon already stressed military families.

This chapter reviews the most common examples of each of these stressors in the lives of military families, the effects of these stressors upon their children, and the influence of these stressors on assessments and treatments by therapists who work with this population.

THE ROUTINE MILITARY LIFE STRESSORS

The life of the military family has been described as one of "gilded poverty"—that is, one in which, depending on the rank of the military "sponsor" (the active-duty parent), the family is paid relatively little in terms of direct salary compared to the family's civilian counterpart, but receives many other sources of support. This support comes in the form of housing; medical care; travel opportunities; and low-cost food, entertainment, and other privileges.

In exchange, the military sponsor (and his or her family) effectively gives up total autonomy, in the sense that the military sponsor is on 24-hour duty every day of the year. Unlike civilian workers, who have certain hours and days they are required to work or be available, military sponsors can be called up at any time, without extra pay, to meet a given need or military mission. This might include, for example, being called in for weekend duty, working an extra shift (i.e., 16 hours instead of 8), or going into the field for several weeks straight with no weekends or days off—all without any notice. Holidays can be forfeited at the last minute. A sponsor can receive orders one week before Christmas to be part of a disaster response, or to be shipped off to a remote location on the globe. There is no extra pay associated with extra hours, days, or weeks of work. Overtime pay is not part of military vocabulary.

Although the life of the military family can be positive and broadening, and can result in many uniquely enjoyable experiences not available to other families, the tradeoff is unpredictable and can result in much more stress for a given military family than for another. The variables that determine the impact of these experiences on a family are many. The extent to which a child or family is stressed by these experiences is heavily influenced by the particular job the sponsor has; the family's income level; the locations of assignments and associated schools that the child attends; the degree of both civilian and military community support; surrounding geopolitical times and circumstances; the flexibility and malleability of the parents and children in the family; the presence of already existing mental health, family, and medical problems in the family; and the personality attributes that family members bring with them into the military.

When a therapist performs an evaluation on a military child who is referred because of disruptive behavior in school, it is not uncommon to find that for some time, the remaining parent (still usually—though no longer always—the mother) has been raising this child in the repeated absence of the military parent (still usually the father), who has been away for weeks at a time. In addition, it is not unusual to find that the child has attended eight different schools in the last 6 years. Furthermore, the military parent may have just left again for a 1-year remote assignment. These findings are more common than uncommon in the average military family.

Studies have been conducted to examine the effect of routine separations on the remaining parent, and thus the effect on the children of the military parent (Amen, Jellen, Merves, & Lee, 1988; Hardaway, 1990a; Jensen & Shaw, 1996). School-age children and adolescents typically manifest both externalizing and internalizing symptoms in the form of irritability, home conflict, oppositional behavior, difficulty in concentration and task completion, and deterioration in academic performance. Compounding effects include frequently having to start over at a new school and establish a new set of friends.

In addition, now more than in past decades, the military family finds itself isolated from the extended family. Although this is actually a general phenomenon in the United States (i.e., all families have become more mobile and removed from extended family support), it is more of a problem when a temporarily single parent finds him- or herself isolated, especially overseas. When the family is located overseas, phone calls and visits are expensive and difficult, and the tendency is to move without the expectation of extended family support.

For an intake history, it is important for the therapist to obtain the following information:

- The length and number of separations between the military sponsor and the rest of the family.
- The number of schools the child has attended.
- The child's response to new situations.
- The way the remaining parent disciplines and organizes the family.
- The sponsor's "military occupational specialty" (i.e., his or her specific job within the military).
- Whether or not the family lives in military housing or a military community.
- The extent of other family support systems.
- The length of time the family is expected to remain in the community in which the therapist is practicing.
- The role of religion or place of worship.
- The backgrounds of the parents.

However, practitioners must realize that in addition to the unique features of military children, they experience the same internal development, the same reactions to stress, and the same mental health and medical problems as do all children. Thus a therapist may still be treating ADHD or depression, but it will occur in the context of the military demands on the family. Treatment recommendations must take account of the demands upon the military parent in order to be feasible and to achieve compliance. In one instance I encountered, a therapist recommended that a child's anxiety would be reduced if the sponsor would no longer go into the field or be separated from the family, and that there should be no more geographical moves. This basically served as the "kiss of death" for the sponsor's career and the family's only reliable source of income. The sponsor could even have been discharged from the military because of the restriction that he or she could not be deployed or receive training away from the family.

On the other hand, certain requests can be made of the sponsor's military command (e.g., to allow the sponsor's participation in the child's therapy, to stabilize the sponsor for a year without moves, or other specific requests), if they are framed in such a way as to indicate that the military's support for the sponsor to participate in therapy will improve the sponsor's functioning and actually make him or her more predictably deployable. The improved function of a sponsor's family member, or of the sponsor's family as a whole, is frequently regarded as a factor that improves the key functioning and "deployability" of the sponsor, because improvement in family functioning reduces the likelihood that the sponsor will be preoccupied with family problems.

All children's problems must be considered in the context of the child's surrounding family circumstances. This is especially true in assessing the problems of a military child. Treatment will be ineffective and possibly destructive unless the factors pertinent to the status of the child's military family constitute an integral part of the treatment plan.

ACUTE, SEVERE STRESSORS OF WARTIME DEPLOYMENT

One would think that with all the experience the U.S. military has had, its members would have an intrinsic understanding of the impact of wartime deployment on military children, and commanders would promote behavior in military sponsors that would minimize the negative impact on their families. However, like many other lessons of war, these frequently need to be relearned at the beginning of every new wartime conflict.

One lesson that seems to be very difficult to learn is the need for the military sponsor and the family to come together, to discuss, and to prepare for the upcoming wartime deployment. Unfortunately, great resistance to and denial of this need exist. Denial is a helpful defense initially for any loss or anticipated loss or separation. However, it is a very short-lived and ultimately ineffective defense or tool for dealing with the stress brought about by an upcoming extended separation, especially one posing risks to life and limb.

As a military sponsor and his or her military unit prepare to go to war, the intensity of the everyday mission rises exponentially; there is suddenly a demand to be mobilizing supplies, equipment, and personnel, and to have extensive, prolonged, and stressful planning meetings. These activities translate into much harder and demanding tasks, performed over 12- to 16-hour workdays, after which the soldier, sailor, or airman/airwoman returns home late at night, physically and emotionally exhausted, and not in the mood to discuss the upcoming separation with his or her family. The family, in turn, stressed in its own fantasies of the worst-case scenarios, is happy to collude with the military member's reluctance to discuss the deployment. It is not uncommon to find that families have not discussed even the rudiments of preparations, such as powers of attorney for financial and legal issues, wills, budgeting, or even arrangements for paying the rent. Even less frequently discussed are the more important issues regarding how family members will stay in communication, how the family will work together in the absence of the military parent, how the remaining parent will reconfigure supporting the family emotionally, or how the parents can help the children to process and grow from the upcoming deployment. And this assumes that there are not complicating problems, such as preexisting family problems, medical and developmental disorders in family members, or financial hardships.

When a child is referred for treatment, his or her behavior and emotional status may have been severely affected by the deployment of one or both of the parents. The therapist must consider the same military contextual issues that were discussed previously (the sponsor's military job, the extent of his or her absence, the child's previous moving and school experience, etc.). In addition, the potential impact of a much more severe stressor inherent in the context of wartime deployment now must be considered. In order to help the child with the presenting behavioral or mental health problem, an understanding of the military demands upon the family is critical. The practitioner may need to explain to the school (which may have no other children with deployed parents) the impact of this situation. The remaining parent may need help to begin processing in a constructive way his or her feelings regarding the deployment, his or her ability to engage in planning activities and discipline at home, and other factors that should have been addressed before the deployment but were not.

Phases of Deployment

In a study of the impact of deployment separation on children of 13,000 troops, Amen et al. (1988) divided the deployment experience into three phases: (1) predeployment, (2) deployment, and (3) redeployment. In the first phase, predeployment, Amen et al. noted that parents were in a "double bind"—wanting to be close, but needing to distance themselves as a defense against the pain of separation. They also noted the barriers caused by the long hours worked by the military sponsor in preparation for the deployment. Furthermore, there was the attempt by parents to "protect" the children by not allowing discussion of impending departure. Guilt feelings were noted in the children: "If I behave better, Dad won't have to go."

The second phase, or deployment proper, revealed some sense of relief as well as anxiety on the part of sponsors' spouses, one of whom stated, "Now I can get on with it." Some depressive symptoms were noted among the spouses, such as tearfulness, withdrawal from sources of support, sleep disturbance, sleep deprivation, and physical complaints. Anxiety was manifested by overprotectiveness of the children. There was an increase in "busy" activities—caring for other spouses and families. This increase was also noted by some military children in a small-group curriculum I developed (Hardaway, 1990b). At some point, many spouses even seemed pleased with their new-found independence, which later represented a problem upon the return of the deployed parents in the redeployment phase.

During the deployment phase, Amen et al. (1988) noted children's reactions as well. Developmental progression in many stopped or regressed. There was limited availability of caregivers at a time when the children needed the most nurturing. There was a "father hunger" syndrome manifested by grief reactions, sleep and eating disturbances, changes in mood and personality (including intense irritability), and wetting and soiling in younger children. In addition, there was preoccupation with the remaining parents, as I also noted (Hardaway, 1990b).

The redeployment phase, or time of return by the military sponsors, was also fraught with difficulties. Especially in extended and wartime deployments, military parents were not adequately briefed before returning home. They had developed somewhat distorted senses of entitlement as returning victorious warriors, with the expectation that there would be loving and devoted families and children just waiting to jump into their arms upon their return. These were very unrealistic expectations, as it was common for children to be guarded and quiet upon the return of their deployed parents. Families had learned to function without the deployed parents. The remaining parents' newfound independence was threatened. The remaining parents actually even felt some resentment and hostility, since they had had to deal alone with an array of discipline, school, financial, and other stressors.

At Fort Hood, Texas—the largest U.S. Army installation in the free world, where I practiced during and at the end of Desert Storm—there was a jump in spouse and child abuse rates when 30,000 soldiers returned home from the Persian Gulf. Much family turmoil ensued, and certainly much disillusionment was felt by both the families and the returning parents. Whatever family difficulties had been present prior to deployment became magnified. There had been instances of infidelity. It took a significant amount of time to bring families back to equilibrium. Two sessions of the small-group curriculum I developed for this situation (Hardaway, 1990b) addressed the children's expectations and worries, which helped them anticipate possible feelings and actions so that they would not be as stressed upon the return of their military parents. Unless these factors are addressed with the family of an index patient or client, focus on a behavioral or emotional disorder will be ineffective, or at least seriously compromised.

Supporting the Child Whose Military Parent Is Deploying

The most important way to address the severe stressors associated with deployment of a military parent is to engage the family beforehand in preventive actions. It is much more difficult to treat a problem after the deployment has begun and the military member is gone. A therapist can use the following guidelines to help parents before and after a deployment.

1. *Encourage family members to talk as a family before deployment.* Before a deployment, military parents are usually preoccupied with many preparatory activities at their military unit, requiring extended hours and increased workload. As noted earlier, these parents thus come home tired,

perhaps late, and are reluctant to address painful issues of impending separation. Other family members frequently collude in this. It is important to encourage families to overcome this resistance and make plans for a family conference as far ahead as possible.

2. *Have parents bestow, rather than "dump," new responsibilities on children.* Among the concerns often expressed by a child after a parent has been deployed are that everything has changed at home and the child now has to do "everything" that the deployed parent used to do. Discussions before deployment, in which trust and faith in a child's ability to carry out a responsibility are expressed, help the child to feel that he or she is important to the family and to the deployed parent, and that the child can help share a potential burden with the remaining parent. Although the child's perception is that "everything" has been left to him or her to accomplish, the reality is that a few selected responsibilities (chosen with regard to the child's age and ability to perform them) can be "bestowed" formally upon the child as an honor, rather than left for the child by default. As a result, the remaining parent will have more time and energy for all the children.

3. *Help the family make plans to continue to progress together, and to include the deployed parent in ongoing projects.* It is important that the family not put "life on hold" in anticipation of the return of the deployed parent. This will result in stagnation, loss of direction, and burnout. The family should make plans for specific goals to be reached by each of the children and the remaining parent, as well as family projects to work on. The remaining parent should help children design ways to communicate with the deployed parent, and to relate the progress they have made, so that the deployed parent can be part of that progress. For example, the children can send pictures and report cards, to which the deployed parent can respond and provide encouragement. The remaining parent and deployed parent need to make specific plans about how to communicate. Communication should be regular, but not too frequent. The remaining parent should keep the deployed parent informed and involved, but should not discuss problems and issues about which the absent parent cannot do anything.

4. *Family should continue existing traditions and develop new ones.* Very stabilizing factors in a family are routines and traditions. Friday pizza night or Saturday outings should not stop because a parent has deployed. If anything, traditions should become even more predictable. Family bowling night, attendance at and fellowship at places of worship, and involvement in events with other families are important ways to maintain a sense of stability and continuity. If the family has not previously had regular family traditions, now is a good time to start them. The remaining parent should encourage children to talk about these events and activities to the deployed parent in their communications.

5. *Parents should help children understand the finite nature of a deployment by devising developmentally appropriate timelines.* Although the parents may not always know the exact time that the deployment will start or end, it is still helpful to make an estimate and then to help a child craft a calendar of some type, illustrated and punctuated with events that help to define time for him or her. Examples of events to include are holidays, birthdays, special family and extended family events, school events, vacations, and other "markers" that help to divide up the time of deployment absence into short and finite episodes. A family can create a paper timeline, which extends around a room and can be illustrated by a child, or a chain made of illustrated paper links that are dated and illustrated. These links can be cut ceremoniously on a daily basis.

6. *To children, no news is worse than bad news.* Studies with children of deployed parents (described in more detail below) reveal that the children's main preoccupation from day to day is not with their absent parents, but with their remaining parents. At some level, a child is concerned about what is going on with the remaining parent. If that parent becomes tense, cross, self-absorbed, and/or tearful, with no explanation, the child's fantasies about that parent's ability to function are worse than what the reality is. Thus the remaining parent should be relatively open about sharing concerns and news about the deployed parent. If the child has an explanation as to why the parent is irritable, tearful, or preoccupied, it is much easier to accept. Parents should not use their children as surrogate adults and load all of their concerns on the children, but should use judgment in sharing enough to ease the children's worries.

7. *The remaining parent should listen to a child's worries about the deployed parent, and answer questions as truthfully as possible.* A child's questions can be followed up with further questions as to what prompted him or her to bring up an issue. Encourage the remaining parent to listen carefully first, before trying to dispel what may seem to be false notions on the part of the child; to explore as far as possible a child's questions and concerns, to show that the parent is trying to understand the child's worries; to refrain from pursuing the issue after a child appears to be satisfied; and to be reassuring about protective measures and training designed to protect the deployed parent, but to avoid false reassurances about the absent parent's not getting hurt or not dying.

8. *Firm routine and discipline should be maintained in the home.* Under the best of circumstances, maintaining order and routine for children in the home is difficult. It is even more difficult when one parent is suddenly absent. A child will manifest anxiety about this new separation, and the concerns over the remaining parent's ability to function, by testing the remaining parent's resolve, bending or breaking rules, and flouting routines. With the increase in responsibilities, numbers of tasks; and new

stresses, it will be tempting not to pursue and enforce limits. The remaining parent should be proactive and discuss with the child the intent to have very firm routines related to bedtimes, morning routines, room cleanup, chore accountability, and homework. The parent should then follow through with a clear and predictable set of consequences and rewards to keep the program going.

9. *The family should initiate and maintain a close relationship with the school and the child's teacher.* There should be a conference with the significant figures in the child's school, depending on the child's level. This may involve the child's classroom teacher for a young child, or several teachers, a counselor, and the principal for an older child or special-needs child. The remaining parent should make clear that the child's military parent has been deployed, and that there may be an increase in stress at home. Signs of vulnerability and stress in the child may include deteriorating academic performance, behavioral problems in the classroom, problems in peer relationships, unexplained mood changes, tearfulness or irritability, or worsening of previously existing behavioral problems. A plan should be devised with the school authorities for constructive and helpful responses to support the child and redirect him or her to previous levels of successful function. The remaining parent should be ready to have further conferences if necessary, and to be proactive and take the lead.

10. *The remaining parent needs to take care of him- or herself.* If one is interested in the well-being of a child, the dictum is always "Take care of the caretaker." Unfortunately, because of the many demands upon the remaining parent, it is difficult to make this happen. Parental self-care must be seen as a necessity and given high priority in planning. Frequently, the remaining parent is basically a working single parent. Such a parent can be told, "Let your child know that you will be much better able to take care of him or her, will be much more fun to be with, and will have more energy if you can take time to get out and exercise, take a scheduled nap, have alone time, or take time with a supportive friend. The time periods can be short, but should be planned, so that you are not feeling guilty. Express appreciation to your child when you take the time for yourself, and let him/her know how much better you feel."

Children's Responses to Separation in Wartime Deployment

Studies looking at the impact of war upon U.S. military children are limited, because much of the literature deals with the devastation of children who have been directly exposed to war situations. Examples are the direct or indirect exposure of children to violence in Israel and other Middle East countries (Baker, 1990; DeShalit, 1970), African wars (Shaw & Harris, 1989, 1994), Central American warfare (Arroyo & Eth, 1985), and religious conflicts in Northern Ireland (Fee, 1980). Because very few American children have been directly exposed to war, these studies seem less relevant to understand their responses to wartime deployment, which involve concerns about separation from and possible loss of or injury to a parent

The few studies looking at the effect of wartime deployment on U.S. military children reveal some predictable behaviors and responses. My observations (Hardaway, 1990a), when I administered a small-group curriculum to assist military children in public and Department of Defense (DoD) elementary schools with wartime deployment, were that the main preoccupation of the children was not with their deployed parents, but with their remaining parents (as noted above). They made frequent references to changes that had taken place at home, including these:

1. An increase in the amount of work and chores that had to be done.
2. Anxiety and friction with siblings.
3. Concern about their remaining parents' being tense, worried, impatient, or emotionally or physically unavailable to them.
4. Worries about their remaining parents' ability to cope or function.

Many of these observations were based on the children's fears rather than reality. But perceptions such as these cause anxiety and therefore constitute the grist of therapy.

Some additional observations in my study of children of deployed parents (Hardaway, 1990a) were that grade school children had bizarre fantasies about the activities of their deployed parents, where the parents had gone, and what it was like in the parents' new location. For example, when asked to draw where their deployed parents had gone, one child drew a picture of another planet; another drew a picture of an area of land right next to his home state of Texas, because "it's sandy in the desert, and when we went to Oklahoma, it was sandy there too." No child was able to identify the location in the world of the Middle East, Kuwait, or Iraq. One educational intervention included instructing the children in geography, and having them measure how many miles it was to their parents' deployment location. It was important to explain distance to the children in terms they could comprehend. For example, identifying that it took a day to drive 500 miles, the children took turns plotting 500-mile trips and connecting them on a world map to show how many days it would take to drive to the Middle East (without accounting for the ocean).

When asked about the people in the area where their deployed parents were going, the children spoke of those people as if they were menacing aliens, not humans. One drew a picture of Saddam Hussein in a blimp, drifting over the playground at her school, dropping bombs. Another was surprised to know that there were other children living in the area where the parent was. Treatment again included educating the children regarding the culture of the people in that area—what clothes they wore, what their schools were like, what activities the children were engaged in, and what food they ate. Humanizing the people in the foreign area was key to increasing the children's understanding and acceptance of the deployed parents' situation.

When the children were asked about what they thought their deployed parents were doing, one girl drew a picture of her father in a bathing suit, lying on a chaise lounge under the sun on the beach, sipping a drink. She knew her father was going where there was a lot of sand. She never knew what her father did at his job at home before, and she just made up something to fill in the gaps as to what he was doing now.

The remainder of the small-group curriculum used activities to help the children identify feelings in others, and their own feelings, through role playing and storytelling. They identified ways to put the feelings into words, so that they could communicate their concerns to others in more positive ways than acting out or getting into trouble. Involving the remaining parents in "homework" for these sessions helped these parents to become sensitive to their children's fantasies, worries, and occasional inability to find the words to express feelings accurately. The ultimate goal was to have the children identify constructive ways to elicit support from the environment (authority figures and peers), rather than acting out in ways that would create a nonsupportive or hostile response.

Another study noted that spouses of deployed military personnel became overwhelmed during separation and were consequently indulgent, somewhat numb, and inconsistent with routines and discipline (Amen et al., 1988). The same study indicated that other mothers whose husbands were deployed became overprotective toward their children. This study confirmed some observations noted in my study—that mothers generally had less patience, and that some just withdrew completely.

Other studies have reported behavioral responses in children of fighting, defiance, fear, depression, anxiety, and school difficulties (Crumley & Blumenthal, 1973). These are the behaviors my colleagues and I attempted to decrease through the therapeutic curriculum. In a comparison study of children and families of military personnel deployed during peacetime versus wartime, Kelley (1994) noted that families that experienced *peacetime* separation reported higher levels of family togetherness after the fathers' return. Previously disrupted family interactions during the separation improved with more family closeness upon the fathers' return. In contrast, Kelley (1994) noted that wives of husbands deployed during the 1990–1991 Persian Gulf War reported less ability to maintain nurturing, cohesive family environments. In these circumstances, it was more difficult to regain the initial family closeness after the reunion. Kelley speculated that this could be due to the war-related anxiety and uncertainty, and perhaps the fathers' changed behavior upon return from war.

Kelley's (1994) study revealed that "in contrast to the behavior of peacetime children, which exhibited fewer problems over time, [the behavior] of children with fathers in the Persian Gulf War did not improve" (p. 109). This probably reflected the additional stress experienced by the families, and also the observation (as noted in the curriculum small groups) that children may be particularly sensitive to maternal behavior and family closeness during a stressful deployment. With the added dimension of television coverage, the children in the study had considerable difficulty interpreting events, and the distorted and threatening perceptions appeared to affect their behavior adversely.

These findings and observations underscore the need to provide support and education to children and remaining parents in processing the separation, the concerns over death and dying, and the marked changes in their households and families upon deployment. This kind of support can be part of therapy when used to deal with problem behaviors or emotional conditions. This support can also be provided in a more routine and less stigmatizing way through educational activities in small groups of children with deployed parents. This can be done with an entire classroom or in small groups of children with or without recognized problem behaviors.

MILITARY CHILDREN EXPERIENCING DEATH OF A MILITARY PARENT

Although an extensive literature exists addressing the issues of grief in children experiencing traumatic loss or death of a parent, there is very little written about the grief experienced by children in military families who lose a parent as a wartime casualty. As in other issues involving military children, there are unique factors involved in assisting them—some of which are negative, others positive.

When a parent dies as a wartime casualty, there are many built-in financial and support benefits that attempt to recognize, if not compensate for, the tremendous sacrifice made by the military parent and the family. There are associated honors, which usually are spelled out publicly in many ways, so that the family knows that this parent's death is respected by peers, coworkers, other students at school, school staff, and the community at large. This reverence and outpouring of appreciation add a helpful dimension not usually afforded to children who lose a parent to other causes.

A military burial at a national cemetery further assists the family regarding decisions about the burial location and arrangements. The military honors bestowed upon the military member, spouse, and family are an outward demonstration of national appreciation for the soldier, sailor, or pilot who makes the supreme sacrifice for the country's freedom.

Although there is some financial death benefit in this situation, it is relatively small in terms of compensation for lost future wages, or of the family's future financial needs. Unless the military member has made extra life insurance arrangements, the family is usually left with relatively little to live on subsequent to the death.

What is especially difficult is the usually sudden manner in which everything happens. The notification is by definition abrupt—not insensitive, but certainly unexpected. A casualty office team of representatives from the command of the military member's unit, along with a chaplain, is dispatched to the home. The news is given in person to the family, and further support is provided by members of the military unit who subsequently assist and comfort the family. However, one can only imagine what it is like for a child sitting in class to receive this news, especially where there are other military children whose parents are deployed to war. This experience is conveyed by Carroll and Mathewson (2000):

> The classroom door opens and the school nurse steps in. Everyone is tense and fears the worst. A name is called, but it's not yours. Susan collects her books and heads for the door. She glances back and you do your best to give her a reassuring smile. You don't see her again, because the news that came that day was that her father had been killed in a land you can't even pronounce, near where your own dad is serving. You have a mixed reaction of sadness for her and fear for yourself. How close it was to being you! You hear later that Susan left quickly with her mom and little brother for the States for a funeral at Arlington National Cemetery. They came back to Germany only long enough to pack up their belongings and figure out where to go. Rumor had it they wound up back in the little Midwestern town where Susan's mom had grown up, to live with Grandma for a while and try to "sort things out" (p. 250)

One of the main difficulties in treating military children who have experienced such a massive and sudden loss is that they do not stay in the military. Their families have a certain amount of time (weeks or months) to move out of their quarters or military housing; the children must leave their DoD dependent school, if the families have been assigned overseas; and they get only acute initial support from their peers and community, because they must leave that community. If a family's members live stateside in a civilian community, there are issues as to whether they can still afford to live in their home, whether they need to move in with extended family members while the surviving parent regroups and looks for other work, and whether the family's civilian peers can truly understand the nature of what they are going through. If the family is more enlightened, its members may be fortunate enough to have been plugged into a supportive church or synagogue, or to have established a network of social contacts in the community. However, in the majority of instances, the family is relatively young and not particularly sophisticated in having established prior networks of support. Thus the initial devastation of the death and loss is compounded by the ensuing social, educational, and financial disruption and isolation.

Carroll and Mathewson (2000) describe a successful organization known as Tragedy Assistance Program for Survivors (TAPS), which provides support for military families who experience this kind of tragedy and loss. TAPS sponsors an annual Kids Camp in Washington, D.C., which provides a group setting for children of deceased military parents. There are multiple group and individual activities to assist the children in expressing feelings that may not be appreciated by others who cannot relate to their experience. The camp has the normal social and outdoors activities to promote peer support, in addition to group sessions that allow the children to do important processing and grieving–not only with respect to their past loss, but regarding ways they deal with their grief now, and their plans for future development of full and productive lives. They have field trips through the D.C. area that serve to promote pride in the values of the country that their parents died defending. Along with the children's program, there is a program enabling the surviving spouses to do similar therapeutic work with other spouses, while the children are engaged at their camp. This gives the parents much-needed respite and the opportunity to engage in necessary and constructive grieving with the help of facilitators and other grieving spouses.

When a therapist is consulted because of the loss suffered by a child of a deceased military member, the therapist must once again consider all the variables that can complicate an already traumatic loss. That is, a careful history must clarify previous stressors associated with the child's military life (e.g., moves, schools, assignments to remote areas), as well as previously existing emotional, behavioral, and family problems. The effects of loss and subsequent grief never occur in a vacuum; they are always complicated by the context. In these cases, it is important not only to know the personal context, but the impact of the military context as previously described, in order to address all the complications that may act as barriers to the grieving process. Local military support resources can serve as vital aids to enhance therapy.

Specific guidance in the assessment of children who have experienced death of a parent, along with the assessment of the distinction between "normal" and "disabling" grief, is provided by Webb (2002). Further descriptions of helpful specific modalities of treatment are given in the same work. Art, storytelling, and groups are valuable ways to assist children in general with the grieving that is so necessary to restore their functioning and optimal continued development. With military children, it is important to add that the makeup of bereavement groups should be as homogeneous as possible. That is, they should have the same contextual background: They should be composed of children from military families, who have experienced the death of a parent in military action.

Finally, if the always feared loss of a parent in war does happen, it need not bring a child's life and development to a stop. When a civilian practitioner is aware of the military issues described above, and is sensitive to the impact of this loss, such a therapist can provide much-needed relief by assisting the child and family to engage constructively in the grieving process so that there can be personal and family growth and healthy development.

TERRORISM THREATS AND LIVING IN HOSTILE ENVIRONMENTS

The events of September 11, 2001 brought issues of terrorism into the forefront of professional efforts to assist children and adults with the impact of trauma. This was because the threat of terrorism had actually come onto U.S. soil and become real for the general population. However, for decades prior to "9/11," the threat of terrorism and actual acts of terrorism have been certain and concrete reality for families of government workers and military personnel overseas.

While conducting small-group assessments and therapy in DoD elementary schools in Germany during Operation Desert Shield/Desert Storm, I (Hardaway, 1990c) included sessions on terrorism because of the imminent threat and actual acts of terrorism that had occurred in the geographical area where these children lived. A few years previously, an American Army general had been killed in a terrorist bombing in the U.S. military area of Heidelberg. The same month that the small groups were held, a bomb exploded at the local train station in Frankfurt. Children at that time were being subject to searches of their cars when their parents drove them off the housing areas to school, or even to get groceries on base. There were armored personnel carriers with 50-millimeter machine guns in front of their schools, and there were armed military guards patrolling the school halls.

For U.S. embassy personnel, both military and nonmilitary, terrorist acts at home and at the workplace are not new. Rigamer (1986) noted the reactions of children of government workers at the U.S. embassy in Kabul, Afghanistan. These military and nonmilitary families actually lived in the embassy compound when the U.S. ambassador was assassinated, and there were further subsequent terrorist threats from the Palestine

Liberation Organization. In addition, there was a simultaneous threat of a Soviet political coup of the regime. The children of the embassy personnel were, in this case, directly exposed to the terrorism threat and acts. The reactions and questions by the children included these: "Will we get bombed, too? Can we get out of here, or do we stay here like the Afghans? Will they kill more Americans? Could Daddy or Mommy be killed?"

So it is clear that the anxiety associated with 9/11 was not new for the children of military families—especially those assigned to remote areas, or to even areas considered friendly, such as in European host nations. However, the 9/11 acts were of such a magnitude that the reaction by adults raised great anxiety and concern in children.

Military Children's Reactions to 9/11

In the aftermath of 9/11, I again worked with small groups of elementary-age children in the DoD schools in Germany. The following unexpected phenomena were noted: First, children manifested an acute awareness and understanding of the facts and issues surrounding the 9/11 act. They were especially stressed by two issues. First, they were very worried by the initial reactions of their caregiving adults. One second grader stated that one adult had shaken her when she did not seem to be very concerned, and stated, "You're not concerned at all! Don't you know what just happened?" The child described that event as having been the most upsetting moment of the whole ordeal.

The other stressful issue was the repetitive nature of the events as broadcast on TV. One boy in the third- to fifth-grade group described having had repetitive dreams that the "plane keeps flying into the building." Another boy in the group looked at him and said, "That's because the plane keeps flying into the building over and over again on TV!" Although the first boy probably was describing some mild manifestations of posttraumatic stress, the second boy did have an important point: The television coverage tended to be all-consuming and took up every moment of the broadcast time for a long time after the event.

An additional unexpected phenomenon that I found upon preparing to implement a small-group curriculum for children to assist in dealing with terrorism and 9/11 issues was that ultimately they did not need it. Although there had been understandable panic, anxiety, and grief reactions on the parts of adults initially, the surrounding family, school, and military community had done a remarkable job in tending to the children in very important ways.

Families had felt the need to come together, because they were in a relatively isolated environment. Schools had developed well-organized plans to structure the children's experience and perceptions. They had developed reassuring security plans, as well as plans to communicate quickly with all families and school staff. The schools had coordinated very closely with the surrounding military community and leadership to come in and brief the children on what was being done to keep the community safe and secure. Children could recite all the security precautions with each threat level. When I asked a group of first and second graders what all the guards and barricades were about, one second-grade girl looked incredulously at me and asked, "Where have you been? Don't you know about 9/11? This is much better now that we're at 'threatcom Charlie.' You should have seen us when we were at 'Delta'!"

Military leadership came in and gave realistic but reassuring briefings; these educated the children not only on security issues, but on measures that were being taken to combat the terrorists. One Air Force pilot came and let the children go through some of the relief packs to see what food and other necessities were being dropped to the Afghan people who were suffering. This provided a human element to the otherwise nebulous perceptions of where their Air Force parents were being sent on their missions.

For these children living on military installations in Germany after 9/11, there was no "return to normal" as there was for nonmilitary children back home, where people returned to their routines of visiting malls, going to school, and basically living life as usual. These military children were well aware that they were still potential targets, and that they had to be vigilant when traveling with their families. They had to walk long distances to buy groceries with their families at the base commissary, because there were concrete barriers that kept them from parking within 100 yards. In addition, they were still being checked on their school buses for an identification badge that even kindergartners had to have around their necks. They had to be prepared to leave the bus if they didn't have their passes. They still experienced the daily routine of having their school bus checked for bombs upon coming in through a special entrance to the base, and they saw weapons trained at the gate they were entering. Yet these children were not in need of the curriculum I had thought they would need. This was because appropriate security and reassurance practices were in place.

Terrorism-Related Treatment Planning for Military Children

Therapists who work with military children around issues of terrorism should utilize measures parallel to those taken by the community and schools as described above.

In a paper on developing treatment strategies for children in dealing with terrorism (Hardaway, 2001), I recommended that a therapist should work from some basic principles to build an individual treatment plan or preventive education plan. These include the following (Hardaway, 2001):

1. Children's concerns and fears regarding terrorism should be addressed in a child's everyday setting, rather than in a therapist's office or clinic setting, if possible.
2. Fears and concerns are best addressed in a child's group of peers.
3. Clear information should be delivered in a developmentally appropriate and sensitive way, with further clarifications as requested by children if necessary. "No news is far worse than bad news."

The next step is to define the actual problem to be addressed. It is one thing to speak in general terms; it is another to have a child in therapy for a given problem and to address it directly. The following problems are typical of school-age children:

1. Unspoken, undefined, and frightening thoughts and fears.
2. The perception that fears should not be mentioned, due to the possibility of worrying or angering parents or other potentially supportive adults.
3. Confusion about whether police checkpoints, guard patrols, car searches, or evacuation drills are sources of comfort and protection or signs of imminent danger.
4. Concern that terrorist acts can happen at any time, right away, in play areas, schools, and homes.
5. Lack of knowledge about the actual geographical location and frequency of terrorist attacks. Children infer the frequency of attacks proportionately from the amount of time these are given on TV. For instance, if these actions and threats are being addressed for 60% of the TV time, then it must follow to children that there is a 60% chance of the actions' taking place again. In the children's minds, the attacks are imminently likely to occur daily at their schools and dwellings.

A focused treatment plan moves from the assumptions and specific problems noted, and formulates individual or mass education objectives. Objectives for treatment of individual children with behavioral and emotional difficulties, and also for populations of military school children, are as follows (Hardaway, 2001):

1. The children will be aware of their specific fears regarding the nature, possible times, and possible places of terrorist attacks.
2. They will communicate these fears to trusted adults and peers.
3. They will be able to demonstrate awareness of the fears of their siblings, friends, and school peers.
4. They will be able to state a more realistic incidence rate and likeli-

hood (in their own terms and understanding of time and frequency) of forthcoming and possible attacks.

5. They will be able to list common-sense measures to take as reasonable and prudent precautions to avoid becoming targets and to avoid provoking nonsupportive responses from peers and authority figures in the environment.

6. The children will be able to explain the obvious protective roles played by the police and security provided by the military "threatcom" procedures that they see daily; furthermore, they will know that these measures do not constitute evidence of imminent attack.

7. The children will be able to use common-sense precautions with a sense of control over their lives, to the point where they can work, play, and otherwise function without undue emotional burden or distress related to terrorism fears.

Lenore Terr (personal communication, December 2001; see also Terr, 1990)—who has closely studied the effects of trauma in children, most notably in the kidnapped children in Chowchilla, California—has distilled four major principles to consider in planning an intervention to assist a child with either anticipated, ongoing, or past trauma:

1. Discern the *affect* of the child first. In this case, "affect" refers to the nature of the child's emotional, visceral, or "gut" reaction to the threat. Observe the child's behaviors, reactions, and verbal responses, which provide clues as to how emotionally affected the child is by the threat. Without colluding in the child's perceptions, attempt to validate the child's feelings, emphasize that he or she has a right to them, and state that they certainly are understandable, given the child's experience and memory. The child must feel that the therapist, or group facilitator, understands and accepts the child's feelings and worries.

2. Evaluate the child's understanding of *context*. That is, a helper must know (based on the child's cognitive, emotional, and psychological developmental level) the child's perceptions of the significance of a terrorist event, the immediacy of the threat, the nature of the threat, and the resulting perception of the direct relevance of the threat in the child's life. The child's perceptions of context have to do with the cognitive understanding of issues related to time, geography, and cultural/political situation, as well as more personal issues related to understanding reasons for the behavior of significant adults in the child's life, such as parents, teachers, and others. These must be understood before any meaningful intervention can be planned.

3. Based on the understanding of the child's affect and perceptions of context, *education* is provided to address the distortions and mis-

perceptions causing the anxiety that is impairing the child's ability to function. The education is very effective in a group setting when possible, so that the child does not feel somehow abnormal or defective because of his or her feelings or worries. The same principle applies in individual therapy, where these worries are part of a larger clinical problem that is being treated. The education should be at an appropriate developmental level, and should be simple and as short as possible. Questions should be addressed, but without going into detail that is distracting to the child. Education can be verbal or can be provided in various activities, such as drawing, videos, or discussion. Verbal discussion is more likely to be effective for middle and high school students, while younger children will require learning activities such as drawings to focus their attention and to help them to comprehend and remember what they have learned.

4. The final step is to provide the child with ways to alter *behavior* that will give the child the genuine sense of being in control of his or her life. This is where interventions are designed to help the child to change behavior to accomplish this objective. We know that children who experience severe trauma, and whose function is impaired as a result, have a sense that they have no control. Thus, in play therapy, these children will repeat certain situations over and over without ever achieving the sense of mastery. The goal here is to assist a child to achieve this sense of mastery and ability to conquer a threat. Most play addresses the need to do this all the time. Cops and robbers, cowboys and Indians, and video games all present a threat, and although there is an illusory component to the sense of omnipotence, playing such games does develop some skills that are reassuring to the child. In therapy, the child uses play to express feelings and experience validation from the play therapist (Webb, 1999, 2002).

For a military child, answering the following specific questions can increase the child's sense of security and mastery:

1. What are grownups already doing around us to protect us and make our lives safe and secure?
2. What do our moms and dads do at home to protect us?
3. What do our teachers do, and what kind of rules do they give us, so that we can learn in a safe and predictable environment?
4. What are our schools and principals already doing to keep us safe, and to help us focus on our primary job of learning and living with each other?
5. What does the military do around us to protect us?
6. What can we do as individuals to stay safe?
7. What can we do to make things safe for others and for our friends?
8. What are common-sense approaches to handling mail when there

are concerns over anthrax? (Examples: opening only mail we recognize, and allowing Mom and Dad to open up all other mail.)

9. Why is it important to learn effective ways to solve problems and
conflicts with each other?

10. Why do certain individuals sometimes grow up wanting to hurt
others?

11. Some children who feel excluded, who feel less smart or less
good at athletics, or who don't know how to make friends grow
up and become angry with everyone. What are ways we can help
others who don't have as many skills to become part of our
groups?

12. What is the difference between tattling, and telling a grownup if
someone is harassing or bullying? What must grownups be willing to do with children who are angry, who are bullies, and who
harm others?

Helping a child formulate behaviors to address these concerns, or to be
able to verbalize behaviors that supportive adults engage or should engage in, will decrease behavioral and emotional dysfunction based on the
anxiety associated with terrorism.

Terrorism may become less of a problem for the general population
in the United States, depending on the effectiveness of the Department of
Homeland Security and military efforts. However, the threat will always
exist for military children and families, because they will always be considered as targets by whatever group of terrorism is carrying out its agenda.
Thus understanding and being able to address these concerns in military
children will always be important in addressing the context in which they
live, and in planning treatment for their emotional and behavioral problems.

CONCLUSION

In this era of new threats and challenges to children and to their parents,
counselors, therapists, and mental health professionals have an additional
dimension that they must be able to address. Mass trauma and psychological casualties are now no longer just the realm of military personnel, police officers, or firefighters. They are now part and parcel of the entire
population.

In order to treat these new kinds of casualties, practitioners must be
well educated not only in the common developmental and mental health
entities, but in the contexts in which their patients function. The contextual issues may be racially and ethnically based, socioeconomically based,
or geographically based. The contexts may overlap. Because historically

initial psychological interventions in response to disaster trauma, such as critical incident debriefings, were administered in a "one kind fits all" manner, there have been recent challenges to the usefulness of these interventions (Haraway, 2002).

This chapter was written to help providers become familiar with the unique characteristics of military children and families. It is important to be familiar with their unique nature to treat them successfully, and to be aware of the military support resources available to aid in the treatment process. It is also important to understand that although children in military families live in a unique world, they share the same human strengths and vulnerabilities as their civilian peers. Attentive practitioners will utilize all these principles in providing relief and successful treatment to military children and families.

REFERENCES

Arroyo, W., & Eth, S. (1985). Children traumatized by Central American warfare. In S. Eth & R. S. Pynoos (Eds.), *Posttraumatic stress disorder in children* (pp. 101–120). Washington, DC: American Psychiatric Press.

Amen, D. G., Jellen, L., Merves, E., & Lee, R. E. (1988). Minimizing the impact of deployment separation on military children: Stages, current preventive efforts, and system recommendations. *Military Medicine, 153,* 141–146.

Baker, A. A. (1990). The psychological impact of the Intifada on Palestinian children in the occupied West Bank and Gaza: An exploratory study. *American Journal of Orthopsychiatry, 60,* 496–505.

Carroll, B., & Mathewson, J. (2000). The military model for children and grief. In K. J. Doka (Ed.), *Living with grief: Children, adolescents, and loss* (pp. 249–260). Washington, DC: Hospice Foundation of America and Brunner/Mazel.

Crumley, F. E., & Blumenthal, R. S. (1973). Children's reactions to temporary loss of father. *American Journal of Psychiatry, 130,* 778–782.

DeShalit, N. (1970). Children in war. In A. Jarus, J. Marcus, J. Oren, et al. (Eds.), *Children and families in Israel: Some mental health perspectives* (pp. 151–182). New York: Gordon & Breach.

Fee, F. (1980). Responses to a behavioral questionnaire of a group of Belfast children. In J. Harbison & J. Harbison (Eds.), *A society under stress: Children and young people in northern Ireland* (pp. 31–42). Shepton Mallet, England: Open Books.

Hardaway, T. G. (1990a, January). *Curriculum for children of deployed parents.* Curiculum implemented in the Killeen Independent School System, the San Antonio Northside Independent School System, and the Department of Defense Dependent Schools in Europe.

Hardaway, T. G. (1990b, January). *Curriculum on issues in reunification: Treatment program for families and children reuniting with soldiers returning from war.*

Hardaway, T. G. (1990c, January). *Curriculum on terrorism: Assisting children and schools in dealing with ongoing terrorist incidents.*

Hardaway, T. G. (2001, December). *Crafting and tailoring a terrorism curriculum for children of American soldiers overseas.* Paper presented to mental health practitioners in the Department of Defense Dependent Schools (DoDDS) in Europe at the Annual DoDDS Symposium, Moerfelden, Germany.

Hardaway, T. G. (2002, December). *Is immediate post-trauma debriefing helpful or counterproductive?* Paper presented at the 46th Winter Meeting of the American Academy of Psychoanalysis and Dynamic Psychiatry, San Antonio, TX.

Jensen, P. S., & Shaw, J. A. (1996). The effects of war and parental deployment upon children and adolescents. In R. J. Ursano & A. E. Norwood (Eds.), *Emotional aftermath of the Persian Gulf War: Veterans, families, communities, and nations* (pp. 83–109). Washington, DC: American Psychiatric Press.

Kelley, M. L. (1994). The effects of military-induced separation on family factors and child behavior. *American Journal of Orthopsychiatry, 64,* 103–111.

Rigamer, E. (1986). Psychiatric management of children in a national crisis. *Journal of the American Academy of Child and Adolescent Psychiatry, 25,* 364–369.

Shaw, J., & Harris, J. (1989, October). *A prevention–intervention program for children of war in Mozambique.* Paper presented at the annual meeting of the American Academy of Child and Adolescent Psychiatry, New York.

Shaw, J., & Harris, J. (1994). Children of war and children at war: Child victims of terrorism in Mozambique. In R. J. Ursano, B. G. McCaughey, & C. S. Fullerton (Eds.), *Individual and community responses to trauma and disaster: The structure of human chaos* (pp. 287–305). Cambridge, England: Cambridge University Press.

Terr, L. C. (1990). *Too scared to cry.* New York: Harper & Row.

Webb, N. B. (Ed.). (1999). *Play therapy with children in crisis* (2nd ed.). *Individual, family, and group treatment.* New York: Guilford Press.

Webb, N. B. (Ed.). (2002). *Helping bereaved children. A handbook for practitioners* (2nd ed.). New York: Guilford Press.

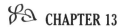

CHAPTER 13

A Drawing Technique for Diagnosis and Therapy of Adolescents Suffering Traumatic Stress and Loss Related to Terrorism

TOVA YEDIDIA
HAYA ITZHAKY

The theoretical and research literature indicates a relationship between difficult life events such as exposure to terror, and traumatic symptoms such as psychological, behavioral, and social disorders (Herman, 1992; Neumann, 1995). Exposure to terror in adolescence leads to a traumatic reaction similar to that of adults, but in the case of the former it comes at a time when the victims are already vulnerable, because their development is in process. An adolescent's personality and coping mechanisms are the most important factors in restoring his or her functioning following traumatic exposure (Tiano, 1997).

In this chapter we discuss adolescents who were exposed to terror and consequently suffered physical and/or psychological traumatic injury, in addition to the loss of a close person. We present a model for diagnosing this population, focusing on the main parameters cited in the literature and indicated by our own clinical experience in coping with trauma. The diagnosis includes evaluation of the magnitude of the event, the traumatic symptoms, the style of coping with the trauma, and the level of use of denial. We suggest therapeutic goals based on the diagnosis. The main tool in the diagnosis is an art therapy technique called the "bridge drawing."

The diagnostic model proposed here is unique, in that it uses an artistic tool to diagnose parameters of adjustment to trauma. The use of art was chosen because of the difficulty adolescents have in accepting therapists; this stage of development is characterized by resistance to dependence on parents, and consequently fear of developing a relationship with a therapist, who is considered as an authoritative adult.

THE TRAUMATIC EVENT AND STRESS REACTIONS

Terrorist attacks are traumatic experiences. As such, they cause suffering and distress outside the range of normative life experience (American Psychiatric Association, 2000; Neumann, 1995). Trauma causes emotional shock, which an individual interprets as endangering his or her essential needs for security, self-esteem, and physical wholeness; it may also be a threat to life itself. The event is followed by disturbance of the victim's emotional balance with possible onset of neurotic symptoms, which vary among individuals in magnitude and character (Neumann, 1995).

The most common disorder among adults following a traumatic event is known as posttraumatic stress disorder (PTSD). PTSD is characterized by reexperiencing of the traumatic event in nightmares, flashbacks, persistent memories, and reactions to stimuli that are reminiscent of the event, as well as by anxiety-driven avoidance of thoughts, memories, places, situations, or anything associated with the traumatic event. PTSD also includes symptoms of arousal, such as irritability, oversensitivity, sleeping disturbances, and general hypervigilance (American Psychiatric Association, 2000). The literature indicates that PTSD can occur not only in survivors of traumatic events, but also among relatives and therapists who have close contact with the survivors. This is known as "secondary traumatization" (McCann & Pearlman, 1990; Figley, 1995).

An individual's stress reaction is determined by (1) the magnitude of the objective threat, and (2) the strength of the individual's strategies for coping with the threat. The cognitive approach considers the magnitude of the event in evaluating the individual's response (Lazarus, 1966). Herman (1992) suggests that traumatic events place individuals in extreme situations of helplessness and fear that arouse catastrophic reactions. In her opinion, they generate deep and persistent changes in physical alertness, emotions, consciousness, and memory. Some people may experience powerful emotions, but be unable to recall the event clearly; others may remember the event in minute detail but feel nothing. Traumatized individuals are constantly on guard and nervous, but cannot understand why. The symptoms may have no apparent connection with the traumatic event that caused them. The trauma may actually destroy an individual's psychological defenses.

Neumann (1995) discusses the split between a client's inner and outer worlds as a result of trauma: Massive trauma interferes with the ability to register the event. The victim's mechanisms of observing and recording are impaired and temporarily cease to function. Even though the event actually occurred in reality, it seems to have happened outside the parameters of "normal" reality—that is, without connection to place, time, continuum, and logic. Therefore, it exists outside the range of understanding and control. Traumatized persons are not grappling with memories, but with an event that cannot be contained. Therefore, from their point of view, the event continues to be present in all senses.

ADOLESCENCE AND TRAUMA

Children, adolescents, and adults experience posttraumatic stress reactions, but youth are more vulnerable than adults when they are exposed to mental pressure that they cannot control (Weissman, Schwartzwald, Solomon, & Klingman, 1992). Among other causes, teenagers' vulnerability stems from the special characteristics of the separation–individuation process of adolescence. Blos (1962) discusses the relative weakness of the adolescent ego, due to the intensification of urges and weakening of the absolute ego—especially in the phase of individuation, in which the individual strives for self-definition and ego maturity. This phase is characterized by adolescents' resistance to parental support in their development of self-identity.

During adolescence, young people devote themselves to the dual process of separation and individuation by strengthening their personal boundaries and developing a sense of personal and sexual identity (Masterson & Costello, 1980). This period is frequently characterized by anger, difficulties in creating emotional relationships, and acting out. While an adolescent attends to the task of consolidating his or her identity, we can observe a variety of phenomena that are normative to this period but would be unacceptable in functioning adults: regression, merging of boundaries, sharp shifts in opinions, and decision making based on unrealistic grounds.

In normal circumstances, the ego continues to function even though it is diminished. However, the greatest threat to adolescents' mental health is coping with stress. The disturbance in functioning that results from stress is likely to create a setback in an adolescent's normal development. One of the danger signs during this process is adolescents' difficulty in experiencing and expressing feelings associated with events they have experienced (Laufer & Laufer, 1984). Against this background, a terror attack (or any other traumatic event) intensifies the storm and the pressure, and may upset an adolescent's already fragile mental balance.

Adolescents' ability to cope with the traumatic situation is related to the level of their defenses and coping strengths. One of the main defense mechanisms in coping with traumatic situations is denial, which enables an individual to ignore information related to the traumatic experience, thereby reducing anxiety. According to research, mental health in some situations requires repression, denial, and illusion (Breznitz, 1988). Accordingly, Breznitz (1988) describes different levels of denial:

1. Denial of the significance of existing feelings about the threat.
2. Denial of the existence of feelings related to the threat.
3. Denial of responsibility and of ability to have an impact by coping with the threat.
4. Denial of the urgency of coping with the threat.
5. Denial of the existence of a personal threat to the individual.
6. Denial of the existence of a threat at all.
7. Denial of information or of the general reality.

As the graded list indicates, the use of denial as a defense is liable to lead an adolescent to total denial of reality.

However, caution should be taken in treating denial. According to Breznitz (1988), direct and invasive therapy aimed at eliminating denial structures is liable to lead to more distorted use of these structures. In his view, a supportive, indirect approach is preferable for the purpose of reducing the sense of threat and the need to employ denial.

Rofe and Lewin (1979) also refer to the defense styles of adolescents and young adults who are exposed to traumatic events. They classify the following four different styles of coping with trauma, and suggest an appropriate method of treatment for each style:

1. "Repressors" tend to repress anxiety rigidly, and are incapable of coping with the threat in an adaptive manner because of distortions. The proposed treatment is gradual and focused on moderate elimination of the denial to enable short-term coping.
2. "Suppressors" regulate their self-exposure by involving themselves in activities that are adaptive to the danger. The proposed treatment is immediate brief crisis intervention.
3. "Synthesizers" seek a transition to immediate adaptive activity in the face of threat, as well as self-awareness, integration of the meaning of the experience, and resolution of the associated conflicts. The proposed treatment is immediate crisis intervention followed by ongoing psychotherapy.
4. "Sensitizers" experience a flooding of thoughts and feelings, with a resultant inability to act adaptively. The proposed treatment is psychotherapy that includes support for strengthening defenses.

Because of the special characteristics of adolescence as discussed above, an adolescent's willingness to engage in therapy is key. The very therapy process and the formation of a therapist–client relationship are the main challenges in therapy with an adolescent. Esman (1983) notes that at their stage of development, adolescents have not yet evolved cognitive and self-observing capacities that permit the use of free association, such as that used in analytic therapy. Adolescents are more oriented toward action than toward reflection as a means of reducing tension and coping with anxiety.

In Israel, terrorism has created a state of ongoing anxiety. A survey of residents in an area subject to an ongoing threat of terrorist attacks indicates that posttraumatic symptoms are very common among those exposed to such a threat (Shalev, Adski, Boker, Fridman, & Koper, 2002). However, in most cases, these symptoms do not necessarily indicate dysfunction. Fears that arise because of the situation are likely to be focused and realistic, thus protecting an individual and preventing exposure to danger. Therefore, in situations of ongoing exposure to danger, it is difficult to differentiate between normal reactions and pathological responses that require therapeutic intervention (Shalev et al., 2002).

Research has shown that early psychotherapy is likely to reduce the long-term effects of exposure to stress situations (Solomon, 1993). Therefore, in countries where there is extensive exposure to trauma, it is important to find accessible, simple-to-use diagnostic tools for identifying cases that require therapeutic intervention (Shalev et al., 2002).

METHODS FOR ENGAGING ADOLESCENTS

Among the most common projective means for examining traumatic situations among children and adolescents are drawing and storytelling. Nader and Pynoos (1991) have adapted Winnicott's and Piaget's methods of drawing in work with traumatized children. The present model combines Rofe and Lewin's (1979) classification of styles of coping with trauma, and Breznitz's (1988) diagnosis of denial level, with the projective tool of the bridge drawing (to be described below).

The description of the bridge drawing is followed by presentation of three cases in which this model was applied, illustrating the use of this tool with adolescents exposed to trauma.

THE BRIDGE DRAWING AS A TOOL
FOR DIAGNOSING TRAUMATIZED ADOLESCENTS

The bridge drawing is a structured tool from the field of art therapy that has been found to be effective in diagnosis and therapy of adolescents (Yedidia, 1993). It is used in diagnosing the mental state of adolescents as part of the process of therapeutic invention (Hays & Lyons, 1981; Yedidia,

1993). The bridge symbolizes an individual's perception of the world (dangerous or safe) and of his or her level of control over the environment (low or high). Each client is first asked to draw a bridge and then to place him- or herself in the picture. The size, placement, and grounding of the bridge; the scenery on either side of the bridge; and the position of the client in relation to the bridge are all important factors in the analysis of the bridge drawing. In the second stage, the client is asked the following questions: "What type of bridge is it? How strong is the bridge? How fragile is the bridge? Where does the bridge originate? Where does it lead? What is on either side of the bridge? What is under the bridge? What is the person's location on the bridge?"

The adolescent is then diagnosed on the basis of the drawing, according to the following parameters. These are based on tests by Hays and Lyons (1981), who pioneered the use of this tool through examining 72 female and 78 male high school students aged 14–18, in the United States, and by Yedidia (1993), who studied 34 adolescents aged 15–18 being treated in youth treatment centers in Israel:

1. *Appearance of the bridge.* A bridge drawn as a narrow, dotted, or broken strip represents the artist's lack of self-confidence. A thick bridge that seems stable represents the artist's sense of confidence in him- or herself.

2. *The materials of which the bridge is made.* A bridge made of flimsy material, such as rope, represents the artist's sense of lacking security and control. A bridge made of sturdy materials, such as metal or wood, represents the artist's sense of having security and control.

3. *Grounding of the bridge.* A bridge that is not connected to the ground represents the artist's sense of detachment from reality. A bridge that is grounded represents the artist's sense of stability and connection to reality.

4. *Bridge railing.* A bridge drawn without a railing represents the artist's sense of being unprotected. A bridge with a railing represents the artist's defenses.

5. *The location of the person on the bridge.* Location of the person off the bridge represents anxiety about coping with danger. A person positioned in the middle of the bridge represents the artist's feeling of being stuck. Location of the person on the bridge, walking toward the end, represents the artist's sense of ability to cope with the danger.

6. *The area surrounding the bridge.* Depiction of the surrounding area as dangerous represents the artist's sense of exposure to a dangerous environment. Description of pleasant surroundings represents the artist's sense of security in the environment.

As noted above, a therapist evaluates a client's coping style, as expressed in the bridge drawing, on the basis of Rofe and Lewin's (1979) classification of adolescents' styles of coping with trauma. On the basis of our clinical experience with dozens of adolescents victimized by terror and other traumatic events, we have developed the following guidelines to serve as the basis for mapping young clients' coping styles:

1. *Repressors* draw a bridge made of stable materials, give this bridge high railings, and depict themselves as imprisoned on the bridge.
2. *Suppressors* draw a stable bridge with railings, but portray themselves in an unstable position on the bridge (or off the bridge altogether), and they depict the surroundings as dangerous.
3. *Synthesizers* draw an unstable bridge or place the human figure above the bridge; they also add railings to the bridge and portray dangerous surroundings.
4. *Sensitizers* draw an unstable bridge that is not grounded, and they draw themselves in an unstable position on the bridge or off it; the bridge has no railings, and the environment is depicted as very dangerous.

This classification of the styles of coping with traumatic situations and construction of parameters for diagnosing the level of defenses on the basis of the bridge drawing is then applied to establishing a therapy plan that may include further use of creative tools.

Figure 13.1 illustrates the model as a three-part structure. The first part (at the upper left of the figure) describes the aspects of the bridge drawing that are considered in diagnosing the level of defenses. The second part (at upper right) includes the other parameters for diagnosis that

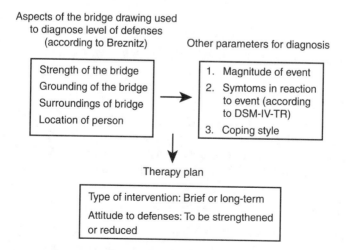

FIGURE 13.1. Model for diagnosis and therapy with adolescents in trauma.

can be evaluated during intake and on the basis of observation and discussion of the bridge drawing with the client. Finally (at the bottom of the figure), following diagnosis of the level of denial, magnitude of the event, symptoms, and coping style, a therapy program is developed; this includes choice of therapy method, attitude to be taken toward defenses, and consideration of the use of creative methods in therapy.

The proposed model was developed after extensive experience in treating adolescents, as part of a private therapy practice that serves adolescents. One of the most instructive cases in which the model was applied involved community and group interventions following a terror attack on a high school. In this event, a suicide terrorist fired on teenagers and then blew himself up among a group of them. About a week later, we applied the bridge drawing model to ascertain the influence of the trauma on the teenagers. This method enabled us quickly to obtain preliminary information about how the adolescents were coping, and, on this basis, to recommend suitable crisis intervention and other treatment.

Furthermore, the bridge drawing helps legitimize the feelings and symptoms the adolescents are having as a result of their shared traumatic experience. Sometimes these feelings and symptoms are unfamiliar to them and are therefore perceived as embarrassing. In the group, the adolescents realize that others share similar feelings. This is a single-session group model.

In order to demonstrate the use of the model, we present descriptions of the diagnosis and therapy of three young people who were exposed to traumatic events and who requested therapy a few months later. The third of these examples involved a teenage girl who sought therapy after being diagnosed in a group as suffering severe posttraumatic symptoms.

CASE EXAMPLES OF ISRAELI ADOLESCENTS WHO EXPERIENCED TRAUMATIC STRESS AND LOSS

Case 1: Karen, Age 20

Karen had completed high school and national service, and was working in computerized graphics, when she requested therapy. She was the younger child of Ben, an engineer, and Yael, a teacher. Karen had an older sister, Dana, who was married and had completed her studies in psychology.

The Traumatic Event

Six months earlier, Karen had been traveling on a bus that was attacked by a suicide bomber. In the explosion, 2 people were killed and about 10 were injured. Karen herself was not injured physically, but she was affected emotionally. According to the intake, the magnitude of the event that Karen experienced was very high—it was a terrorist attack on a bus.

Symptoms Following the Trauma

Karen continued to function fairly well at work and in her social life. She even resumed traveling on buses, but she had flashbacks of the traumatic event and obsessive memories in reaction to stimuli that reminded her of the trauma. Every time another terror attack occurred in Israel, Karen was overwhelmed with fear; she experienced a sense of catastrophe and helplessness; and she was unable to function for several days.

Karen requested therapy from Tova Yedidia (who is the "I" in the case description that follows) because of these intense emotional reactions she was having to other terrorist attacks in Israel. She agreed to the inclusion of art in the therapy after clarifying exactly what this meant. At the beginning of the therapy, I asked Karen to draw a bridge.

Analysis of the Bridge Drawing

Karen drew a stable bridge with a railing that looked like window grating (see Figure 13.2). The bridge was not grounded. She drew herself standing at the middle of the bridge. When asked, she said that the bridge was made of wood, and that the surroundings at one side were inhabited, while at the other side of the bridge there was nothing. Stormy waters

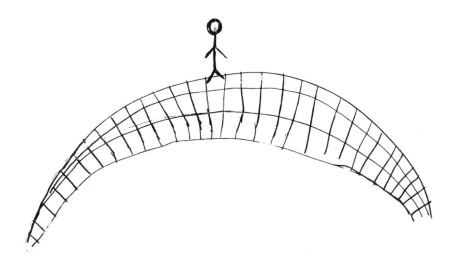

FIGURE 13.2. Karen's bridge drawing.

flowed under the bridge. Anyone who fell from the bridge was liable to drown or be eaten by sharks, but the high railing prevented falling.

On the basis of the drawing, the following conclusions were drawn about Karen's coping style and defenses:

Coping Style. According to Rope and Lewin's (1979) classification, it seems that Karen belonged to the group of suppressors. She regulated her exposure to death fears by busying herself with activity adapted to the danger. This could be seen in the drawing of the stable bridge, with Karen located at the beginning of the ascent onto the bridge.

Defenses. Karen managed to repress her anxiety during her daily routine. According to Breznitz's (1988) scale of levels of denial, she denied her feelings connected to threat. She expressed her level of denial in the drawing by means of the high grated railing, which, as noted earlier, indicated defensiveness. However, when terrorist events took place, Karen lost her ability to regulate her exposure and was overwhelmed by anxiety, as shown in the drawing by the ungrounded bridge and the stormy waters with sharks.

Further Comments

After gaining these insights by examining and discussing the bridge drawing, Karen was able to get in touch with the traumatic event itself. She drew a terror attack involving a bus split in half, surrounded by flames and smoke, and with body parts dispersed all around. Karen actually depicted the inner picture that overwhelmed her with anxiety every time an attack took place. In observing this picture, Karen said, "This is the first time I can look at the atrocity with my own eyes." It is hoped that this drawing activity will help to reduce her anxiety.

Case 2: Jonathan, Age 18

Traumatic Event

Jonathan lived in an isolated village. On the road to his home, there had been several fatal shootings. A neighbor whom he knew was killed, and several people who resided in or near his village were injured. Rocks had been thrown at a car in which Jonathan himself was traveling, although there were no injuries in that event. Jonathan had three sisters; his father was a banker, and his mother a secretary. According to Jonathan, he had been functioning normally during the Intifada (Palestinian uprising against Israel): He studied for his matriculation exams and went out with friends, traveling on the dangerous highway with no means of protection.

Symptoms Following the Trauma

Jonathan requested therapy because of headaches that could not be explained medically, which began a few months after the Intifada broke out. Jonathan rejected any attempts on the part of those close to him to get him to confront his denial of the danger directly. When he came to therapy, he demonstrated fear and caution. He said that he didn't believe in psychotherapy, but agreed to try it because the medical system had given up on helping him. He responded to the suggestion of using creative work in the diagnosis and therapy with some reservations, but agreed after some explanation was provided that the art projects were not complicated, that we would interpret them together, and I would share my understanding of the picture with him. Jonathan received my assurance that he could stop using art in the therapy at any point he chose, after we discussed the reasons for this wish.

According to the information obtained at the intake, the magnitude of Jonathan's exposure to trauma was moderate. He was not personally injured in an attack. The symptoms following the trauma were headaches that Jonathan did not associate with traumatic exposure. Jonathan perceived my request that he draw the bridge picture as curious, but easy to execute.

Analysis of the Bridge Drawing

As Figure 13.3 shows, Jonathan drew a very stable bridge, which took up the entire page (he left no room for the surroundings). According to Jonathan, a highway ran under the bridge. He indicated the directions of travel on the highway with arrows. The bridge had a strong, safe railing. Jonathan drew himself wearing dark glasses and coming off the bridge, with his back to the bridge. A woman was lying under the bridge. When I asked Jonathan what the bridge was made of, he said it was iron. According to him, the bridge was safe. He explained that the highway below was dangerous to anyone falling from the bridge, because cars traveled there at very high speed, but there was no danger of falling off the bridge onto the highway. I called his attention to the woman he had drawn. According to him, she hadn't fallen from the bridge, but was lying injured on the highway.

On the basis of the drawing, I drew these conclusions about Jonathan's coping style and defenses:

Coping Style. Jonathan was characterized by anxious avoidance of thoughts related to traumatic events. On the basis of Rope and Lewin's (1979) classification, Jonathan seemed to belong to the group of re-

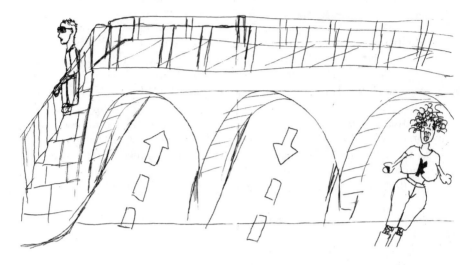

FIGURE 13.3. Jonathan's bridge drawing.

pressors. This was indicated in the drawing by the stable bridge, and in the subsequent discussion by Jonathan's very high sense of control (his claim that there was no danger of falling off the bridge). The arrows in the drawing were directed straight to the target.

Defenses. According to Breznitz's (1988) scale, Jonathan displayed a very high level of denial. In the picture, he depicted himself with his back to the injured woman, his eyes covered. According to him, there was no room in the picture for the surroundings of the bridge.

Despite his denial, Jonathan was in a state of alertness and sensitivity (as represented by his headaches), but he did not associate this with the trauma-related anxiety. The defense mechanism that Jonathan used put his life in danger, because he did not take any measures of precaution as required by the real danger.

Further Comments

The externalization of the emotional conflict by means of the drawing enabled the beginning of therapy that centered (1) on getting Jonathan to recognize the dangerous situation and his anxiety about it; and (2) on regulating the anxiety so that Jonathan could function in his daily life, but could also sense the threat in dangerous situations and protect himself accordingly.

Case 3: Jasmine, Age 15

The Traumatic Event

Jasmine applied for therapy 4 months after her mother had incurred moderate injuries during a terrorist attack on a shopping center. Jasmine lived with her father; she had an older brother who was a soldier. She was a nice-looking, very quiet girl. Jasmine participated in brief group therapy at her school because of problems with functioning in school—namely, lack of concentration and fatigue. The group was set up by the school counselor after several students displayed different problems in reaction to the terror attacks. The aims were to identify the participants who needed further therapeutic intervention on an individual basis, and to help all participants cope with anxiety related to the security situation. The group facilitator (Tova Yedidia, who is again the "I" here) used the bridge drawing tool; it was on this basis that Jasmine was diagnosed and offered individual treatment. In the group meeting and in the first therapy session, Jasmine answered the questions asked briefly. She did not expand on any subject at her own initiative.

Symptoms Following the Trauma

Jasmine said that she had trouble falling asleep at night and concentrating on her studies, and that this had led to a decline in her achievement.

   According to the intake, the magnitude of Jasmine's exposure to trauma was moderate (relative, for instance, to Karen's experience and to the general situation in Israel). In fact, she had not been exposed to an event directly, but only through her mother. The traumatic symptoms were sleeping disturbance, oversensitivity, difficulty concentrating, and social avoidance.

Analysis of the Bridge Drawing

Jasmine drew the bridge on a small portion of the page that was offered her (see Figure 13.4). Her bridge consisted of only a thin line and looked unstable. She placed herself slightly above the bridge, as though hanging on a restraint. When I asked Jasmine what the bridge was made of, she said it was made of ropes. When I asked how safe it was to walk on the bridge, she replied that it was easy to fall off. Falling meant being shattered, since the bridge was very high, and under it was a highway. Jasmine did not know what to answer when I asked what was at either end of the bridge and where it led.

   On the basis of the drawing, I reached these conclusions about Jasmine's coping style and defenses:

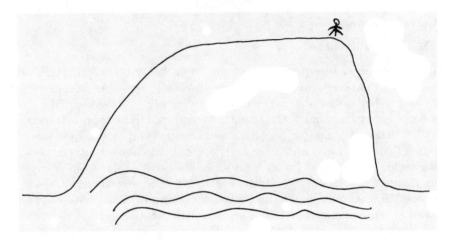

FIGURE 13.4. Jasmine's bridge drawing.

Coping Style. According to Rope and Lewin's (1979) classification, Jasmine seemed to belong to the group of sensitizers. She was overwhelmed by emotions and thoughts that prevented her from functioning adaptively. Her depression was evident in the minimalist drawing. Her anxiety was represented by the flimsy bridge; according to her, it was easy to fall from the bridge and be smashed. She expressed her sense of helplessness in the picture by depicting herself as a tiny figure, disconnected and unstable, dangling over the bridge.

Defenses. Jasmine used only a minimal degree of denial or repression, as indicated by the absence of a rail on the bridge and the drawing of the figure as seemingly hanging from a restraint.

Further Comments

The bridge drawing helped Jasmine admit the depression and anxiety that she felt, which were causing her to close up to those around her; to be fatigued and uninterested in the daily life of her peers, which had previously given her pleasure; and to live in fear of the next catastrophe. Jasmine felt very lonely, depressed, and anxious. Emotionally, the trauma compounded the state of upheaval associated with the process of adolescence. Thus the pain and anxiety regarding her mother's injuries were all the more difficult for Jasmine to contain, because she was an adolescent. Like every teenager fighting dependency on his or her parents, she had difficulty seeking her father's support. Moreover, the situation affected all members of the family, so that each one was overwhelmed with his or her own pain. It was clear that Jasmine needed help in working through the trauma, and supportive therapy to help her build a flexible defense system that would allow her to continue functioning.

DISCUSSION

We have presented a model for intervention in situations of stress that is based on a creative tool for diagnosis and therapy with adolescents who are exposed to traumatic events. The unique feature of this technique is its effective use in diagnosing the coping styles and defenses of adolescents and young adults who are exposed to the ongoing stress of a war-like environment, in forming a therapy contract, and in formulating a therapy plan.

The cases presented here show that three adolescents exposed to traumatic events at different levels reacted to the trauma not only according to the magnitude of their exposure, but mainly according to their subjective reactions to the event, which were related to their emotional state and to the level and quality of their defenses. Table 13.1 presents the individual differences among the adolescents in their objective exposure to a traumatic event, their subjective reaction to the trauma, and its reflection in the bridge drawing.

The table shows that Karen was exposed to the most powerful trauma, which involved the death of other people and a genuine threat to her life. Jonathan was indirectly exposed to traumatic events that involved death, and because of the security situation, he was repeatedly exposed to life-threatening situations. Jasmine experienced a secondary trauma involving her mother's injury in a terror attack, as well as the general situation of terrorist attacks in Israel.

According to the magnitude of the traumatic event, we might expect Karen to have the greatest difficulty coping. However, as noted in the literature, stress reaction is determined not only by the magnitude of the objective threat, but also by the strength of the strategies used to cope with the threat (Lazarus, 1966). Karen, who experienced the most serious event, demonstrated good coping strengths; Jonathan, who experienced a lesser degree of danger than Karen, refrained from confronting his anxiety and coped as though there were no danger; and Jasmine had little strength to cope with the trauma. The three young people also developed different symptoms in the wake of their respective experiences. Karen experienced flashbacks and memories in reaction to subsequent terror events, which triggered a reliving of her traumatic experience; however, she functioned normally in her routine life. Jonathan was characterized by anxious avoidance of thoughts about the trauma, and Jasmine overreacted to the trauma she had experienced, impairing her ability to function in her daily routine.

TABLE 13.1. Case Analysis According to the Diagnostic Model

	Karen	Jonathan	Jasmine
Magnitude of the event	Very high: Karen was physically exposed to an event in which people were killed.	Moderate exposure: Jonathan was exposed indirectly to traumatic events.	Moderate exposure: Jasmine's mother was injured, but she lived in an area that was not considered exposed to terror.
Reaction to event according to DSM-IV-TR	Flashbacks and memories in reaction to stimuli that reminded her of the trauma.	Headaches and anxious avoidance of thoughts related to trauma.	Sleep disturbance, oversensitivity, difficulty concentrating, social avoidance.
Coping style	Suppressor	Repressor	Synthesizer
Level of denial	Level 2—denial of the existence of feelings related to threat.	Level 5—denial of the existence of a personal threat.	Very low—difficulty employing the denial mechanism.
Characteristics of the bridge drawing	Dangerous surroundings; stable but ungrounded bridge.	Dangerous surroundings; stable bridge with railing; Jonathan turning his back to the danger and wearing dark glasses.	Dangerous surrounding; unstable bridge with no railing; Jasmine hanging from a restraint.
Therapy plan	Immediate brief crisis intervention; use of art in the therapy; work on repressed memories.	Help with gradual reduction of denial; use of art to build the therapeutic relationship and increase awareness.	Supportive psychotherapy to strengthen defenses; possibility of employing art in the therapy.

Herman (1992) explains that traumatic symptoms are likely to be cut off from their origin and to develop a life of their own. This can be seen in the case of Jonathan, who denied any relationship between the headaches he suffered and the trauma he experienced. Another familiar phenomenon in situations of trauma (Herman, 1992) occurred with Karen, who clearly remembered the traumatic event, but whose memories were devoid of related feelings.

The results of research on coping with stress suggest that denial and repression are sometimes effective mechanisms for healthy emotional adjustment to traumatic situations (Breznitz, 1988; Rofe & Lewin, 1979). An example of this can be seen in the way Karen coped. Even though the danger of a recurrent event continued, her level of denial enabled her to continue functioning in her daily life. However, it did not protect her from anxiety when traumatic events occurred subsequently.

We have seen that Karen, according to her classification in the group of suppressors, regulated exposure in her daily life by engaging in adaptive activity in the face of danger. By contrast, Jonathan's level of denial was so high that it did not allow him healthy mental adjustment. Classified in the group of repressors, Jonathan rigidly denied feeling any anxiety. He was incapable of coping with the threat in an adaptive manner, and consequently exposed himself to existential danger. Jasmine's response was at the opposite end of the continuum of defense levels from Jonathan's. Her traumatic event aroused high levels of fear, making her unable to function because of her weak ability to deny, as characteristic of the group of sensitizers. Jasmine was in a constant state of emotional hyperarousal and anxiety, overwhelmed by thoughts and feelings to the point of being unable to act adaptively.

It is significant that in all three cases reported here, the traumatic events occurred during adolescence; this affected both the magnitude of their reaction and their coping ability. As noted earlier, the adolescent stage of development is characterized by a relatively weak ego, related to stronger urges and weakening of the absolute ego, due to the adolescent's resistance to parental support (Blos, 1962). Even though we did not examine the clients' ego strengths and coping patterns prior to the traumas, they all reported normative functioning before the traumatic event. Jasmine's case most clearly illustrates the relationship between the process of adolescence and reaction to trauma. Her ego weakness, and her difficulty in relying on her family for support, were clearly evident. Dadia (2002) notes that injury or loss sometimes creates a sense that a family is "falling apart." In this situation, an adolescent is mobilized to support his or her family and draw closer to the parent(s). This closeness is likely to cause regression in the process of adolescence and to cut off the process of individuation and self-development. Because of her mother's injury, such intimacy between Jasmine and her mother was liable to delay Jasmine's process of individuation.

Jonathan displayed typical adolescent behavior, such as making decisions based on estimation rather then on the real situation (Masterson & Costello, 1980). The trauma led Jonathan to extreme use of denial and unrealistic decision making (e.g., his decision to travel in an unprotected vehicle in a dangerous area).

All the adolescents described here were able to use the bridge drawing to help them better understand the emotional impact of the traumatic event and sharpen their awareness of how they coped with trauma. Karen used the defense of denial (the railing) effectively, but the unstable bridge she drew indicated the fragility of this mechanism in confronting future terror events. Jonathan expressed his denial of danger in his picture by depicting himself with his back to it and drawing a very stable bridge. Jasmine drew a bridge that, like her feelings, seemed unstable and dangerous as she stood on it, unprotected.

THE THERAPY PLAN

Construction of a therapy plan for an adolescent who has experienced traumatic stress is based upon evaluation of the adolescent's level of denial and coping style. Both of these factors influence the adolescent's ability to function normally in his or her routine life. Her denial enabled Karen to function relatively well in routine life, and thus it constituted an effective coping mechanism. Like other trauma survivors, however, Karen was living with an event that could not be contained, and therefore it was impossible for her to progress toward its closure. The symptoms that arose with the repeated terror incidents indicated Karen's need for help in containing her difficult memories of the event. Karen needed brief therapy. According to Pynoos (1990), in cases of PTSD such therapy enables the client to rework the details of the traumatic event; understand its meaning; identify positions that express feelings of helplessness, anger, and guilt that appeared during the event; and generate change in them.

In contrast, Jonathan's level of denial endangered him. For him, therapy had to help him bring the denied feelings of trauma to the surface, understand them, associate them with his coping style, and gradually reduce his use of denial.

For Jasmine, it was necessary to create a long-term therapy plan. In the first stage, the therapy would help strengthen her defenses, enable her to control her thoughts about the event, and reduce the overanxiety that resulted from the trauma. Next, she needed to work through her feelings of loss because of her mother's injury and strengthen her family support, taking into account the adolescent dilemmas regarding dependence on parents. The overall aim was to help Jasmine function more adaptively, increase her well-being, and continue the normal process of identity development.

Clearly, the pretrauma personality is also important in developing the course and plan of therapy (Tiano, 1997). However, a discussion of all the personality components of the cases described is beyond the scope of the chapter. Therefore, we have chosen the central parameters presented in the literature regarding diagnosis and therapy of traumatized youth.

The three cases described here share in common the use of a projective technique that enabled the clients, as adolescents, to accept the therapist's mirroring, which had a strong emotional effect (Oaklander, 1997).

Structured drawing is an activity that minimizes resistance and gives adolescents a sense of control over their exposure in the therapy process. This enables positive therapist–client exchanges, which constitute a basis for a continued therapeutic relationship.

These assertions are supported by the cases of these three adolescents. Karen agreed to cooperate when she realized that this technique was a structured tool that provided a sense of control. Jonathan, who resisted therapy and was the most threatened by it, lowered his resistance. Jasmine, who spoke minimally about her feelings, was able, through the bridge drawing, to express her overwhelming anxiety.

According to the literature, plastic arts techniques such as the bridge drawing enable externalization of conflicts and emotions, so that adolescents can observe them from the outside and lower their level of denial (Carlson, 1997). Jonathan, whose level of denial was very high, managed to see the parallel between his drawing—where he depicted himself as wearing dark glasses and turning his back on what was happening—and his defensive denial of anxiety regarding the threat of terror.

The fact that a bridge drawing is relatively easy to execute reduced the adolescents' level of resistance to using a creative tool for diagnosis and therapy. For example, after the initial experience with drawing, Jonathan, who was very reserved about therapy and the use of art, cooperated willingly in creating and analyzing a collage. Similarly, Karen asked to draw the traumatic event she had experienced.

Finally, we would like to point out once again that although this chapter focuses mainly on the use of the bridge drawing as a tool in individual therapy, we have also discussed its use in groups of adolescents who have experienced a traumatic event, to identify those in need of one-on-one intervention. For example, Jasmine's difficulty was discovered in group work with high school students who had been exposed to terror attacks. Nader and Pynoos (1991) claim that group work following a traumatic event enables brief therapy aimed at working through the traumatic event and helping restore a sense of control. For some individuals in such groups, the duration and force of the reaction to the traumatic event are extreme, indicating a need for long-term therapy. In Jasmine's case, brief therapy was not adequate, and she needed long-term individual therapy because of the traumatic symptoms she described.

CONCLUSIONS

In summary, we have presented a unique diagnostic model based on the use of a simple creative tool to encourage the cooperation of adolescents traumatized by terror, and to obtain diagnostic information needed for therapy with such adolescents. The bridge drawing can also be used in therapy with younger children suffering stress, whose verbal skills and ability to express emotions are relatively lower.

It would be interesting to conduct empirical research on the connection between the exposure of adolescents to traumatic events and their coping strengths, as expressed in the bridge drawing and with other artistic tools.

In Israel and elsewhere, we have witnessed mass terror attacks on locations with a high concentration of adolescents, such as educational institutions and entertainment venues. On the basis of our experience with this tool in the case of a mass attack on a school, we recommend the use of the proposed model for community intervention with adolescents following terror attacks.

REFERENCES

American Psychiatric Association. (2000). *Diagnostic and statistical manual of mental disorders* (4th ed., text rev.). Washington, DC: Author.

Blos, P. (1962). *On adolescence: A psychoanalytic interpretation*. New York: Free Press.

Breznitz, S. (1988). The seven kinds of denial. In P. B. Defares (Ed.), *Stress and anxiety: The series in clinical and community psychology* (pp. 73–90). New York: Harper & Row.

Carlson, T. D. (1997). Using art therapy: Enhancing therapeutic possibilities. *American Journal of Family Therapy, 25*(3), 271–282.

Dadia, M. (2002). *Immediate and postponed disclosure in sexual assault victims: Trauma, psychiatric symptoms and dissociation*. Unpublished master's thesis, Bar-Ilan University, Ramat Gan, Israel.

Esman, A. (1983). *The psychiatric treatment of adolescents*. New York: International Universities Press.

Figley, C. R. (Ed.). (1995). *Compassion fatigue: Coping with secondary traumatic stress disorder in those who treat the traumatized*. New York: Brunner/Mazel.

Hays, R. E., & Lyons, S. J. (1981). The bridge drawing: A projective technique for assessment in art therapy. *The Arts in Psychotherapy, 8*, 207–217.

Herman, J. L. (1992). *Trauma and recovery*. New York: Basic Books.

Laufer, M., & Laufer, M. E. (1984). *Adolescence and developmental breakdown*. New Haven, CT: Yale University Press.

Lazarus, R. S. (1966). *Psychological stress and the coping process*. New York: McGraw-Hill.

Masterson, J. E., & Costello, J. L. (1980). *From borderline adolescent to functional adult: The test of time*. New York: Brunner/Mazel.

McCann, I. L., & Pearlman, L. A. (1990). Vicarious traumatization: A framework for understanding psychological effects of working with victims. *Journal of Traumatic Stress, 3*, 131–151.

Nader, K., & Pynoos, R. (1991). Play and drawing as tools for interviewing traumatized children. In C. Schaefer, K. Gitlin, & A. Sandgrund (Eds.), *Play, diagnosis and assessment* (pp. 375–389). New York: Wiley.

Neumann, M. (1995). Reactional emotional situations. In C. Monitz. (Ed.), *Selected chapters in psychiatry* (pp. 257–286). Tel Aviv: Papyrus. [In Hebrew]

Oaklander, V. (1997). The therapeutic process with children and adolescents. *The Gestalt Review, 1,* 292–317.

Pynoos, R. (1990). PTSD in children and adolescents. In B. Garfinkel, G. Carlson, & E. Weller (Eds.), *Psychiatric disorders in children and adolescents* (pp. 48–53). Philadelphia: Saunders.

Rofe, Y., & Lewin, I. (1979). Who adjusts better: Repressors or sensitizers? *Clinical Psychology, 35,* 875–879.

Shalev, A., Adski, R., Boker, R., Fridman, S., & Koper, R. (2002). Clinical interventions in ongoing stress events. *Sihot, 17,* 5–19.

Solomon, Z. (1993). *Combat stress reaction.* New York: Plenum Press.

Tiano, S. (1997). Posttrauma stress disorder. In S. Tiano (Ed.), *Child and adolescent psychiatry* (pp. 235–240). Tel Aviv: Dionon. [In Hebrew]

Weissman, M., Schwartzwald, Y., Solomon, Z., & Klingman, A. (1992). Emotional stress reactions among students following the Gulf War. *Sihot, 6*(3), 256–263.

Yedidia, T. (1993). *Developing diagnostic tools from expressive therapy for diagnosing youth in distress.* Unpublished doctoral dissertation, Union Institute and University, Cincinnati, OH.

CHAPTER 14

Living in the Shadow of Community Violence in Northern Ireland

A Therapeutic Response

ISOBEL REILLY
MATT McDERMOTT
STEPHEN COULTER

The context for the therapeutic work with children and their families in Northern Ireland described in this chapter is a specialist mental health service, the Family Trauma Centre. It is a community-based facility situated in Belfast (the capital city of Northern Ireland) and run under the aegis of the U.K. public health and welfare system, the National Health Service. The Family Trauma Centre was opened in early 2000, following the recommendations of the Victims' Commissioner (Bloomfield, 1998), as a Northern-Ireland-wide regional service for children, young people, and families affected by the civil conflict of the last 30-plus years. This conflict is often euphemistically referred to as the "Troubles." Two of us (Isobel Reilly and Stephen Coulter) are employed as family therapists and trauma specialists in the Family Trauma Centre. The other author (Matt McDermott) is a social worker and play therapist based in a child and family psychiatric department of a large Dublin teaching hospital. The three of us share an interest in using nonverbal approaches in the treatment of trauma experienced by children and adolescents.

This chapter begins with a description of our work in terms of the experience of community violence that has continued in Northern Ireland for over 30 years, including some of the changes in emphasis before and after the peace settlement of 1998 (the "Good Friday" agreement). The next section reviews key aspects of posttraumatic stress reactions in children and the application of the diagnostic category of posttraumatic stress disorder (PTSD), discussing its utility in the context of multiple traumas and continuing threats such as those experienced by many children and families in Northern Ireland. A family-oriented systemic approach to trauma recovery is proposed and developed through a case study, and some implications for therapists working and living in the shadow of community violence are described.

THE WORK OF THE FAMILY TRAUMA CENTRE

Our practice in the Family Trauma Centre is strongly influenced by systemic thinking, and we employ a range of therapeutic approaches, including family therapy, cognitive-behavioral therapy, child psychotherapy, and individual trauma treatments (e.g., imaginal exposure, eye movement desensitization and reprocessing). We receive referrals from a number of sources—family physicians, community nursing services, social workers in both health care and community settings, victims' groups, police, and the justice sector—as well as self-referrals. The core staff group is drawn from experienced mental health professionals (social workers, psychologists) who specialize in the child and adolescent psychiatric field and who have undertaken further professional training in traumatology.

THE TROUBLES, PAST AND PRESENT

The Nature of the Conflict

The context for our therapeutic work in the Family Trauma Centre is the civil conflict that has lasted for over three decades and resulted in over 3,600 deaths. According to Fay, Morrissey, and Smyth (1999), 40,000 people had sustained injuries as of the late 1990s; however, this is probably about one-third of the true number, as many injuries were unreported or minimized. The first half of the 1970s had the highest number of deaths, approximately 50% of the total number; 1972 was the worst year, with 496 deaths and the particular events of "Bloody Sunday" and "Bloody Friday." One of Northern Ireland's most horrifying statistics is that 91% of those killed were male. Of these, half were in the 14–29 age range, peaking in the late teens and early 20s. Even with a peace process underway, and new institutions already well established to address and correct previous injustices, the period after the cease-fires from the mid-1990s to the present day has been marked by continuing violence and strife (but to a less intense degree).

The conflict has also been notable for its geographic specificity. For this reason, it is possible in many areas of Northern Ireland to be relatively unaffected by the Troubles. In areas of highest communal strife, however, poverty, marginalization, and social exclusion are significant. Also evident in these areas is the sectarian dimension of the conflict. This has always been directly expressed in community violence, riots, and invasions of territory perceived as belonging exclusively to one particular "side" or the other. In many towns and villages throughout Northern Ireland, the overt and explicit trappings of sectarian prejudice are apparent in the slogans and wall murals depicting revered heroes and significant historical events, the flying of flags, and the emblematic colors painted on the sidewalks. Bigotry and sectarianism-fueled tensions are entrenched, and their expression is bitter. They range from name calling and taunts to the throwing of missiles such as stones, fireworks, and various types of bombs. Vehicles are hijacked, used as barricades, and burned. Such activities became increasingly common as the peace process got underway—a paradox also apparent in other postconflict societies (Hamber, 1998). Often included in these phenomena are rises in criminality, racketeering, and gang activity, as paramilitary groups try to keep control of their areas and diversify their activities from armed struggle to marketing drugs and counterfeit goods.

The communities most affected by the conflict and continuing violence have also suffered major population changes, as these areas have become less religiously "mixed" (Protestant and Catholic) and correspondingly more polarized. The first so-called "peace lines" were erected in August and September 1969—either by communities as barricades, or by the police and soldiers to contain rioting and incursion and to protect the warring communities. Despite the expectation that they were temporary, they have now become permanent fixtures and are bounded by areas known as "interfaces." Interfaces occur where one community lives in close proximity to the other but assiduously avoids any contact. However, when tensions are running high (such as over disputatious memorials and parades), conflict regularly ignites (Bryan, 2004).

Children's Experience of the Troubles

Children and Young People's Proximity to a Traumatic Event

An early piece of research in Northern Ireland (McGrath & Wilson, 1985) found that one in five (20%) of 522 children aged 10–11 randomly sampled across Northern Ireland reported being exposed to or near a bombing, or knew a relative or friend who had been injured. Later, McAuley (1988) found that among children in a similar age range in a socially deprived area, there was much more significant experience of conflict. She found that 37% had experience of bombs exploding, and high propor-

tions had also witnessed the throwing of stones (98%), searches by soldiers (91%), and the firing of plastic bullets (74%).

A more recent study found that a group of nearly 700 children aged
8–11 in Northern Ireland had frequently experienced conflict-related
traumatic events (Muldoon & Trew, 2000). Although exposure to such
events did not reach the levels in areas as Israel and the former Yugosla-
via, this research revealed that one in four children had witnessed shootings and street riots. In the minds of professionals in a range of children's
services, there is little doubt that children in the interface areas (i.e., those
living close to a "peace line") are particularly exposed to violence, whether
they are directly injured or are "merely" witnesses. The family described
in the case study later in the chapter lived until recently in a notorious interface area; the family members were affected daily by a barrage of missiles and experienced very real threat to their home.

Children and Young People's Relationship to the Violence

Children have also been actively involved in the Troubles as both participants and perpetrators. Although the armed conflict and the terrible
death rates at the height of the Troubles decreased, children are still involved today in jeers and taunts, stone throwing, and rioting. In some
communities, this involvement is accepted and even sanctioned by the
adults. Though Jarman and O'Halloran (2001) have described such activities as "recreational rioting," children do get hurt and are seen regularly
in the Family Trauma Centre with posttraumatic stress reactions. We also
encounter children who have been injured as a result of being attacked by
other members of their own community for misdemeanors such as petty
crime, joy riding, and drug use. This type of vigilante law enforcement is
commonly described as "punishment attacks," principally carried out by
paramilitary groups (Kennedy, 2001). The punishment meted out can be
brutal. The amount of force and weapons used—for example, guns fired at
close range into the knee, elbow, and ankle joints; baseball bats studded
with nails—leave crippling long-term injuries.

Children, Young People, and Resilience

The literature discusses coping with stressful life events, protective factors, and resilience in the face of adversity (Haggerty, Garmezy, Rutter, &
Sherrod, 1994; Fonagy, Steele, Steele, Higgit, & Target, 1994; Rutter,
2000). Cairns (1996) reviews the weak and conflicting evidence regarding
the effect of political violence on children. He suggests that it is not inevitable that children will suffer serious psychological consequences. At the
same time, those who do suffer in this way experience a wide variety of
symptoms, which tend to get worse over time rather than better. This situation is exacerbated by the fact that the degree of family support available

may diminish as political violence increases and families find it increasingly difficult to function.

Research is still required to accurately evaluate the complex relationship between vulnerability and resilience, particularly in the context of children and political violence. Resilience also must be considered at a societal and cultural level. People in Northern Ireland, of whatever religion or community identity, are described as stoical and forbearing. Recovery from crises is enabled by such traits, but the question remains: At what price? Are the characteristics of fortitude and defenses such as minimization more closely related to dissociation than is helpful for healthy adaptation? Whatever analysis is brought to the question of resilience, in the meantime clinicians continue to work with children and their families to address current crises and presenting problems—taking into account the part played by past traumas, and building resources for the future that strengthen coping responses, and, we hope, resilience.

THE TROUBLES AND THERAPY

The Troubles, past and present, are the backdrop to the range of work done at the Family Trauma Centre. In any one week, we may see people affected by the legacies of past traumas, on which the peace process has lifted the veil of silence and denial that has helped people survive and get by. We may also work with those caught up in more recent traumatic events and atrocities, such as the bomb in Omagh in 1998. Since September 2001, referrals to the Family Trauma Centre have included a rising number of children and families affected by current community violence. This includes both sectarian-inspired violence as one community fights it out on the streets with the other, and violent acts associated with the "rough justice" dealt to those who threaten the new social order in paramilitary-controlled areas. Many of the families we see have stories of much hurt and pain, but so too there are stories of stoicism and fortitude. The present trauma can combine in a toxic mix with past, often previously untreated traumas, to provide unique challenges for therapists.

Children, Trauma, and PTSD in the Context of Continuing Threat

Exposure to Trauma and Posttraumatic Stress Reactions

A traumatic event or a psychic trauma can be defined as occurring when "a sudden, unexpected, overwhelming intense emotional blow or series of blows assaults the person from outside" (Terr, 1990, p. 8). However, external traumatic events can quickly become incorporated into the mind;

consequently, a traumatic association can trigger a traumatic remembrance. Furthermore, for children as for adults, such traumatic reminders can be embedded and cued both internally and externally (Pynoos, Steinberg, & Goenjian, 1996). James (1994) argues that the basis for a diagnosis of traumatization should be the context and meaning of a child's experience, and not just the event alone or itself. She also states that it may not be the number or even the kinds of fears that are important, but rather their intensity.

For a child, fear is not only a worry about what may happen in the future, but also an immediate sensation—physiological as much as emotional and cognitive—that signals danger and threat (Greenfield, 2000). The degree of the child's fear may be determined by the absence of personal inner resources or associations that help the child make sense of the situation. Perry (1997) found that persisting fear and the neuropsychological adaptations to this fear can alter the development of the child's brain, resulting in changes in physiological, emotional, behavioral, cognitive, and social functioning. Possibly linked to this finding, and depending on the severity of the trauma and the availability of treatment, is the risk that the trauma may promote major character or personality change in the child. For example, in her study of 26 children kidnapped from their school bus in Chowchilla, California, Terr (1990) concluded that

> despite the fact that psychiatry is becoming increasingly biological and genetic, here is a place that the environment continues to rule. Nobody is born with a genetic diathesis to psychic trauma. If you scare a child badly enough, he will be traumatized—plain and simple. (p. 107)

There is evidence that psychic numbing due to repeated abuses and/or trauma may occur as a psychological defense to protect the ego from being overwhelmed (Karr-Morse & Wiley, 1997). Yet reliance on this coping mechanism may eventually distort the child's personality, resulting in difficulties in relating to others and managing feelings.

Posttraumatic Stress Disorder

Historically, it has been common for clinicians to use broad categories in classifying a child's traumatic experience. Contemporary thinking and research (e.g., Perrin, Smith, & Yule, 2000) suggest a more precise delineation of the specific objective features of traumatic experiences associated with more severe posttraumatic reactions. A child need not personally be subjected to a traumatic event to experience a posttraumatic reaction (Pynoos et al., 1996). The presence of such factors as being exposed to direct life threat; hearing unanswered screams for help and cries of distress; smelling noxious odors; being trapped or without assistance; being in proximity to threats of violence; witnessing atrocities; having a relationship to the assailant or to other victims; and being exposed to physical coercion and violation can be sufficient (Pynoos et al., 1996). Indeed, McFarlane (1988) considers that a person is victimized primarily by his or her *memories* of the event, and not necessarily by the event itself.

The diagnostic category PTSD was introduced in the *Diagnostic and Statistical Manual of Mental Disorders*, third edition (DSM-III; American Psychiatric Association, 1980) to describe the existence of a chronic clinical disorder in people exposed to traumatic stressors. Its definition has been expanded in the subsequent versions of the DSM (American Psychiatric Association, 1987, 1994, 2000) and has become a well-established category in research, the literature, and general professional usage.

PTSD is a diagnostic category that specifies a requirement of exposure to a particular type of etiological factor—that is, a traumatic event (American Psychiatric Association, 2000). PTSD initially tended to be portrayed as a "normal" reaction of an otherwise psychologically healthy person to a traumatic event. Although this has been seen as a useful stance from a therapeutic point of view, it may not stand up to statistical analysis. For example, Yehuda and Giller (1996) suggest:

> The fact that the majority of individuals do not develop chronic PTSD following a traumatic event is information recently acquired from epidemiological and longitudinal studies that compels us to reconsider the premise that exposure to trauma is not only necessary but also a sufficient condition for the development of PTSD. . . . There are obviously risk factors for PTSD *other* than trauma exposure. (p. 234; emphasis added)

The original concept of PTSD as "a normal response to an abnormal event" (Shalev, 1996, p. 78) and the implication that it does not depend on an individual's constitution, have been called into question. A more comprehensive analysis of the historical, political, and social forces that influenced the original construction of PTSD is presented by Yehuda and McFarlane (1995).

Pynoos et al. (1996), in considering the presence of factors that can precipitate a posttraumatic reaction in children, cogently argue:

> From a developmental perspective, we would urge that the concept of "traumatic memory" be placed within the broader concept of "traumatic expectation." In general, childhood traumatic experiences contribute to a schematization of the world, especially of security, safety, risk, injury, loss, protection, and intervention. The importance of traumatic memories lies in their role in shaping expectations of the recurrence of threat, of failure of protective intervention, and/or helplessness, which govern the child's emotional life and behavior. "Traumatic expectation"

provides a more powerful explanatory concept for understanding the long-term consequences of trauma on the child's emerging personality. (pp. 349–350)

These reminders, if sufficiently persistent and intrusive, can be associated with the development of secondary stresses and increase the risk of childhood comorbidity (i.e., negative changes in school performance, familial relationships, and peer relationships). Comorbidity is more likely to occur if a child has been exposed to repeated or long-standing trauma, or lives within an atmosphere of ongoing threat or unpredictability (Goenjian et al., 1995; Hubbard, Realmuto, Northwood, & Masten, 1995) . Parts of Northern Ireland have provided such an atmosphere for more than 30 years.

Beyond PTSD

Green, Wilson, and Lindy (1985) propose a psychosocial framework as a way of understanding the process by which "a particular traumatic event leads to a particular psychological process, and finally to some symptomatic or functional outcome" (p. 57). Essentially, this framework conceptualizes the traumatic experience as being cognitively processed by the victim in a way that results in a particular adaptation. This adaptation may be in the direction of stabilization and growth or, alternatively, a variety of pathological outcomes. The framework indicates that the two major factors affecting this cognitive processing (and therefore the resulting adaptation to the traumatic event) are the individual characteristics of the traumatized person and the person's recovery environment. According to this model, then, whether a particular traumatic event leads to PTSD is mediated by the individual's experiences of the event, his or her personal characteristics, and the social environment in which the individual lives. (See Webb's tripartite assessment model as described in Chapter 2 of this book for further discussion of interacting factors.)

The PTSD category, by definition, refers to situations in which the exposure to the traumatic stressor is no longer occurring (i.e., the disorder is "*post*traumatic"). It cannot, therefore, be uncritically applied to situations in which the trauma is prolonged and/or ongoing. We can appreciate how the recovery environment will be significantly different in these circumstances. In respect to the situation of ongoing low-level intercommunity and intracommunity civil conflict (with periodic high-level flare-ups) in Northern Ireland, every factor in the recovery environment may be adversely affected.

Herman (1992a, 1992b) has argued the case for recognition of a complex form of PTSD, to take account of the wider range of symptoms experienced by victims/survivors of prolonged and repeated trauma, including victims of political violence and low-intensity conflict sustained over years. Herman has referred to this as "disorders of extreme stress not otherwise specified" (DESNOS), and it was termed simply "disorders of extreme stress" (DES) for the purposes of the DSM-lV field trials. Herman (1992b) writes:

> Clinical observation identify three broad areas of disturbance which transcend simple PTSD. The first is symptomatic: the symptom picture in survivors of prolonged trauma often appears to be more complex, diffuse, and tenacious than in simple PTSD. The second is characterological: survivors of prolonged abuse develop characteristic personality changes, including deformations of relatedness and identity. The third area involves the survivor's vulnerability to repeated harm, both self-inflicted and at the hands of others. (p. 379)

van der Kolk (1996), in reviewing the complexity of adaptation to trauma, refers to the field trials conducted on this new category of DES for the DSM-IV (van der Kolk, Roth, Pelcovitz, & Mandel, 1993). Although DES was not formally incorporated into DSM-IV, the trials "confirmed that trauma has its most profound impact during the first decade of life, and that its effects become less pervasive in more mature individuals" (van der Kolk, 1996, p. 202). Such a conclusion lends support to our commitment to work actively with traumatized children, and our working hypothesis that such treatment will have potentially long-lasting effects on the lives of the children we see.

Underpinning Herman's proposal for a revision of PTSD to include more acknowledgment of the complexity of human experience and presentation of reactions to trauma is the assumption that trauma can also be experienced as continuing. We find this construction helpful, given that more than 30 years have passed since the start of the Troubles in Northern Ireland, and thus a whole generation has known nothing other than a context of ongoing civil conflict. For this generation, a peaceful society would be an aberration of their normal experience.

Jenkins and Bell (1997), writing about the urban United States, provide an apt description of children's experience that also applies in parts of Northern Ireland:

> Many children, particularly those in urban areas, are exposed to considerable amounts of life-threatening violence in their homes and communities. Such exposure may be a result of direct victimization or, more likely and more difficult to document, [may consist of] witnessing . . . violence and having friends and family members victimized by violence. Often the violence is chronic, with children existing in milieus where violence and threat of violence are constant. (p. 9)

Establishing safety is usually a prerequisite for treatment of PTSD. In situations of ongoing civil conflict, the establishment of safety is an equally important consideration, but is much more relative in nature (Coulter, 2001). Most of the children and families we work with live in communities characterized by low-level chronic conflict, with periodic exacerbations affecting the families or localities. The memory of one trauma can be activated by news of similar incidents involving others in the community and/or by a further trauma to the same individual or family. In this regard, perhaps due to the increased vulnerability to harm by self or others (referred to by Herman, 1992b, above), the "world is ill divided." Our experience is that multiple traumas tend to affect particular family networks cumulatively.

Bringing a Systemic Approach to Trauma Recovery

In making a connection between childhood trauma and troubled development, Garbarino, Dubrow, Kostelny, and Pardo (1992) state:

> Children draw maps of their world and their place in it and move forward on paths they believe exist. If the child's map is of a hostile world and self as insignificant we must expect troubled development. (p. 10)

This is the concern we are seeking to address. The organizing principles of our work are to create an experience of mastery for children and to help open as many alternative positive paths for children and their families as possible.

We describe our approach as multimodal. It includes a variety of methods and techniques to treat the effects of traumatic events. From the internal and intrapsychic aspects to the more relational aspects of human functioning and promotion of well-being, we keep each individual's context and lived experience in mind. We may work directly with the other agencies and services involved with our clients' lives toward the development of more empowering experiences that enable our clients to continue to survive in the community.

Figley (1986) proposes the following four tasks to help a family integrate the impact of a traumatic experience:

1. To determine how the catastrophic experiences and the family problem(s) in which it may be embedded are affecting each individual family member.
2. To explore how this problematic behavior may be reinforcing or exacerbating the difficulties.

3. To assess the family's understanding of the effects of trauma, in terms of both immediate and long-term consequences.
4. To establish strategies that family members can use to deal with their trauma-associated problems and difficulties.

Figley (1988) also identifies a paradox for family members seeking mutual support, in the following terms:

> Families attempting to cope with an extraordinarily stressful event, for example, tend to draw together for mutual comfort and emotional assistance. Yet at the same time, because family interaction under stressful conditions often increases stress, there is also a tendency to separate, to avoid interaction, particularly discussions of the trauma. (p. 93)

It is our experience that many of the families we see require professional help in facilitating these kinds of conversations, so they can achieve better communication and ameliorate the effects of this paradox.

As noted above, in addition to the effects of any specific traumatic event, the chronic effect on families of living in a society/area characterized by continual violence must be considered. Osofsky, Wewers, Hann, and Fick (1993) found a significant relationship between exposure to chronic community violence and stress reactions in young children. Reactions included sadness, anger, aggressiveness, sleep disturbance, uncaring behavior, and erratic behavior. There is also evidence that due to young children's less developed psychological concepts, they struggle more to make sense of traumatic events and suffer more PTSD. For example, Davidson and Smith (1990) found that traumatic events experienced before age 11 were three times more likely to result in PTSD than events experienced after age 12.

Therapists must provide children with specialized and developmentally informed input. Marans and Adelman (1997) for example, make the following observation:

> What sets childhood trauma apart from adulthood trauma is that, for children, the adaptive capacities, defensive structures, and internal resources—as these are determined by developmental processes—are vastly different than those potentially available to adults. In the throes of the maturational process, children have fewer and more uneven psychological resources at their disposal: their developing defensive organization is acutely vulnerable to traumatic disruptions, derailments and impingements from the environment. (p. 205)

Frederick and Sheltren (2000) put the therapeutic situation more forcefully. They note that children are unlikely to do well in therapy if they are forced to lie on the procrustean bed of adult communication. The child's verbal skills are not fully formed. Children tend to express their feelings and the meanings of their interactions metaphorically, through play and games, story-telling and art. (p. 187)

Play therapy, therefore, is the preferred method of treatment for children under age 12 (Webb, 1999).

At the same time, a family-oriented systemic approach needs to take account of the interactions between parents and children (Dyregrov, 2001). Thus a combined systemic and developmental understanding informs our practice and leads to a therapeutic mixture of art, enactment, writing, and story for processing the traumatic events, as illustrated in the case study below. These methods run counter to the traumatic experiences and the environment of chronic civil conflict, in that they may be both pleasurable experiences in themselves as well as cathartic, placing children and their parents in a position of control over the output (Hanney & Kozlowska, 2002).

CASE STUDY: THE MCGARRY FAMILY[1]

Background

The family (Catholics) consists of Margaret, mother, age 28 at the time of intake; Kevin, father, age 30; elder daughter, Maria, age 9; elder son, Kevin, named after his father and age 8; younger son, Conor, age 7; and younger daughter, Megan, age 3. The McGarrys came to the Family Trauma Centre during the summer of 2001, a time when community tensions were running high in several of the interface areas in Belfast. The family home was adjacent to a high "peace wall" dividing a loyalist/Protestant community from its nationalist/Catholic neighbors. For many years the two communities had existed side by side, sharing commercial facilities and shops. Some streets were mixed, with Protestant and Catholic families living close by. However, over the course of the Troubles, a creeping "ghettoization" developed. In the year previous to the referral, a bitter internal loyalist paramilitary feud caused families from a more hard-line loyalist area a kilometer away to be relocated to the area where the McGarrys lived.

The fragile coexistence escalated into violent confrontations toward the end of the 2000–2001 school year, when Protestants objected to Catholic parents' walking their children to school along the street through

---

[1]The family members signed a release granting permission to write about their experience; however, their names have been changed to preserve confidentiality.

which both the Protestant and Catholic primary schools are accessed. The loyalist/Protestant residents described their protest as a desperate measure to draw attention to their sense of being systematically pressured to move out of the neighborhood so that Catholics could take over their houses. The end of the school year brought no lessening of tension. The barrage of missiles thrown over the "peace wall" continued, and families like the McGarrys, whose yard backed onto the wall, were particularly vulnerable.

The Referral

Two of us (Isobel Reilly and Stephen Coulter) worked together with the McGarrys following their referral to the Family Trauma Centre. For several weeks, stones and missiles had been thrown at the back of their house, and the parents had been struggling with the walk to school with Maria, the oldest child. The McGarrys were not being specifically singled out. Many of their neighbors' houses were suffering the same fate, and many had metal bars fixed to the windows. On one particular night, a petrol (gasoline) bomb struck the McGarrys' house. The children's toys were destroyed, and Conor, the 7-year-old son, was so distressed his parents couldn't calm him down. He was brought to the emergency room of the local hospital, where it was recommended that the family physician seek specialist help for the boy and support for the family as a whole. In her referral to the Family Trauma Centre, the family physician also said that all the children were feeling unsafe, and that the mother had been prescribed medication to help lower her level of anxiety.

The Therapeutic Process

Initial Family Session

The aim of the initial family session was threefold:

- First, to engage all the family members so we could support them through the difficult and frightening time they were experiencing.
- Second, to specifically assess Conor's trauma reactions.
- Third, to provide the parents with psychoeducational information and material that would assist them in managing the children's reactions to the ongoing stress.

The creation of a genogram revealed some of the Troubles-related trauma stories from the past, as well as information about the mother's miscarriages and a baby who had survived only a few days and was still much remembered and mourned. The children participated with great enthusiasm, making sure that we accurately recorded all their cousins and where they lived. They spoke of how much they loved their grandparents, and also conveyed their awareness of their maternal grandmother's deteriorating health. After a short break, when Conor was seen individually, the treatment plan was discussed with the parents. We saw this as combining general support to the family as a whole and a specific focus on Conor (with whom Stephen Coulter would conduct a series of individual sessions).

Response to Individual Needs

After the first few individual sessions with Conor, it became clear that Margaret, his mother, was also suffering from the accumulated effects of the recent stressful events in the community. The family had applied for emergency accommodation and, on fleeing their home, were put up in a local hotel for a few days. Margaret's mental state deteriorated sharply; she confided feelings that life was not worth living, and expressed suicidal intent that also included the children. This constituted a mental health emergency, and an appointment was quickly arranged for her assessment at the local psychiatric outpatient clinic. The assessment was followed by an emergency admission and a 2-week hospital stay. Margaret's recovery was assisted by support from extended family members, who helped Kevin take care of the children. In addition, Margaret was motivated to be well enough to cope with her own mother's terminal illness.

Some months later (after the grandmother had died), the older son, Kevin, now age 9, refused to go to school and was described as very upset and difficult. He too required some individual therapy (again with Stephen Coulter). Individual sessions have been a recurring feature of our work with the McGarry family, as each new crisis has called for specific attention. Maria, the older daughter, has also been seen (by Isobel Reilly) both separately and with her mother, when exam stress was high and her appetite and eating habits were giving concern.

Seeing the Bigger Picture

At the time of this writing, therapeutic involvement with the family has continued for 18 months. The work has been a mixture of individual therapy with the two boys, the elder daughter, and the mother; regularly convened family sessions every few months (including several conducted in the family's old and new homes); and occasional couple sessions with a focus on parenting issues. Interventions in the wider system have been undertaken by a number of different professionals. For example, the school principal joined in our recommendation for rehousing (which needed police confirmation of intimidation), and we worked with the family doctor when the mother's mental health crisis precipitated her emergency hospital admission. In the background was the maternal grandmother's terminal illness. The family history also revealed traumatic deaths and injuries associated with the Troubles, as well as stories of emigration by some members in order to make better lives for themselves.

Our work with the family has focused on individual therapy within an overall context of ongoing family support. Over the time of our contact, the pattern that has evolved is one of episodic periods of specific involvement and interventions against the backdrop of longer-term continuing support. Critical times when involvement has increased noticeably have centered around the house move and the deaths of the maternal grandparents.

Taking the Longer View

We have learned from this family the importance of staying in touch and its value in the context of complex and continuing trauma. The work has also brought a much greater appreciation of the vulnerability of families in trauma and crisis, and the corresponding need to accompany the highs and lows as events unfold. One example of this was the maternal grandfather's diagnosis of and death from lung cancer, less than a year after his wife's death.

We bring to our work knowledge of the impact of traumatic events and the potential erosion of families' abilities to adapt and go forward. We have noted the relative speed with which the impact of traumatic stress can ricochet around a family, with presentations for particular help surfacing episodically in relation to unfolding events. Shamai (2001), working in Israel, studied parental perceptions of children in a context of shared political uncertainty. She found that "children are often a channel for expression of their parents' emotion, and that the feelings evoked by the uncertainty are negative emotions such as fear, anger, hate, the desire for revenge, and avoidance" (p. 249). Families can become "trauma-organized systems" (Banyard, Englund, & Rozelle, 2001; Bentovim, 1992), alerting us to the way in which trauma can contaminate family relations.

In addition to being sensitive to these dimensions of trauma recovery, we need to review our plans regularly and to encompass a more flexible clinical approach, rather than one dominated by conventions such as contracts with endpoints and fixed appointments. Very often as other events intervene, cancellations and rescheduling are recurrent features; these are normal and are not seen as disruptions or nuisances.

Working with continuing trauma in a context where normal, yet stressful, life events (e.g., house moves, school examinations, and class changes) exacerbate an already tense situation is both complex and challenging. Our multimodal approach allows us to bring together disparate treatment methodologies and to change pace and focus as needed.

Writing and Witnessing: The Use of Writing as an Archival and Therapeutic Tool

One aspect of our involvement with the McGarry family has been the use made of writing. Several authors have attested to the mental health benefits of writing (Pennebaker, 1993, 1997; Esterling, L'Abate, Murray, & Pennebaker, 1999), while others have used writing to help clients give voice to painful memories and experiences (Penn, 2001; Weingarten & Worthern, 1997; Weingarten, 2000). In Northern Ireland, several victims' groups have harnessed the power of stories to give expression to people's experiences through the Troubles, using both the written word and video (An Crann/The Tree, 2000; Smyth & Fay, 2000). Radio has also been a fruitful medium utilized by many to bear witness to private loss and pain (Reilly, 2000). With the McGarry family, writing became a very powerful medium and a significant element of our work. Some pieces were initiated by us as therapists, such as Conor's "List of Things a 7-Year-Old Shouldn't See" (August 2001):

1. bricks thrown at our windows
2. gun-man running up the alley
3. car getting smashed up
4. men shooting at the wall
5. nail/tennis ball bomb thrown over and banged
6. a brick hit me on back of head
7. pipe bomb—kitchen windows smashed
8. petrol bomb × 2—toys burnt
9. blast bombs in area

This was followed by a sequel 1 month later—"More Things a 7-Year-Old Shouldn't See (but I've Seen)"—which included seeing a man with a big gun; his father and older sister hit by bricks; fireworks exploding over the family's shed; and a friend hit by the police. Counterbalancing these lists was one entitled "Things I Am Looking Forward To":

1. when they stop throwing fireworks
2. stop throwing bricks
3. getting a new house

Other examples of therapist-initiated writing have included Maria's food diary and, more recently, Margaret's daily 15-minute freestyle diary entry.

Some writing has been initiated by family members themselves and is seen as therapeutically beneficial. The chief example of this has been Margaret's book, which she titled after the song "Something Inside So Strong." In this she wrote about herself, her upbringing, and the values she derived from her parents—a legacy that was (and still is) helping her to keep going. In her book she recorded the day-to-day details of things happening to her family, her neighbors, and her friends, in a mixture of observations and reflections. Here is an excerpt:

> I heard a bang and my kitchen smashed into pieces. I stood in shock I dont remember much after that but I do remember Conor squealing, he was shouting, give me a knife so I can kill them. Somebody tried to hold him back and calm him down. I was taken to hospital by ambulance along with my neighbour. It was my next door neighbour's house which was hit by a pipe bomb but my windows came in.

Maria also kept notes that she brought for us to read. Her school had been receiving lots of letters from sympathetic people all over the world, especially the United States, and this draft was stimulated by those letters to the school:

> One day me and my friend were playing out my back garden having lots of fun. . . . a brick came over, we never bothered until more came . . . we came running into my mother and told her. She went out, there was nothing there, we went back to see . . . it was quiet, you could have heard a leaf fall. We were afraid of something happening so we went in. . . . I forgot to tell who I am, well I am . . . my name is Maria and I am in primary 5, I am 10 years old and one other thing is my Granny died before Christmas, well 20 November 2001.

Margaret was still writing her book 6 to 8 months after her mother's death, and well after the McGarrys had moved house and were settled in a more peaceful area. When asked about the value in writing about such difficult times, Margaret replied with a paradox: "Writing about the bad is good." Maria was party to this conversation, and she agreed with her mother. Margaret's reason was that while the bad times were awful and frightening, they also included her last few weeks with her mother before she died, and she derived comfort from those memories. Furthermore, the act of writing was in itself cathartic; she could later read over her story, and the words on the page were an affirmation that what happened was really true.

The family made a scrapbook full of press cuttings of the summer of 2001, some featuring photographs of Maria and Megan. Together with Margaret's book, these constitute an archive of an important point in the family's history, when against many odds (community violence, family ill health and death, school problems and worries) the family pulled through.

Other pieces of writing by the family came as requirements from outside. One of these was a letter written by Margaret to the education authority to request that Maria be considered favorably for a transfer to a particular high school, as her marks for her last year in primary school were adversely affected by the community violence. Another example is Kevin's poem about his grandmother, which was written in schoolwork and went on to be published locally:

> When all the others are away watching football,
> I was all hers. We spring-cleaned the rooms.
> The fresh smell of polish sprayed on the furniture,
> The silence broken as we poured water into the bucket.
> The steam billowing up from the heat of the water
> spreading across the room.
>
> Sitting for hours beside her hospice bed,
> I watch, just in case she needs something done.
> Waiting, hoping.
> Mummy cries with some of her brothers,
> Others just stand and stare.
> Daddy has to go a message[2] with grandad.
> I remember putting her cross and chain back
> On her bedside table and dusting her ornamental jar;
> Thinking about the special time I spent with her.

Witnessing, with its several dimensions and interactive aspects—telling, being heard; listening, and hearing—is essential to the therapeutic process. In agreeing what details of the family's story and extracts from members' writings to include in this chapter, Margaret has said how pleased she is to have the opportunity to share her experiences.

IMPACT ON THE THERAPISTS

Like our clients, we ourselves live in the shadow of community violence. Although it is possible to avoid flashpoints, such as along the interface areas, sometimes our work takes us close to danger. As individuals, we also have our own stories—fleeing from bombs, losing our cars to "joy riders," being stuck for hours unable to get home because of security alerts, enduring checkpoints in shopping areas, and being body-searched at airport terminals.

Pearlman and Saakvitne (1995) and Figley (2002) alert us to the effects of vicarious or secondary traumatization on therapists engaged in

---

[2]"Message" is a colloquialism for "shopping."

psychotherapy with trauma survivors. To ameliorate the negative effects of the toxicity of trauma, we have found it crucial to have some balance in our working lives. We achieve this through having other interests and responsibilities such as teaching, research, and writing. These afford us with opportunities both to "stand back" and to process the work and its impact. Other opportunities, such as those mentioned in Chapter 15 of this book, include supervision and study days. Working in teams has proved immensely valuable—not just for sharing clinical management but for debriefing and psychological support. Team composition reflects the two different communities (Protestant and Catholic), and it also ensures that we bring a breadth and depth of understanding to our practice.

LOOKING FORWARD

In this chapter, we have described the context for trauma recovery in Northern Ireland, where the nature of the community violence affecting society is described as ongoing, low-level conflict with high-level exacerbations. The particular effect of this is to sensitize people and make them less able to cope with the developmental and predictable life crises. The shadow cast by this context has implications for both treatment and recovery. Sluzki (1993) argues that such politically motivated violence has a "devastating and long-lasting effect on its victims" (p. 178). There is a fundamental dissonance between the social contract that binds us as human beings to care for and about each other, and community violence that threatens to erode this commitment. Assumptions we normally have about being able to protect our children and ourselves are challenged. Violence destroys the meanings we hold dear about stability and predictability, and "mystifies meanings so that recognition of that shift from protection to violence is blurred" (Sluzki, 1993, p. 178). This is the "interface" where we work as therapists in the Northern Ireland context. Using our expertise in facilitating healing and transformative practices, and contributing in this way alongside the wider process of community relations, conflict resolution, mediation, and peace-building work, constitute the challenge we face in countering the effects of political and community violence.

REFERENCES

American Psychiatric Association. (1980). *Diagnostic and statistical manual of mental disorders* (3rd ed.). Washington, DC: Author.
American Psychiatric Association. (1987). *Diagnostic and statistical manual of mental disorders* (3rd ed., rev.). Washington, DC: Author.

American Psychiatric Association. (1994). *Diagnostic and statistical manual of mental disorders* (4th ed.). Washington, DC: Author.

American Psychiatric Association. (2000). *Diagnostic and statistical manual of mental disorders* (4th ed, text rev.). Washington, DC: Author.

An Crann/The Tree. (2000). *Bear in mind: Stories of the Troubles.* Belfast: Lagan Press.

Banyard, V. L., Englund, D. W., & Rozelle, D. (2001). Parenting the traumatised child: Attending to the need of nonoffending caregivers of traumatised children. *Psychotherapy, 38,* 74–87.

Bentovim, A. (1992). *Trauma organized systems: Physical and sexual abuse in families.* London: Karnac Books.

Bloomfield, K. (1998). *We will remember them: Report of the Northern Ireland Victims' Commissioner.* Belfast: Her Majesty's Stationery Office.

Bryan, D. (2004). Belfast: Urban space, 'policing' and sectarian polarisation. In J. Schneider & I. Susser (Eds.), *Wounded cities.* Oxford: Berg.

Cairns, E. (1996). *Children and political violence.* Oxford: Blackwell.

Coulter, S. (2001). Creating safety for trauma survivors: What can therapists do? *Child Care in Practice, 7*(1), 45–56.

Davidson, J., & Smith, R. (1990). Traumatic experiences in psychiatric outpatients. *Journal of Traumatic Stress Studies, 3*(3), 459–475.

Dyregrov, A. (2001). Early intervention: A family perspective. *Advances in Mind–Body Medicine, 17,* 9–17.

Esterling, B. A., L'Abate, L., Muray, E. J., & Pennebaker, J. W. (1999). Empirical foundations for writing in prevention and psychotherapy: Mental and physical health outcomes. *Clinical Psychology Review, 19*(1), 79–96.

Fay, M. T., Morrissey, M., & Smyth, M. (1999). *Northern Ireland's Troubles: The human costs.* London: Pluto Press.

Figley, C. R. (Ed.). (1986). *Trauma and its wake: Vol. 2. Traumatic stress theory, research, and intervention.* New York: Brunner/Mazel.

Figley, C. R. (1988). Post-traumatic family therapy. In F. M. Ochberg (Ed.), *Post-traumatic therapy and victims of violence* (pp. 83–109). New York: Brunner/Mazel.

Figley, C. R. (Ed.). (2002). *Treating compassion fatigue.* New York: Brunner-Routledge

Fonagy, P., Steele, M., Steele, H., Higitt, A., & Target, M. (1994). The Emanuel Miller Memorial Lecture 1992: The theory and practice of resilience. *Journal of Child Psychology and Psychiatry, 35,* 231–257.

Frederick, C., & Sheltren, C. (2000). All in the family: Therapy for the families of traumatised children and adolescents. In K. N. Dwivedi (Ed.), *Post traumatic stress disorder in children and adolescents* (pp. 184–197). London: Whurr.

Garbarino, J., Dubrow, N., Kostelny, K., & Pardo, C. (1992). *Children in danger: coping with the consequences of community violence.* San Francisco: Jossey-Bass.

Goenjian, A., Pynoos, R. S., Steinberg, A. M., Najarian, L. M., Asarnow, J. R., Karayan, I., Ghurabi, M., & Fairbanks, L. A. (1995). Psychiatric co-morbidity in children after the 1988 earthquake in Armenia. *Journal of the American Academy of Child and Adolescent Psychiatry, 34,* 1174–1184.

Green, B., Wilson, J., & Lindy, J. (1985). Conceptualizing post-traumatic stress disorder: A psychosocial framework. In C. Figley (Ed.), *Trauma and its wake: Vol. 1. The study and treatment of post-traumatic stress disorder* (pp. 53–69). New York: Brunner/Mazel.

Greenfield, S. (2000). *The private life of the brain.* London: Penguin.

Haggerty, R. J., Garmezy, N., Rutter, M., & Sherrod, L. (Eds.). (1994). *Stress, risk and resilience in children and adolescents: Process mechanisms and interventions.* Cambridge, England: Cambridge University Press.

Hamber, B. (Ed.). (1998). *Past imperfect: Dealing with the past in Northern Ireland.* Derry/Londonderry, Northern Ireland: INCORE (University of Ulster and the United Nations University).

Hanney, L., & Kozlowska, K. (2002). Healing traumatized children: Creating illustrated storybooks in family therapy. *Family Process, 11*(1), 37–65.

Herman, J. L. (1992a). *Trauma and recovery: From domestic abuse to political power.* London: Pandora.

Herman, J. L. (1992b). Complex PTSD: A syndrome in survivors of prolonged and repeated trauma. *Journal of Traumatic Stress, 5,* 377–391.

Hubbard, J., Realmuto, G. M., Northwood, A. K., & Masten, A. S. (1995). Comorbidity of psychiatric diagnoses with posttraumatic stress disorder in survivors of childhood trauma. *Journal of the American Academy of Child and Adolescent Psychiatry, 34*(9), 1167–1173.

James, B. (1994). *Handbook for treatment of attachment-trauma problems in children.* New York: Lexington Books.

Jarman, N., & O'Halloran, C. (2001). Recreational rioting: Young people, interface areas and violence. *Child Care in Practice, 7*(1), 2–16.

Jenkins, E. J., & Bell, C. C. (1997). Exposure and response to community violence among children and adolescents. In J. D. Osofsky (Ed.), *Children in a violent society* (pp. 9–31). New York: Guilford Press.

Karr-Morse, R., & Wiley, M. S. (1997). *Ghosts from the nursery: Tracing the roots of violence.* New York: Atlantic Monthly Press.

Kennedy, L. (2001). *They shoot children, don't they?: An analysis of the age and gender of victims of paramilitary 'punishments' in Northern Ireland* (Report prepared for the Northern Ireland Committee against Terror and the Northern Ireland Affairs Committee of the House of Commons) [Online]. Available: http://cain.ulst.ac.uk/issues/violence/docs/kennedy01.htm

Marans, S., & Adelman, A. (1997). Experiencing violence in a developmental context. In J. D. Osofsky (Ed.), *Children in a violent society* (pp. 202–222). New York: Guilford Press.

McAuley, P. (1988). *On the fringes of society: Adults and children in a disadvantaged Belfast community.* Unpublished doctoral thesis, Queen's University, Belfast.

McFarlane, A. C. (1988). The phenomenology of posttraumatic stress disorders following a natural disaster. *Journal of Nervous and Mental Disease, 176*(1), 22–29.

McGrath, A., & Wilson, R. (1985, September). *Factors which influence the prevalence and variation of psychological problems in children in Northern Ireland.* Paper presented at the annual conference of the Development Section of the British Psychological Society, Belfast.

Muldoon, O., & Trew, K. (2000). Children's experience and adjustment to political conflict in Northern Ireland. *Peace and Conflict, 6*(2), 157–176.

Osofsky, J. D., Wewers, S., Hann, D. M., & Fick, A. C. (1993). Chronic community violence: What is happening to our children? *Psychiatry: Interpersonal and Biological Processes, 56,* 36–45.

Pearlman, L. A., & Saakvitne, K. W. (1995). *Trauma and the therapist.* New York: Norton.

Penn, P. (2001). Chronic illness, trauma, language and writing: Breaking the silence. *Family Process, 40*(1), 33–52.

Pennebaker, J. W. (1993). Putting stress into words: Health, linguistic, and therapeutic implications. *Behaviour Research and Therapy, 31*, 539–547.

Pennebaker, J. W. (1997). Writing about emotional experiences as a therapeutic process. *Psychological Science, 8*(3), 162–163.

Perrin, S., Smith, P., & Yule, W. (2000). The assessment and treatment of posttraumatic stress disorder in children and adolescents. *Journal of Child Psychology and Psychiatry, 41*(3), 277–290.

Perry, B. D. (1997). Incubated in terror: Neurodevelopmental factors in the "cycle of violence." In J. D. Osofsky (Ed.), *Children in a violent society* (pp. 124–148). New York: Guilford Press.

Pynoos, R., Steinberg, A., & Goenjian, A. (1996). Traumatic stress in childhood and adolescence: Recent developments and current controversies. In B. A. van der Kolk, A. C. McFarlane, & L. Weisaeth (Eds.), *Traumatic stress: The effects of overwhelming experience on mind, body, and society* (pp. 331–358). New York: Guilford Press.

Reilly, I. (2000). Legacy: People and poets in Northern Ireland. *Australian and New Zealand Journal of Family Therapy, 21*(3), 162–166.

Rutter, M. (2000). Resilience reconsidered: Conceptual considerations, empirical findings and policy implications. In J. P. Shonkoff & S. J. Meisels (Eds.), *Handbook of early childhood intervention* (pp. 651–682). New York: Cambridge University Press.

Shalev, A. Y. (1996). Stress versus traumatic stress: From acute homeostatic reactions to chronic psychopathology. In B. A. van der Kolk, A. C. McFarlane, & L. Weisaeth (Eds.), *Traumatic stress: The effects of overwhelming experience on mind, body, and society* (pp. 77–101). New York: Guilford Press.

Shamai, M. (2001). Parents' perceptions of their children in a context of shared political uncertainty, *Child and Family Social Work, 6*, 249–260.

Sluzki, C. (1993). Toward a model of family and political victimisation: Implications for treatment and recovery. *Psychiatry, 56*, 178–187.

Smyth, M., & Fay, M. T. (2000). *Personal accounts from Northern Ireland's Troubles: Public conflict, private loss.* London: Pluto Press.

Terr, L. (1990). *Too scared to cry.* New York: Harper & Row.

van der Kolk, B. A. (1996). The complexity of adaptation to trauma: Self-regulation, stimulus discrimination, and characterological development. In B. A. van der Kolk, A. C. McFarlane, & L. Weisaeth (Eds.), *Traumatic stress: The effects of overwhelming experience on mind, body, and society* (pp. 182–213). New York: Guilford Press.

van der Kolk, B. A., Roth, S., Pelcovitz, D., & Mandel, F. (1993). *Disorders of extreme stress: Results of the DSM-IV field trials for PTSD.* Washington, DC: American Psychiatric Association.

Webb, N. B. (Ed.). (1999). *Play therapy with children in crisis* (2nd ed.): *Individual, group, and family treatment.* New York: Guilford Press.

Weingarten, K. (2000). Witnessing, wonder and hope. *Family Process, 39*(4), 389–402.

Weingarten, K., & Worthern, M. E. W. (1997). A narrative approach to understanding the illness experience of a mother and daughter. *Families, Systems and Health, 15,* 41–54.

Yehuda, R., & Giller, E. L., Jr. (1996). Diagnosis and assessment of individuals who have experienced traumatic events: a review of the conceptual and practice issues. *Baillière's Clinical Psychiatry, 2*(2), 229–243.

Yehuda, R., & McFarlane, A. C. (1995). Conflict between current knowledge about posttraumatic stress disorder and its original conceptual basis. *American Journal of Psychiatry, 152*(12), 1705–1713.

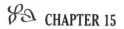 CHAPTER 15

Avoiding Vicarious Traumatization

Support, Spirituality, and Self-Care

MADDY CUNNINGHAM

> Trauma is like a pebble thrown into a pool: just as the circles of water
> spread further and further to the perimeter of the pool, the anxiety
> generated by a traumatic event can have a rippling effect on families, on
> communities, and even on future generations.
>
> —TERR (1989, p. 15)

Those of us who treat terrorized children are exposed to traumatic events
and the painful consequences of those events vicariously. As we listen to
the children's stories, watch their play, and witness the accompanying
painful feelings of rage, anguish, and fear, we often find ourselves having
some of the same reactions. Using the concept of "vicarious traumatization" (McCann & Pearlman, 1990a; Pearlman & Saakvitne, 1995a) as a
framework, this chapter focuses on the "rippling effect" of terrorism on
therapists treating children affected by large-scale traumatic events, such
as the attacks of September 11, 2001, or the Oklahoma City bombing. I
present a discussion of vicarious traumatization, its evolution, and its
symptoms; I then focus on a variety of ways to limit and alleviate its deleterious effects.

September 11, 2001 dawned warm and clear in New York City. It was
the kind of late summer day everyone cherishes, knowing the cool winds
of autumn are not far away. As we busied ourselves getting ready for a
normal day of work or school, we had no idea that within a few short
hours we would experience unspeakable horror. At approximately 8:46
A.M., American Airlines Flight 11, bound for Los Angeles, struck the
South Tower of the World Trade Center (WTC). It was first believed to be
an awful accident, and the media rushed to the scene. Shortly afterward,
"live" on television, the North Tower was hit by a second plane. Ulti-

mately, both towers collapsed into a heap of rubble as stunned Americans watched on their television screens. Meanwhile, in Washington, D.C., a plane struck the Pentagon; another hijacked plane, targeting the White House, crashed in a field in Pennsylvania. Within a short period of time, it was clear that an unprecedented event was occurring: The United States was under a wide-scale attack by terrorists. Airports were shut down, and in-air flights were ordered to land. Bridges and tunnels were closed, and the U.S. borders with Canada and Mexico were secured. Many schools were "locked down," only releasing children when parents contacted school personnel. Chaos and confusion reigned. In the attacks of that day, it is estimated that a total of over 3,000 people lost their lives. Images of people fleeing the WTC scene, the planes hitting the towers, and the collapse of the buildings were played repeatedly on the television screen and in our minds. Fear of more attacks filled us with fear, and grief gripped our hearts as we learned of lost lives and shattered families.

On April 19, 1995, in Oklahoma City, the Murrah Federal Building was bombed, leaving 168 people dead, including 19 children who attended a day care center in the building. In addition, 219 children lost a parent in the bombing, and 3 of these children were left parentless. Fifty children were injured (Oklahoma State Department of Health, 1996). Prior to 9/11, this was the largest terrorist attack in the United States.

THE DIRECT AND INDIRECT IMPACT OF TERRORISM

When wide-scale, highly publicized events such as these occur, we experience confusion, fear, disorientation, grief, sadness, anger, and terror. It is difficult to understand what is happening, or to make sense out of the horror. It is even more difficult for children, whose cognitive and emotional capacities are still developing. Terror renders individuals helpless; overwhelms their capacity to adapt; and affects their sense of control, connection, and meaning (Herman, 1992). The intent of terrorism is not only to kill, maim, and destroy, but specifically to create overwhelming fear. Terrorists seek to destroy individuals from within, so that they are no longer free to live their lives as they once knew them. As Kastenbaum (2001) states, terrorism "changes the way a society thinks about itself" (p. 236).

Moreover, those who witness the pain and suffering of other human beings are at risk of being affected by the same traumatic events (Figley, 1995). A growing body of research indicates that families and friends of victims (Terr, 1989), disaster rescue personnel (Ursano & Fullerton, 1990; Fullerton, McCarroll, Ursano, & Wright, 1992; Beaton & Murphy, 1995), and therapists treating traumatized clients (Cunningham, 2003; Follette, Polusny, & Milbeck, 1994; Pearlman & MacIan, 1995) are all adversely affected by the victims' experiences. Therefore, terrorism affects not only the direct victims, but also those who are able to identify with these victims through a shared sense of community, value, or meaning of the event (Gurwitch, Sitterle, Young, & Pfefferbaum, 2002; Wright, Ursano, Bartone, & Ingraham, 1990). For instance, when the Murrah Building was bombed in Oklahoma City, a client of mine was distraught, even though she knew no one in Oklahoma. Her distress was related to her ability to identify with the grieving parents of the children who were killed in the blast because they attended an on-site day care center. This client had a young daughter in day care and felt very frightened and vulnerable.

THERAPISTS AND TRAUMA WORK: WHY THERAPISTS ARE AT RISK

Historically, the concepts of "countertransference" and "burnout" have been used to describe the experiences of a therapist in the therapeutic encounter. The classical definition of "countertransference" focuses on the individual characteristics of the clinician, often assuming that unresolved personal conflicts account for the therapist's reactions (Gorkin, 1987; McCann & Pearlman, 1990a; Pearlman & Saakvitne, 1995a). However, the nature of countertransference in working with a traumatized child appears to have a distinctive quality related to the content presented by the client, rather than unresolved personal conflicts in the worker (McCann & Pearlman, 1990a; Herman, 1992). Therapists working with traumatized clients may experience reactions similar to those of their clients, including despair, rage, terror, feelings of being overwhelmed, nightmares, and concerns for personal safety (Danieli, 1985; Courtois, 1988, Briere, 1989). In addition, they may feel overwhelmed in their role as witnesses to others' horrific pain and suffering (Herman, 1992).

"Burnout" is another concept used to describe the deleterious affect of demanding therapeutic work. Factors frequently cited in the development of burnout include the isolation of the work, difficult or demanding clients, excessive workload, the need to be constantly empathetic, and bureaucratic and administrative factors (Freudenberger & Robbins, 1979; Farber & Heifetz, 1982; Maslach, 1982). Although many of these factors may also relate to therapists working with terrorized children, the concept of burnout does not adequately capture the experience of therapists exposed to the horrific details of trauma and terrorism (McCann & Pearlman, 1990a; Pearlman & Saakvitne, 1995a).

Since the concepts of countertransference and burnout are insufficient in understanding the impact of therapeutic work with clients such as terrorized children, McCann and Pearlman (1990a) developed a new concept, "vicarious traumatization." They propose that working with these populations can be distinguished from working with other "difficult populations" because of the worker's exposure "to the emotionally shocking images of horror and suffering that are characteristic of serious trauma" (McCann & Pearlman, 1990a, p. 134). Vicarious traumatization is a transformative process that develops over time and accounts for the interaction of personal characteristics of the therapist, the work environment, and the traumatic material and behavior a client presents in sessions (McCann & Pearlman, 1990a; Pearlman & Saakvitne, 1995a).

The hallmark of trauma is the disruptions in people's world views or the assumptions they make about the world. Individuals use these cognitive structures or schemas to organize experience and to function with a certain amount of confidence on a daily basis (Janoff-Bulman, 1992; Epstein, 1991). Common theories people have about themselves and their world include the assumptions that the world is a safe place (Janoff-Bulman, 1989), that they themselves are invulnerable (Perloff, 1983), that other people are basically good, and that events are meaningful (Janoff-Bulman & Frieze, 1983; Janoff-Bulman, 1989; McCann & Pearlman, 1990a).

According to McCann and Pearlman (1990b), schemas are cognitive manifestations of psychological needs and develop in each of the following areas: safety, trust, esteem, control, and intimacy. Experiences shape and reinforce the development of negative or positive schemas in each of these areas, which in turn serve as lenses through which events are interpreted. Certain life events, such as trauma or terrorism, may disrupt positive schemas or reinforce negative ones (McCann & Pearlman, 1990b; Janoff-Bulman, 1992).

The experience of victimization challenges people's positive assumptions and beliefs about themselves and the world (Janoff-Bulman, 1989). Victims question the orderliness, safety, and meaning of the world (Silver, Boon, & Stones, 1983). In fact, it is proposed that much of the anguish people experience following traumatic events stems from the fact that their assumptions and illusions about themselves and the world are "shattered" (Janoff-Bulman, 1992). Therefore, therapists who are vicariously exposed to the horrors of terrorism are at risk of having their world views, disrupted. This disruption may be accompanied by feelings of depression, hopelessness, and inadequacy. Therapists may have difficulty getting images of their clients' trauma out of their minds, and these images may persist or come upon them unexpectedly between sessions. They may have nightmares, feel anxious, and have less regard for humanity, because they are witnesses to the shocking horror other human beings can cause. Therapists may feel vulnerable, have difficulty trusting, or be flooded by strong emotions such as grief or anguish. They may defend themselves against the pain by feeling numb or even callous. These reactions are personally unsettling and may lead a therapist to question his or her professional identity (McCann & Pearlman, 1990a; Pearlman & Saakvitne, 1995a).

Key to understanding the development of vicarious traumatization are the concepts of "exposure" and "empathy" (Figley, 1995; Pearlman & Saakvitne, 1995a). A therapist's capacity to engage empathically with a traumatized client is a chief source of his or her vulnerability (Pearlman & Saakvitne, 1995a). Moreover, working with traumatized clients involves being exposed to and "absorbing information that is about suffering," and frequently this process "includes absorbing the suffering as well" (Figley, 1995, p. 2).

THERAPISTS AND TERRORIZED CHILDREN

There are several reasons why therapists who treat terrorized children may be at particular risk of developing vicarious traumatization. Therapists often find child trauma "provocative" (Figley, 1995, p. 16) and tend to have a stronger identification with child clients (Dyregrov & Mitchell, 1992). The images presented by a traumatized child also tend to be more intrusive and vivid (Brady, Guy, Poelstra, & Brokaw, 1999). Therapists working with traumatized children may experience the same sense of helplessness the children feel, and may become overwhelmed and feel ineffectual (Nader, 1994).

Furthermore, therapeutic work with these children can be especially difficult, due to some of the damaging sequelae of terrorism. These effects include aggression, trauma-related fears, trust problems, pessimism, and irritability (Terr, 1991; Koplewicz et al., 2002; Silverman & La Greca, 2002; Nader & Pynoos, 1993; Garbarino, 1991). A child's reactions to terror, including helplessness, rage, and the desire for retaliation (Coppenhall, 1995; Nader, 1994), may be difficult for a therapist to tolerate.

Overwhelmed therapists may question their ability to provide relief. Rachel, a therapist with many years of experience in treating traumatized children, struggled in the treatment of a young child who lost her cousin in the WTC attack. As the child grieved for the loss, Rachel questioned how one "consoles the inconsolable." Grace, another therapist with years of experience in working with children and families, stated that she "suddenly" did not "feel like an expert on anything." Previously, parents would ask her advice on dealing with their children; however, in the uncertainty and confusion following the collapse of the WTC, she struggled to advise parents on what to tell children whose relatives were missing and how to answer questions such as "Where is Uncle John?"

Because acts of terrorism are brought about by human intention, they leave insidious marks—loss of positive esteem for others, and an inability to trust (Terr, 1991; McCann & Pearlman, 1990a; Janoff-Bulman, 1992). Terrorized children need to heal within the context of a healthy therapeutic relationship (Herman, 1992); however, the impaired relational ability that results from the trauma creates difficulties in the engagement and maintenance of the therapeutic alliance. This difficulty in developing the therapeutic relationship, along with the overwhelming experience of the child, may lead a practitioner to question his or her ability as a therapist.

The play of terrorized children may be especially disturbing and create a great deal of discomfort for therapists witnessing it. Terr (1979, 1983) studied a group of children who were kidnapped and buried underground in a truck trailer for 16 hours. Later, these children reenacted scenes from this experience with their nonkidnapped classmates. The play was accompanied by shrieks and screams, along with visual signs of distress on the children's faces. Terr (1990) states that those observing the play experienced the same sense of helplessness the children experienced during the trauma. The play of traumatized children tends to be morbid, constricted, and joyless, and is not accompanied by relief (Terr, 1981). Since 9/11, there have been numerous stories of children repeatedly reenacting the scenes from that day in their play, whether it was through drawings or through piling blocks up and knocking them down. This was the reported play of children who were not in treatment, and who were believed to be too young to understand what was happening.

The treatment of trauma entails review of the traumatic event, sometimes repeatedly (Pynoos, Nader, & March, 1991). For example, some cognitive-behavioral approaches require that a child describe the event repeatedly, in order to reduce the avoidant symptoms inherent in posttraumatic stress disorder (Cohen, Berliner, & Mannarino, 2000; Cohen, Mannarino, Berliner, & Deblinger, 2000). Using a variety of techniques such as drawing or writing, a terrorized child is often asked to describe the traumatic event, and to provide increasing details and accompanying feelings with each repetition (Cohen, Berliner, & Mannarino, 2000, Nader, 1997; Nader & Mello, 2000). The goal of such treatment is "to hear everything, including the worst aspects of victimization" (Nader, 1994, p. 186). Nader (2001) states that "symptoms may temporarily increase over the course of treatment as the symptoms of numbing and avoidance reduce" (p. 300). This increase in symptoms, along with the request that the child talk about that which is "too horrible to talk about" (Nader, 1994, p. 188), may leave the therapist feeling incompetent and concerned that treatment is causing the symptoms rather than relieving them.

Along with these difficulties inherent in clinical work with terrorized children, the repeated exposure to a child's trauma can leave a therapist vulnerable to vicarious traumatization. Witnessing the experience of the child makes it difficult for the therapist to deny the existence of horror that terrorist events have brought about. "The insidious reality of terrorism is that anyone, anytime, anywhere can be a target" (Gurwitch et al., 2002, p. 327). An additional factor for therapists working with children affected by mass terror attacks, such as the events of 9/11 or the Oklahoma City bombing, is that the therapists are likely to have been affected by the events as well. The content of a child's narrative or play may trigger painful images or feelings of the attacks. As therapists may struggle to comfort and reassure children, they may be unable to comfort or reassure themselves. Likewise, severe trauma affects a child's view of the future (Terr, 1991), and acts of terrorism create fear of more attacks (Silverman & LaGreca, 2002; Webb, 2002), which makes closure difficult (Webb, 2002). A therapist may be concerned about future attacks as well, which may further compromise his or her ability to be reassuring. Grace, one of the experienced child therapists mentioned earlier, found this aspect of her work after 9/11 particularly difficult. She met with many children in group settings and was instructed by her agency administrators to tell the children that "the government is doing everything possible to guarantee our safety," but she felt like a "hypocrite" because she did not believe this herself. "For the first time in my clinical practice, I felt like I was not being myself." Likewise, Rachel worked with a young girl who was so frightened that she would not leave her backyard. She asked Rachel repeatedly, "Where are we safe?" Rachel had the same thoughts and feelings, and wondered how she could possibly help this child feel more secure in such a period of uncertainty.

The work with children affected by terrorism serves as a painful reminder of the devastating effects of horrific events. Along with images of destruction of individuals and property, therapists witness the great emotional toll on young lives. For these children, life has drastically changed, and therapists suffer as they watch the loss of innocence, idealism, and hope in ones so young. In working with these children, therapists must face the "fleeting nature and preciousness of life" (Gamble, 2002, p. 347). Rachel always believed that her work with children would help create a future where these children could live free from the problems that brought them into treatment. However, the children who were affected by the WTC attacks experienced such unbearable sorrow and confusion that she wondered whether she would be able to help them heal from such tragedy.

In summary, work with terrorized children may pose hazards for therapists for a variety of reasons. Among these are the difficulty in engaging and maintaining a therapeutic relationship, the continued exposure to the horrific details of the children's trauma, and the necessity of witnessing the trauma's devastating impact. These factors may leave the therapists feeling overwhelmed and burdened, may trigger feelings and memories of their own experience, and may cause them to question their competence.

SUPPORT, SPIRITUALITY, AND SELF-CARE

Although vicarious traumatization is considered an inevitable reaction to trauma work (McCann & Pearlman, 1990a; Pearlman & Saakvitne, 1995a), its deleterious effects can be ameliorated. In fact, like traumatized clients, therapists can grow through adversity and discover personal strengths they might not have found in a less challenging environment. However, in order to reduce the stress of trauma work, therapists must acknowledge and address the impact the work has on them. A holistic approach to dealing with vicarious traumatization involves addressing its impact both professionally and personally.

Professional Strategies

Training in Trauma Work

Specialized training in trauma theory and its impact increases therapists' effectiveness and may decrease the deleterious effects of the work on them (Danieli, 1994; Pearlman & Saakvitne, 1995a; Yassen, 1995). It provides a theoretical framework that not only helps therapists understand which interventions to use, but "also offers intellectual containment in the face of violence and powerlessness/helplessness it can engender" and "an anchor to assist with feelings or affect" (Yassen, 1995, p. 1998). The Appendix at the end of the book lists some training resources.

Supervision and Support

If we therapists are to provide a safe therapeutic context for our clients to heal, we must also create a safe place for ourselves to deal with the impact of that work on us. We need to be supported in our efforts and be able to discuss our feelings and reactions to trauma work. Ongoing supervision from someone who has knowledge and experience in this area, and who recognizes the effects of trauma work on therapists, is essential (Pearlman & Saakvitne, 1995a). The supervisory relationship can provide a supportive, nonjudgmental environment where a therapist can feel free to discuss the work and how he or she is reacting to it. Furthermore, it is important that agency administrators do not pathologize therapists' reactions, but rather make a continuing commitment to their professional development by providing training in trauma work and good supervision. This can be especially difficult within an environment that emphasizes increased productivity and managed care restraints. However, therapists will heal from vicarious traumatization in a work environment that accepts it as a real and an expected response to trauma work, rather than a problem for an individual;

that focuses on solutions to the dilemma, rather than assigning blame; and that communicates support clearly and directly (Catherall, 1995).

Private practitioners may need to pursue support actively. In addition to seeking regular supervision or case consultation with therapists experienced in the treatment of terrorized children, therapists in private practice can create peer support groups with other such therapists engaged in trauma work. However, peer supervision groups need guidelines and ground rules, particularly in regard to the needs for supportive, nonjudgmental interactions and for confidentiality. Participants can discuss the literature on vicarious traumatization and agree to use it as a framework to process reactions.

Social support is an effective mediator of stress (Ursano & Fullerton, 1990; Fullerton et al., 1992). Some therapists may hesitate to share their reactions to trauma work, especially if they are concerned that these reactions are not professional. However, "One is not 'unprofessional' if haunted or preoccupied by the pain of one's clients" (Gamble, 2002, p. 347). If therapists do not discuss the effects of trauma work, these may become more toxic. This is personally painful and can interfere with the ability to engage in effective treatment (Pearlman & Saakvitne, 1995).

When the effects of trauma work become toxic, therapists may seek support in ways that are inappropriate. I have written elsewhere about the need to be responsible in discussing trauma work with others (Cunningham, 1999). Therapists need outlets to ventilate and process their reactions, but they also need to be aware that what is upsetting to them is likely to be even more distressing to listeners who are not helping professionals themselves. A commitment to discussing the effects of trauma work with an appropriate person, such as a supervisor, one's own therapist, or a trusted colleague, may help lessen the risks of burdening others with strong reactions. The most appropriate person for processing trauma work experience is someone familiar with trauma work and its effects. This will provide a therapist with a supportive, nonjudgmental listener, while also protecting the listener. Supervisors with experience in this area will be more likely to understand their own responses and make a commitment to deal with the impact their supervisory sessions have on them. When time is scheduled on a regular basis, a listener is more prepared for reactions than when they are shared in a casual context.

Some therapists need to be encouraged to discuss reactions and need "permission" to disclose. When I was working in preventive services, I received a phone call from a local school about a referral that included gruesome details of a child's trauma. Shortly after taking the call, I felt exhausted, both physically and emotionally. Not wanting to "burden" anyone else, I kept the details to myself. Years later, when I learned about the concept of vicarious traumatization, I finally understood my reaction and the need to process the experience with someone. Although my concern for my potential listeners was appropriate, my decision to delay sharing the effects the trauma was having on me were misguided. In the time since I processed my feelings about this case, I have thought of the details on occasion; however, the toxicity is gone.

A key to reducing the deleterious effects of vicarious traumatization is balance. For example, a varied caseload that includes some clients who are not traumatized may reduce the risk of vicarious traumatization (Cunningham, 2003). Such a caseload may remind the therapist that not all clients have been traumatized. Furthermore, it is essential to set appropriate and realistic boundaries regarding when a client may contact a therapist between sessions, on weekends, or during longer breaks such as vacations. Therapists need to make arrangements for their clients for the occasions when the therapists are not available; this is a good issue for supervision, especially with novice practitioners. Therapists also need to make a commitment to scheduling some lunch or dinner breaks away from the office, taking sick days when appropriate, and taking a few minutes to connect on a personal basis with coworkers. For many trauma therapists, taking such breaks from the work is difficult. Some feel guilty that they can even think about resting and relaxing when there is little respite for their clients. A commitment to self-care is critical to buffering and healing from vicarious traumatization. Gamble (2002, p. 350) states that this "requires treating our own pain as seriously as we regard the pain of our clients" and involves the development of self-compassion. "Our healing and our clients' healing are interconnected" (Gamble, 2002, p. 350).

In addition to supervision and working in a supportive environment, therapists can try to provide a pleasant work environment for themselves by keeping their desks uncluttered and displaying objects that they find personally meaningful—such as a seashell, a postcard of a beautiful work of art, a meaningful poem or prayer, or a picture of a peaceful place. When I worked in preventive services with children and families at risk for abuse and neglect, I kept a copy of the Prayer of St. Francis of Assisi tucked into the side of my desk blotter. Although I was not particularly spiritual at the time, I found that the words were poetic and the concepts consistent with clinical treatment: " . . . Make me an instrument of your peace. . . . Where there is despair, let me sow hope; . . . and where there is sadness, joy."

A vase of fresh-cut flowers or a beautiful plant can restore the spirit during a long work day. We therapists need to be reminded that there is beauty in life, along with the horrors of trauma. Although therapists usually do not keep personal pictures on their desks, we can keep reminders of loved ones that are more neutral—for example, a picture of the beach as a reminder of a recent family vacation. Remembering our connection to our loved ones is an important way to buffer the stress of the work. Finally, administrative tasks are inevitable, but we can listen to relaxing music while we catch up on paperwork.

Personal Strategies

Since trauma assaults the minds, bodies, and spirits of victims, therapists working with traumatized children need to address each of these aspects in their own healing from vicarious traumatization. Because spirituality may be the most overlooked aspect of such healing, I address it first.

Spirituality

During tumultuous storms at sea, the water 10 feet below the trough of the highest wave is calm (Silf, 1999). Spiritual practice, for some therapists, is a way to access a place of inner calm despite the tumultuous storms of life. Accessing such inner resources is an effective way to buffer the stress of trauma work and heal oneself from its emotional toll.

"Spirituality" can be distinguished from "religion." "Spirituality" may refer in the broadest sense to the ways in which individuals find meaning in the events of their lives (Cunningham, 2000), or to the sense that there is something larger or beyond an individual's own experience. It is "a personal commitment to a process of inner development that engages us in our totality" (Teasdale, 2001, p. 17). "Religion," on the other hand, involves belonging to and belief in and adherence to the doctrines of a formalized institution—for example, Christianity, Judaism, or Hinduism (Cunningham, 2000). Spirituality consists of a contemplative attitude, a commitment to living life fully and searching for meaning. It "originates in the heart, in deep stirrings that may be only beginning to form" (Teasdale, 2001, p. 18), and involves connections to others and the interconnectedness of all beings.

Spirituality may involve belief in a source beyond the self, which some call the "Divine," "God," "Other," or "Higher Power." It is not necessary to believe in God or to belong to a religious tradition in order to be spiritual. Regardless of one's belief, however, there is wisdom in the treasures of many of these traditional pathways, which can be interwoven with one's own personal belief system.

Disruptions in our spiritual framework may be the most painful effect of trauma work for us as therapists. Our exposure to the horrors our clients have endured may leave us, like them, questioning the meaning of life and the why of suffering; such questioning may be accompanied by a loss of hope, idealism, and connection with others (Pearlman & Saakvitne,

1995b). Spirituality may be a way to restore a sense of meaning to life—to help us access our inner resources and connect to others.

"Spiritual practice" refers to the work of inner growth and change and involves profound self-knowledge. Without the inner transformation, the practice is not spiritual (Teasdale, 2001). It includes any attempt to connect to what is beyond us (however we may conceptualize this) and can be drawn from traditional spiritual paths, such as meditation, prayer, or participation in a spiritual community and rituals. Along with or instead of traditional practices, any activity that helps us connect to a purpose in life or a sense of sacredness can be spiritual. This includes a deep connection to nature or humanity, or a commitment to living a compassionate and meaningful life.

We trauma therapists will find many parallels between our clinical practice and the spiritual journey. Pema Chodron (1997, p. 15), a Buddhist nun, states that "the spiritual journey involves going beyond hope and fear, stepping into unknown territory." In fact, she maintains that the most critical issue in spirituality "may be to just keep moving" (p. 15). Our work with terrorized children involves a great deal of uncertainty and moving into the unknown, both for our clients and for us. Faced with overwhelming trauma and the feelings evoked by that experience, we may be unsure of what to do or say, or we may question the effectiveness of our treatment. And yet the most useful thing we can do is to be witnesses—to be with clients in their pain, not to give up, but "to just keep moving." Spiritual wisdom may help us as therapists during this time of questioning.

Therapists trained in psychodynamic therapy have always believed in the need to "trust the process" of therapy. With experience comes the realization that openings for insight will occur and opportunities to raise critical issues will arise, if we wait patiently for them. We learn to rely on our practice wisdom, insight, and intuition built on experience rather than book or empirical knowledge. Spirituality may also lead us to believe that we are instruments for healing and that some "Higher Power" guides our practice. Consistent with good clinical practice, our job is to pay attention to our own inner experience and to listen to our clients with open minds and hearts. As therapists, we may find it helpful to take a few minutes before a session to relax, meditate, or say a short prayer. This helps us to center ourselves and prepare ourselves to be fully present to each client, and to be open to both our client's and our own experience in the encounter. Likewise, taking a few minutes after the session can help us to unwind and prepare for the next task on our agenda.

Grounding. Spiritual wisdom reminds us of the importance of being "grounded" in our own experience—that is, connecting to our true selves. Grounding helps us find meaning in our suffering and a sense of purpose.

It requires that we do not close off painful emotions, but rather use them to grow spiritually (Welwood, 2000). This includes the painful feelings that trauma work evokes. Spiritual practice requires that we accept these feelings and explore them, using them as a springboard for our own work. Much of the anguish associated with trauma work is the recognition that we do not have control over much of what occurs in life—that we are vulnerable. By not closing off the painful feelings that may be evoked by trauma work, we are able to stay fully present to our clients and their pain.

Surrender. Although we need to be grounded in the reality of our experience, we also need to transcend it by releasing attachments and expectations of outcomes (Johanson & Kurtz, 1991)—in other words, to "surrender" to the experience that what is, is. Johanson and Kurtz (1991) note that, in doing this, "we choose to bear witness" (p. 13), rather than to be attached to accomplishing a particular goal or solve problems. They continue, "We enter into the confusion and mystery of whatever is happening with a curious, experimental attitude, not knowing what might be discovered" (p. 13). This goes against our Western tendency "to do something to move people beyond the place where they are stuck" (p. 41).

Surrender may help us be at peace with the limitations of being human, accepting that even though we may not know, we can still be persons of wisdom (Johanson & Kurtz, 1991). Likewise, this allows us to acknowledge that we do not have control over what happened to our child clients or over their healing from the experience. When we truly accept our limitations on the deepest level possible, we become free to be more fully present to children and their pain and suffering. This allows us to approach them in the most respectful manner, and to give them the right to have their own experience.

Awakening the Heart. Another aspect of spiritual practice, "awakening the heart," refers to allowing ourselves to be touched by our clients' stories and pain and to remain open (Welwood, 2000). Pema Chodron (2001, p. 211) states, "To stay with that shakiness—to stay with a broken heart, with a rumbling stomach, with the feeling of hopelessness . . . that is the path of true awakening."

It is natural when we feel emotional pain to want to disconnect from it. In fact, one sign of vicarious traumatization is that therapists become callous or untouched by their clients' story or pain in order to protect themselves. This not only makes treatment ineffective, but is personally painful for the therapists. Being able to connect to our clients' pain without getting lost in it is consistent with Carl Rogers's definition of empathy: the ability to understand another's experience, along with the meaning and feelings of the person, "as if one were the other person, but without ever losing the 'as if' condition" (quoted in Shea, 1998, pp. 14–15).

Mindfulness. "Mindfulness" is the practice of "cultivating some appreciation for the fullness of each moment we are alive" (Kabat-Zinn, 1994, p. 3) and contrasts with taking life for granted. It is a way of becoming more conscious of our lives and our possibilities; it involves being totally present or attentive to what we are engaged in, rather than doing things unconsciously or automatically. In fact, it is more about "being" than "doing." It is not a resignation about life, or a closing off, but a way of waking up to life (Kabat-Zinn, 1994).

I have stated earlier that one of the hazards of trauma work is the disruption in a therapist's spiritual world view and the ultimate questions about meaning and suffering that may be evoked. These "big" or ultimate questions can only be approached spiritually. Psychology has no answer to the "why" of suffering or ultimately to the meaning of life. Spiritual wisdom, especially the practice of mindfulness, reminds us as therapists that we have only the present moment and of the importance of living that moment to the fullest.

Kabat-Zinn (1994, p. 17) poses the question "Where is my mind right now?" Mindfulness practice allows us to be fully present to our clients in sessions, but also helps us balance the rest of our life with our work. When we are mindful, we are able to be genuinely attentive to others in our lives, besides our clients. Since one of the painful consequences of trauma work is that we therapists tend to disconnect from ourselves and others, mindfulness helps counteract this. We become conscious of our relationships with others and our relationship to ourselves. Mindfulness also helps us focus on and appreciate all aspects of our lives: We see, hear, feel, smell, and taste the life around us. When we are mindful, we feel the water splash on our skin as we shower in the morning, rather than think about our caseload for the day; we notice the signs of nature around us on our way to work, and we hear the laughter of a child at play. We taste our coffee or tea in the morning, rather than worry about the mountain of paperwork that awaits us at the office. We become aware that all our worrying never reduced the pile of work, but has kept us from enjoying the small blessings we have in each day. So when we practice mindfulness, we remember to bring our full attention to the task at hand.

Meditation practice is one way of becoming more mindful. There are many different types of meditation, and the practice has both psychological and physical benefits (LeShan, 1974). Meditation "sharpens our intuition" and helps us with the "ups and downs" of life (Gunaratana, 1991, p. 17). Some therapists may not be comfortable with the practice of meditation, but may find a similar effect from any repetitive activity that allows the mind to relax—for example, knitting or other forms of needlework, making bread, or gardening. When we engage in such an activity and do not become attached to the thoughts that enter our minds, but rather allow them to pass by like balloons floating through the air, it has the same effect as meditation practice.

Physical and Psychological Self-Care

There are many activities that can assist therapists in their own physical and psychological self-care. However, one caveat is necessary: It is critically important that each therapist choose what feels comfortable and makes sense to him or her. The commitment to self-care is more important than the particular activity.

Even though there is no bodily assault to us when we engage in trauma work, our bodies hold the stress from hearing the details of our clients' experience and the strong accompanying affect. Basic good nutrition, adequate sleep, and some physical activity are all essential for us as trauma therapists. A walk, jog, or run helps to release some of the tension held in the body from trauma work. A massage as a routine practice or at least as a special treat after a long period of work can help rest the body as well as the mind and spirit. I find walking in nature restorative and restful. At times it is tempting to make it another chore and "speed-walk" to burn calories, but to deal with the stress of vicarious traumatization, I find it most healing to walk at a moderate pace and to pay attention to the sound of birds, the trees in bloom, or the turning colors of autumn. This is a mindful approach to walking. I also find that time at the beach—just watching the ebb and flow of the water, feeling the sea breeze on my arms, and observing the green beach grass against the white sand and the blue of the sky and ocean—is like a mini-retreat.

Gardening may be a way of creating beauty and feeling connected to the earth, or establishing a sense of groundedness. Indeed, any activity that allows us to express our creativity is helpful in healing from vicarious traumatization. Possibilities include writing in a journal, painting, sculpting, drawing, listening to music, or playing a musical instrument. Along with these suggestions, there are many good exercises to help therapists understand and address vicarious traumatization. These can be found in workbooks by Saakvitne and Pearlman (1996) and by Williams and Poijula (2002). The exercises in the Williams and Poijula workbook are designed for direct victims of trauma, but can be modified to address vicarious traumatization. These exercises can be used in conjunction with journaling, and responses and reactions can then be processed in supervision, therapy, or a peer support group.

An important part of self-care is taking time from work to enjoy ourselves. However, we need to be conscious of what we do for entertainment. If we work all week with traumatized children, and then come home and watch only the news or television programs on trauma and terror, it will not provide the needed opportunity for rest and relaxation. A cartoon I found in *The New Yorker* magazine's "Off the Wall Calendar" (January 14, 1997) depicts a television lying on a therapist's couch. The therapist tells the television, "Of course you're depressed. You're tuned to a twenty-four-hour all-news station." We need to find activities that relax us and take our minds off work. This includes being with people who are not traumatized, to remind us that not everyone has endured horrific experiences. We may choose to be physically active, such as dancing or working out, since so much of our time is spent using our minds. We can read things that are uplifting or entertaining, along with the latest journal articles and books on trauma work.

Sociopolitical and professional activities other than direct practice provide opportunities to counterbalance our sense of helplessness. For example, we may give a talk on children and trauma to parents in the local school. This allows us to be helpful professionally, but is not as intense as direct client contact. It also allows us to connect with others and feel a sense of satisfaction in providing a community service. Similarly, we may offer to provide supervision, consultation, or in-service training to a local agency or a workshop at a professional conference.

Awareness of Personal History

A final personal strategy for dealing with vicarious traumatization involves remaining aware of any personal experiences of trauma we have had. It is well documented in the literature that a large number of trauma therapists have a personal history of trauma (Pope & Feldman-Summers, 1992; Pearlman & MacIan, 1995). Mass traumas, such as the Oklahoma City bombing and the events of 9/11, often trigger such therapists' memories of personal trauma. Since the mass events are also shared by the therapists and their clients, therapists are doubly at risk for painful reactions and a reopening of old wounds. For example, Grace worked with a number of children who lost family members in the collapse of the WTC. The realization of how many children would be left without a parent reminded her of her own pain at losing her mother to cancer when she was 11.

CONCLUSION

Acts of terrorism need not be as far-reaching as 9/11 or the Oklahoma City bombing to affect large numbers of children. More local and narrowly focused acts of terror, such as school shootings and random acts of violence, can also take a psychological toll. Therapists working with clients directly affected by acts of violence and terrorism can be expected to find the work difficult and to have it negatively affect them as well as their clients. However, the negative affects of trauma work are augmented by the great satisfactions that accompany witnessing someone heal from traumatic experiences. "There is nothing easy about the work, although through it therapists may deepen their insight into themselves as persons and their wisdom as healers" (Wilson, Friedman, & Lindy, 2001, p. 29).

REFERENCES

Beaton, R. D., & Murphy, S. A. (1995). Working with people in crisis: Research implications. In C. R. Figley (Ed.), *Compassion fatigue: Coping with secondary traumatic stress disorder in those who treat the traumatized* (pp. 51–81). New York: Brunner/Mazel.

Brady, J. L., Guy, J. D., Poelstra, P. L., & Brokaw, B. F. (1999). Vicarious traumatization, spirituality, and the treatment of sexual abuse survivors: A national survey of women psychotherapists. *Professional Psychology: Research and Practice, 30*(4), 386–393.

Briere, J. (1989). *Therapy for adults molested as children: Beyond survival.* New York: Springer.

Catherall, D. (1995). Preventing institutional secondary traumatic stress disorder. In C. R. Figley (Ed.), *Compassion fatigue: Coping with secondary traumatic stress disorder in those who treat the traumatized* (pp. 232–247). New York: Brunner/Mazel.

Chodron, P. (1997). *When things fall apart: Heart advice for difficult times.* Boston: Shambhala.

Chodron, P. (2001). Fear. In C. Willis (Ed.), *Why meditate?: The essential book about how meditation can enrich your life* (pp. 201–230). New York: Marlowe.

Cohen, J. A., Berliner, L., & Mannarino, A. P. (2000). Treatment of traumatized children: A review and synthesis. *Journal of Trauma, Violence and Abuse, 1*(1), 29–46.

Cohen, J. A., Mannarino, A. P., Berliner, L., & Deblinger, E. (2000). Trauma-focused cognitive behavioral therapy: An empirical update. *Journal of Interpersonal Violence, 15*(11), 1203–1223.

Coppenhall, K. (1995). The stresses of working with clients who have been sexually abused. In W. Dryden (Ed.), *The stresses of counseling in action* (pp. 28–43). London: Sage.

Courtois, C. (1988). *Healing the incest wound: Adult survivors in therapy.* New York: Norton.

Cunningham, M. (1999). The impact of sexual abuse treatment on the social work clinician. *Child and Adolescent Social Work Journal, 16*(4), 277–290.

Cunningham, M. (2000). Spirituality, cultural diversity and crisis intervention. *Crisis Intervention, 6*(1), 65–77.

Cunningham, M. (2003). Impact of trauma work on social work clinicians: Empirical findings. *Social Work, 48*, 451–459.

Danieli, Y. (1985). The treatment and prevention of long-term effects and intergenerational transmission of victimization: A lesson from Holocaust survivors and their children. In C. R. Figley (Ed.), *Trauma and its wake: Vol. 1. The study and treatment of post-traumatic stress disorder* (pp. 295–313). New York: Brunner/Mazel.

Danieli, Y. (1994). Countertransference, trauma, and training. In J. Wilson, & J. D. Lindy (Eds.), *Countertransference in the treatment of PTSD* (pp. 368–388). New York: Guilford Press.

Dyregrov, A., & Mitchell, J. T. (1992). Work with traumatized children: Psychological effects and coping strategies. *Journal of Traumatic Stress, 5,* 5–17.

Epstein, S. (1991). The self concept, the traumatic neurosis, and the structure of personality. In R. Hogan (Ed.), *Perspectives in personality* (Vol. 3A, pp. 63–98). London: Jessica Kingsley.

Farber, B. A., & Heifetz, L. (1982). The process and dimension of burnout in psychotherapists. *Professional Psychology, 13*(2), 293–301.

Figley, C. R. (1995). Compassion fatigue as secondary traumatic stress disorder: An overview. In C. R. Figley (Ed.), *Compassion fatigue: Coping with secondary traumatic stress disorder in those who treat the traumatized* (pp. 1–20). New York: Brunner/Mazel.

Follette, V. M., Polusny, M. M., & Milbeck, K. (1994). Mental health and law enforcement professionals: Trauma history, psychological symptoms, and impact of providing services to child sexual abuse survivors. *Professional Psychology, 25,* 275–282.

Freudenberger, H., & Robbins, A. (1979). The hazards of being a psychotherapist. *Psychoanalytic Review, 66*(2), 275–296.

Fullerton, C., McCarroll, J., Ursano, R., & Wright, K. (1992). Psychological responses of rescue workers: Fire fighters and trauma. *American Journal of Ortrhopsychiatry, 62*(3), 371–378.

Gamble, S. J. (2002). Self-care for bereavement counselors. In N. B. Webb (Ed.), *Helping bereaved children: A handbook for practitioners* (2nd ed., pp. 346–362). New York: Guilford Press.

Garbarino, J., Kostelny, L., & Dubrow, N. (1991). What children can tell us about living in danger. *American Psychologist, 46,* 376–383.

Gorkin, M. (1987). *The use of countertransference.* Northvale, NJ: Aronson.

Gunaratana, H. (1991). *Mindfulness in plain English.* Boston: Wisdom.

Gurwitch, R. H., Sitterle, K. A., Young, B. H., & Pfefferbaum, B. (2002). The aftermath of terrorism. In A. M. La Greca, W. K. Silverman, E. M. Vernberg, & M. C. Roberts (Eds.), *Helping children cope with disasters and terrorism* (pp. 327–357). Washington, DC: American Psychological Association.

Herman, J. (1992). *Trauma and recovery.* New York: Basic Books.

Janoff-Bulman, R. (1989). Assumptive worlds and the stress of traumatic events: Applications of the schema construct. *Social Cognition, 7*(2), 113–136.

Janoff-Bulman, R. (1992). *Shattered assumptions: Towards a new psychology of trauma.* New York: Free Press.

Janoff-Bulman, R., & Frieze, I. H. (1983). A theoretical perspective for understanding reactions to victimization. *Journal of Social Issues, 39*(2), 1–18.

Johanson, G., & Kurtz, R. (1991). *Grace unfolding: Psychotherapy in the spirit of the Tao-Te Ching.* New York: Bell Tower.

Kabat-Zinn, J. (1994). *Wherever you go, there you are: Mindfulness meditation in everyday life.* New York: Hyperion.

Kastenbaum, R. J. (2001). *Death, society and human experience* (7th ed.). Boston: Allyn & Bacon.

Koplewicz, H. S., Vogel, J. M., Solanto, M. V., Morrissey, R. F., Alonso, C. M., Abikoff, H., Gallagher, R., & Novick, R. (2002). Child and parent response to the 1993 World Trade Center bombing. *Journal of Traumatic Stress, 15*(1), 77–85.

LeShan, L. (1974). *How to meditate: A guide to self-discovery.* Boston: Little, Brown.

Maslach, C. (1982). *Burnout: The cost of caring.* Englewood Cliffs, NJ: Prentice-Hall.

McCann, L. I., & Pearlman, L. (1990a). Vicarious traumatization: A framework for understanding the psychological effects of working with victims. *Journal of Traumatic Stress, 3*(1), 131–149.

McCann, L. I., & Pearlman, L. (1990b). *Psychological trauma and the adult survivor: Theory, therapy and transformation.* New York: Brunner/Mazel.

Nader, K. (1994). Countertransference in the treatment of acutely traumatized children. In J. P. Wilson & J. D. Lindy (Eds.), *Countertransference in the treatment of PTSD* (pp. 179–205). New York: Guilford Press.

Nader, K. (1997). Treating traumatic grief in systems. In C. R. Figley, B. E. Bride, & N. Mazza (Eds.), *Death and trauma: The traumatology of grieving* (pp. 159–192). Washington, DC: Taylor & Francis.

Nader, K. (2001). Treatment methods for childhood trauma. In J. P. Wilson, M. J. Friedman, & J. D. Lindy (Eds.), *Treating psychological trauma and PTSD* (pp. 278–334). New York: Guilford Press.

Nader, K., & Mello, C. (2000). Interactive trauma/grief-focused therapy. In P. Lehmann & N. F. Coady (Eds.), *Theoretical perspectives for direct social work practice: A generalist–eclectic approach* (pp. 382–401). New York: Springer.

Nader, K., & Pynoos, R. S. (1993). School disaster: Planning and initial interventions. *Journal of Social Behavior and Personality, 8*(5), 299–320.

Oklahoma State Department of Health. (1996). *Injury update: Investigation of physical injuries directly associated with the Oklahoma City bombing. A report to Oklahoma injury surveillance participants.* Oklahoma City, OK: Author.

Pearlman, L. A., & MacIan, P. S. (1995). Vicarious traumatization: An empirical study of the effects of trauma work on trauma therapists. *Professional Psychology: Research and Practice, 26*(6), 558–565.

Pearlman, L. A., & Saakvitne, K. (1995a). *Trauma and the therapist: Countertransference and vicarious traumatization in psychotherapy with incest survivors.* New York: Norton.

Pearlman, L. A., & Saakvitne, K. (1995b). Treating therapists with vicarious traumatization and secondary traumatic stress disorders. In C. R. Figley (Ed.), *Compassion fatigue: Coping with secondary traumatic stress disorder in those who treat the traumatized* (pp. 150–177). New York: Brunner/Mazel.

Perloff, L. (1983). Perceptions and vulnerability to victimization. *Journal of Social Issues, 39*(2), 41–62.

Pope, K. L., & Feldman-Summers, S. (1992). National survey of psychologists' sexual and physical abuse history and their evaluation of training and competence in these areas. *Professional Psychology: Research and Practice, 23*(5), 353–361.

Pynoos, R. S., Nader, K., & March, J. (1991). Post-traumatic stress disorder in children and adolescents. In J. Weiner (Ed.), *Comprehensive textbook of child and adolescent psychiatry* (pp. 339–348). Washington, DC: American Psychiatric Press.

Saakvitne, K., & Pearlman, L. A. (1996). *Transforming the pain: A workbook on vicarious traumatization.* New York: Norton.

Shea, S. C. (1998). *Psychiatric interviewing: The art of understanding* (2nd ed.). Philadelphia: Saunders.

Silf, M. (1999). *Close to the heart: A guide to personal prayer.* Chicago: Loyola Press.

Silver, R. C., Boon, C., & Stones, M. H. (1983). Searching for meaning in misfortune: Making sense of incest. *Journal of Social Issues, 39,* 81–102.

Silverman, W. K., & La Greca, A. M. (2002). Childen experiencing disasters: Definitions, reactions, and predictors of outcomes. In A. M. La Greca, W. K. Silverman, E. M. Vernberg, & M. C. Roberts (Eds.), *Helping children cope with disasters and terrorism* (pp. 327–357). Washington, DC: American Psychological Association.

Teasdale, W. (2001). *The mystic heart: Discovering a universal spirituality in the world's religions.* Novato, CA: New World Library.

Terr, L. C. (1979). Children of Chowchilla: A study of psychic trauma. *Psychoanalytic Study of the Child, 34,* 547–623.

Terr, L. C. (1981). "Forbidden games": Post traumatic child's play. *Journal of the American Academy of Child Psychiatry, 20,* 741–760.

Terr, L. C. (1983). Chowchilla revisited: The effects of psychic trauma four years after a school-bus kidnapping. *American Journal of Psychiatry, 140,* 1543–1550.

Terr, L. C. (1989). Family anxiety after traumatic events. *Journal of Clinical Psychiatry, 50*(11, Suppl.), 15–19.

Terr, L. C. (1990). *Too scared to cry.* New York: Harper & Row.

Terr, L. C. (1991). Childhood traumas: An outline and overview. *American Journal of Psychiatry, 148,*(1), 10–20.

Ursano, R., & Fullerton, C. (1990). Cognitive and behavioral responses to trauma. *Journal of Applied Psychology, 20,* 1766–1775.

Webb, N. B. (2002). September 11, 2001. In N. B. Webb (Ed.), *Helping bereaved children: A handbook for practitioners* (2nd ed., pp. 365–384). New York: Guilford Press.

Welwood, J. (2000). *Toward a psychology of awakening: Buddhism, psychotherapy, and the path of personal and spiritual transformation.* Boston: Shambhala.

Williams, M. B., & Poijula, S. (2002). *PTSD workbook: Simple, effective techniques for overcoming traumatic stress symptoms.* Oakland, CA: New Harbinger.

Wilson, J. P., Friedman, M. J., & Lindy, J. D. (Eds.). (2001). *Treating psychological trauma and PTSD.* New York: Guilford Press.

Wright, K., Ursano, R., Bartone, P., & Ingraham, L. (1990). The shared experience of catastrophe: An expanded classification of the disaster community. *American Journal of Orthopsychiatry, 60*(1), 35–42.

Yassen, J. (1995). Preventing secondary traumatic stress disorder. In C. R. Figley (Ed.), *Compassion fatigue: Coping with secondary traumatic stress disorder in those who treat the traumatized* (pp. 178–208). New York: Brunner/Mazel.

CHAPTER 16

Ongoing Issues and Challenges for Mental Health Professionals Working with Survivors of Mass Trauma

NANCY BOYD WEBB

Traumas come in a variety of forms, including natural disasters, community violence, war, and terrorism. Few if any people escape from having to cope with at least one traumatic event in their lifetimes, whether from firsthand experience or as observers through media accounts of large-scale destruction and deaths. In addition to these actual losses, tens of thousands of people worry about the *possibility* of future devastation related to war or terrorism—affecting not only military personnel and their families, but also civilians in the countries involved.

This book has presented various interventions that have been used to help children, adolescents, and their families cope with their anxiety, grief, and fear following different experiences of mass trauma and loss. Many of these detailed case illustrations depict interventions designed to help people affected by acts of terrorism. Since the terrorist attacks on the United States on September 11, 2001, many people have a sense of fear and foreboding about their safety. When the U.S. government recommended in February 2003 that each family prepare a disaster kit for dealing with possible chemical attacks, the message actually escalated the national mood of anxiety and sense of vulnerability and danger. Mental health professionals, who also felt uncertain about the nation's security, needed to find ways to assist themselves and their clients in dealing with their ongoing anxiety and concerns about future safety.

This book provides many examples that demonstrate how practitioners were able to respond helpfully after the events of "9/11." Although American disaster workers and counselors have had decades of experience in responding to on-the-spot natural disasters, such as hurricanes (Federal Emergency Management Agency [FEMA], 1989; Saylor, Swenson, & Powell, 1992), floods (Ollendick & Hoffman, 1982; Titchener & Kapp, 1976), and earthquakes (Bradburn, 1991; FEMA, 1991), deliberate acts of terrorism have become a relatively "new" focus of concern in the United States—in contrast to several other parts of the world, which have long histories of dealing with civil and political unrest and terrorism. Therefore, in order to give this book a wider, international perspective, I have included two chapters describing methods used by practitioners in two countries—Northern Ireland and Israel—with extensive experience in treating survivors of different forms of terrorism.

The purpose of this chapter is to look toward the future in terms of ongoing issues and challenges that will require our best efforts as we mental health professionals continue trying to understand and deal with the effects of mass traumas on our clients and ourselves. The topics to be addressed include the following:

- Determining whether and when treatment is necessary
- Possible long-term biological effects of trauma
- Culturally sensitive assessments and interventions
- Combining intervention methods
- The traumatized practitioner
- Training practitioners in trauma and grief work
- Integrating research with practice, and vice versa

DETERMINING WHETHER AND WHEN TREATMENT IS NECESSARY

Situations of mass trauma typically create havoc for communities and for their citizens. In the face of extensive destruction of property, breakdowns in communication and transportation, and disruptions in the usual routines of school and employment, many people function automatically, without thinking about their emotional state. Furthermore, when deaths and injuries have occurred, the survivors may feel that professional helpers' top priority must be attending to those who are hurt, hospitalized, or otherwise most in need. Because traumatized people try to avoid remembering their horrible experiences, they are very unlikely to seek help for their anxiety reactions in the immediate aftermath of a traumatic event. Therefore, it is understandable that researchers or clinicians trying to conduct studies or offer services or in the early phases after a traumatic event may encounter "resistance" in the form of denial of problems and/or reluctance to fill out forms. This was confirmed when many mental health agencies in communities surrounding New York City received very low response rates to their publicized offerings of support groups in the first few months following 9/11.

Although the literature recommends a complete multimethod assessment for posttraumatic stress disorder (PTSD) (Drake, Bush, & van Gorp, 2001; Ribbe, Lipovsky, & Freedy, 1995), this may be more practical *after* the first posttrauma month, when the initial shock has subsided and individuals are moving into the recovery phase (Shalev & Ursano, 2003; Gurwitch, Sullivan, & Long, 1998). A comprehensive assessment includes different methods, such as (1) a structured clinical interview, (2) investigation of the individual's pretrauma history and functioning, (3) psychometric assessments, and (4) data about behavioral and physiological responses (Lyons, 1987; Solomon, 1989).

The overall assessment process is complex, time-consuming, and potentially exhausting for the persons involved, who may not see its relevance or necessity, especially in the early weeks after a traumatic event. The literature is inconclusive regarding the timing and type of interventions during the acute posttrauma period, and methods for providing them when large numbers of people are involved need further elaboration (Raphael & Dobson, 2001). In Chapter 2, I have recommended a group screening of children in their school setting, using drawings and narratives to identify children most at risk (Pynoos & Eth, 1986; Nader & Pynoos, 1991, 1993; Nader, 1997). Similar group debriefing methods can be used with adults (see Chapter 6 and Everly & Mitchell, 2001; Mitchell & Everly, 2001) although there is debate in the literature about how helpful these are in actually reducing later symptom development. Psychoeducational approaches are very appropriate to inform parents, teachers, and young people about typical responses that can occur following traumatic experiences. Sometimes people worry about their mental health when they sense their own reactions of disorganization and anxiety.

Since we know that only about 25% of people who experience traumas develop PTSD (Brady, 2001), we need to think about the costs of trying to evaluate *everyone* who has been exposed, when approximately three-quarters will recover spontaneously. The fact that there are more than 160 instruments for assessment of children's fear and anxiety reactions (Barrios & Hartmann, 1997) highlights the tremendous interest among psychologists in studying and learning more about various responses following trauma. Rather than wholesale assessments of entire populations, however, my preference is for more study focused on the efficacy of different types of interventions at different times or phases to help persons who have developed symptoms. Ideally, some kind of psychological "first aid" and/or debriefing should be offered in large groups in the early stages after a traumatic event, with more intensive family and individual treatment later for those who need it. Shalev and Ursano (2003) present the psychological tasks and roles of professional helpers at the four stages of response to traumatic stress, but only in the fourth stage, "Return to life," do they specify the professionals' roles as those of diagnosticians and therapists. Although we do know that some people develop severe and long-lasting symptoms of PTSD for which they require specialized treatment, we must avoid conveying the expectation that *most* people will need extensive or ongoing intervention. An article in the *NASW News* following the sniper attacks in the Washington, D.C. area in October 2002 emphasized the importance of *normalizing* fear responses following trauma, in order to nurture people's resiliency and ability to bounce back (Stoesen, 2003).

POSSIBLE LONG-TERM BIOLOGICAL EFFECTS OF TRAUMA

Although most people who have been exposed to trauma can proceed with their lives without being haunted by memories of what happened, others cannot control their intrusive recollections, and they continue to grapple with the fearful anticipation of similar or worse experiences. In the event that a traumatic event does occur, these people are more prone to develop PTSD. A working hypothesis of why this happens is as follows: Early adverse experiences have created a biological vulnerability that makes it harder for previously exposed persons to reduce their physiological distress in future traumatic experiences (Yehuda, 2001). For example, among the 21 child survivors (ranging in age from 5 months to 12 years) of the 1993 standoff and fire at the Branch Davidian compound in Waco, Texas, "the mean group heart rate at rest was 132 . . . it should have been 90. The children were in a state of chronic low-level fear" (Bruce Perry, quoted in "Children and Families Need Help after Disasters," 1996, p. 1714).

Early experiences of abuse and violence can have a lasting effect on the brain, and the younger the person the more serious the impact, according to Perry (1997), who has studied the persistent physiological hyperarousal and hyperactivity of children exposed to chronic violence in the family and/or in the community. Experiencing chronic physical abuse at the hands of a parent, or watching drug-related fights and murders on the street corner, produces feelings of extreme fear that linger beyond the specific episode. Insofar as such experiences affect the brain, they also influence development and increase vulnerability to future traumas. Studies of adults abused as children have found greater reactions to stress both behaviorally and biologically (Yehuda, Spertus, & Golier, 2001). This is an important area for future study, especially with regard to age and gender factors as these interact with the nature of the violent experience and the later development of PTSD following trauma.

CULTURALLY SENSITIVE ASSESSMENTS AND INTERVENTIONS

Traumas, like birth and death, occur universally, and people from all cultural groups respond with stress reactions when they feel threatened. However, the specific manner of their response is culturally conditioned, and helping methods should be adapted to each culture's particular beliefs about the nature of the problem and how to deal with it. This is a challenge for practitioners in the United States, where approximately 10% of the population is foreign-born, and where both foreign-born and native-born residents come from very diverse groups (Potocky-Tripodi, 2002). In contrast, most practitioners are native-born white persons of Anglo-European heritage (Gibelman & Schervish, 1997). In order to serve clients from diverse backgrounds, mental health practitioners must learn to engage in "culturally friendly" assessments and interventions that respect and incorporate values and beliefs very different from their own. However, people may resist mental health services even when they are provided by practitioners of the same ethnicity and are community-based, as discussed in Chapter 11. In an earlier publication (Webb, 2001, p. 339), I have listed four conditions that can create strains and obstacles in culturally diverse practice:

- Practitioners' lack of understanding about the multidimensional reality and stresses of the clients' individual situation in the context of the clients' specific cultural and family environment
- Difficulties in engaging, communicating, and agreeing about the problem
- Different ideas about seeking help and dealing with the problem situation
- The different values and world views of practitioners and clients

The topic of cultural sensitivity has received a great deal of emphasis in social work over the past decade, following the mandate of the accrediting body of the Council on Social Work Education in 1992 (Council on Social Work Education, 1992a, 1992b) that curricula must contain content on culturally diverse populations. Many social work texts address the challenges of culturally sensitive practice (Lum, 2003; Webb, 2001; Ho, 1987; Fong & Furuto, 2001; Fong, 2004); most of these emphasize the importance of practitioners' self-awareness regarding their *own* cultural beliefs as the starting point for working with clients from different backgrounds. In addition to practitioners' self-awareness, I have recommended the following (Webb, 2001):

- Adhering to culturally expected interactions
- Openly acknowledging cultural differences
- Including members of a client's support network as part of the treatment

Other suggestions to enhance effectiveness in work with people of different backgrounds include using a bicultural approach that combines indigenous and Western interventions in order to facilitate the clients' involvement and participation in treatment (Fong, Boyd, & Browne, 1999). For example, this might involve finding ways to incorporate traditional healing practices into current psychological treatments, so that the efficacy of each may be enhanced (Nader, Dubrow, & Stamm, 1999).

Methods of seeking help are strongly attached to cultural values, and in many cultures the family is the expected resource. In fact, social/cultural norms may consider the family as "a higher value than the welfare of an individual within it, [and this] can increase the reluctance of a traumatized person to reach into a mental health system for help" (Dutton, 1998, p. 1). The following section discusses the use of combined methods and modalities to help traumatized individuals. The interaction of cultural values should guide the selection of both assessment and intervention methods and modalities.

COMBINING INTERVENTION METHODS

In situations of mass trauma, the choice of intervention methods will be strongly influenced by the circumstances of the particular traumatic event. Confusion, anxiety, and panic in the community are typical during the early phases of a mass trauma involving actual or feared loss of lives and destruction of property. Reality-based concerns about survival prevail over worries about mental health.

Choices of intervention typically include different forms of group, family, and individual treatment, but the timing of these varies with the circumstances. The example of the first New York World Trade Center bombing in 1993 illustrates the concept of offering different intervention methods at different times following a crisis event (Webb, 1999). Initially, group interventions were offered to the parents of the two classes of kindergarten children who were trapped in an elevator at the time of the bombing. The school crisis team invited the families to meet as a group as soon as the bus brought the children safely back to their school community. However, only a few families attended this group debriefing session, since many parents wanted to retreat with their children to the safety of their homes. In contrast, a follow-up parent meeting 3 months after the crisis was much better attended; it permitted the parents to discuss how their children were responding, including concerns about some children who were experiencing ongoing anxieties that suggested symptoms of PTSD.

An early intervention for the children took the form of in-class crisis group debriefing the Monday morning after the weekend following the Friday bombing. This debriefing consisted of drawing and play activities; for the play, blocks were provided to permit the children to reenact the explosion and damage to the building that they had witnessed on television replays during the weekend. The crisis team members remained in the classroom only half a day, because they did not identify children who seemed to require more extended interventions at that time. The expectation was that the school social worker and school psychologist would continue to monitor the children in these two classes. Information about how this monitoring was conducted and how children were referred for follow-up mental health services is not available. However, 4½ years following the bombing, an article in *The New York Times* (Martin, 1997) reported that some children were still exhibiting anxiety responses, such as fear of the dark, enuresis, and sleep problems. This would have been the ideal time to make referrals for these children to mental health specialists for follow-up individual services. According to the *Journal of the American Medical Association*, more mental health problems surface 3 months after a disaster than immediately following it ("Children and Families Need Help after Disasters," 1996).

Although schools do not typically provide mental health services, this situation demonstrates how a school can play a pivotal role in identifying children who may need specialized help following a mass trauma. In view of recent shootings and other crisis events in schools, many school districts have moved to provide staff training and to establish emergency procedures. In addition to monitoring pupils, schools are also in an ideal position to identify parents who appear to be extremely anxious, and to suggest referral resources for them. This is clearly justified, since we know that parents' anxiety can have a negative impact on their children. In the aftermath of the 1993 World Trade Center bombing, 8 parents of the 17 children trapped in the elevator were reported as having received counseling (Tabor, 1993).

Family interventions following mass traumas can help deal with issues of grief and loss. Chapters 7 and 8 in this book describe such family-focused bereavement programs, both during the first year after traumatic deaths and over the long term, for families who require ongoing support and assistance to process their feelings.

As emphasized in Chapter 3 and repeated in other chapters of this book, because responses to mass traumas occur in phases and stages, different interventions should be available at different times to meet the varying needs of the affected children and their parents.

THE TRAUMATIZED PRACTITIONER

Mass traumas may affect entire nations (as in situations of war), or their impact may be limited to a specific region, city, or location (as with sniper attacks, terrorist bombings, or school shootings). Mental health practitioners who are themselves bereaved and/or have otherwise been strongly affected by such a trauma may find it difficult to function in a professional capacity and to concentrate on their clients' situations of similar grief and loss. Ideally, these clinicians will have been trained to be self-aware, so that they will recognize their own vulnerabilities and find ways to withdraw temporarily from their professional responsibilities and take care of themselves. Self-care should be considered the foundation of care for others. Chapter 15 deals with the occupational challenge of practitioners' impairment and presents methods to counteract the strain of working with traumatized individuals.

Situations in which the traumatic event is localized, such as the Columbine High School shootings, the Waco fire, and the Oklahoma City bombing, often attract altruistic practitioners from outside the community who volunteer to offer their services. Sometimes large organizations such as the Red Cross or FEMA take charge of the recovery effort and ensure that volunteers have the appropriate background and guidance. The involvement of these large-scale organizations following mass trauma is usually time-limited and can provide an opportunity for traumatized local practitioners to deal with their personal concerns, while less affected outsiders conduct debriefings and help with other necessary tasks. After the initial shock of the traumatic event has begun to subside, 1 week to 3 months after the disaster (Gurwitch et al., 1998), local practitioners may be ready to return to work. Those who continue to work despite being trauma survivors themselves should seek supervision from supervisors/consultants who are knowledgeable about vicarious traumatization (Ryan, 1999; Pearlman & Saakvitne, 1995) and who can assist the counselors in dealing with the personal reactions they experience during the course of their work with trauma survivors.

Although this recommendation appears logical, sometimes survivors of mass trauma resent well-meaning "outsiders" who are trying to help. This happened in a high school in the metropolitan New York City area, when grief counselors who came from outside the school attempted to involve a group of students in debriefing groups following 9/11. Many of the students abruptly walked out of the meeting, thereby indicating either that they were not ready for this level of intimacy with strangers or that it was too soon after the trauma to deal with their feelings (personal communication). Decisions about the timing and type of interventions, and about assignment of helping personnel, all need to be made with sensitivity and understanding that these matters do not conform to a precise formula and therefore flexibility must prevail.

TRAINING PRACTITIONERS IN GRIEF AND TRAUMA WORK

The overlap between grief and trauma makes special demands on practitioners, who may be trained to provide bereavement counseling or crisis counseling, but not both. Whereas all trauma involves loss, all bereavement is not traumatic; thus practitioners who have backgrounds in bereavement counseling may not be knowledgeable about extreme stress responses, and may inadvertently "normalize" some reactions and fail to target them for ongoing attention and reexamination at a later date. Tension sometimes exists between those who believe that traumatic bereavement is a "normal response to an abnormal event" and others who realize that a certain percentage of traumatized people will ultimately develop symptoms of PTSD. Because vulnerable people cannot be identified immediately after a trauma, some practitioners believe that all exposed persons should be monitored, in order to treat those who later develop symptoms at the earliest possible stage. One method for achieving this goal is to give traumatized people psychoeducational materials, with instructions to return for a consultation if they develop symptoms that last longer than 1 month following the traumatic event.

The field of traumatology has grown significantly over the last decade, with various national and international organizations providing training models, standards of education and experience, and certification for trauma counselors. The Appendix lists organizations and other sources that offer this specialized training. In addition to these organized programs, the September 11 Trauma Training Initiative has developed intensive training seminars for psychiatrists, psychologists, social workers, and nurse practitioners. In a full-day format, the training includes a focus on screening and assessment; information about distinguishing normal from pathological responses; information about PTSD; and instruction in front-line interventions using triage, decision trees, and various forms of stress debriefing and symptom management tools (Mental Health Association of New York City, 2003). The ability of the mental health field to deal with mass trauma will increase substantially as more and more practitioners become more knowledgeable about trauma, posttraumatic reactions, assessment, and interventions.

INTEGRATING RESEARCH WITH PRACTICE, AND VICE VERSA

Since the introduction of PTSD as a formal psychiatric diagnosis in 1980 (American Psychiatric Association, 1980), numerous books and research studies have been devoted to learning more about how to assess and treat this distressing outcome of mass trauma events. Much has been learned, but certain difficulties inherent in mass trauma situations prevent the construction of neat research designs. Typically, no standard information is available about people prior to the trauma; therefore, when they later develop symptoms, researchers must rely on their self-reports about their pretrauma histories. In addition, interventions such as debriefing are usually offered in the early stages following a traumatic event, and it can be considered unethical to withhold treatment from a certain group for the purpose of establishing a control group. As with the use of aspirin for headaches, practitioners wish to use interventions they *believe* will be helpful, even when the underlying reasons for effectiveness may be uncertain.

At the beginning of the 21st century, there is a push for "empirically based practice," even as many difficulties in conducting such studies have yet to be resolved. Researchers increasingly must turn to practitioners to learn "what works" with traumatized people, and practitioners must consult researchers about the latest information regarding certain assessment procedures and interventions. If researchers take their cues about what to study from practitioners, and practitioners incorporate new knowledge gleaned from research into their practice, the clients will inevitably be the beneficiaries. The two groups will be more successful if they work together, yet traditionally the two areas of specialization—research and clinical practice—have had minimal cross-fertilization. The key to successful partnership and collaboration is for researchers and practitioners to learn to talk to one another with respect, and to realize that together they will achieve more than either group could accomplish alone.

CONCLUSIONS

We live in an uncertain world where the dangers of war, terrorism, and community violence are ever-present realities. Since 9/11, U.S. families and practitioners alike have had to learn to live with uncertainties and fear about their future safety. Natural disasters have a lifespan and eventually reach a state of closure, no matter how vast the destruction. In contrast, the human-made situations of mass trauma discussed in this book are characterized by a sense of ongoing threat and lack of closure that generates pervasive feelings of anxiety. It remains to be seen whether people will become desensitized and accustomed to this situation, so that it loses some of its forbidding quality.

The helping professions have devised methods to assist people overcome and master some of their frightening experiences, as demonstrated in the numerous examples in this book. We do know about helping interventions that relieve stress, and that aid people in assuming some control and mastery over their lives. Although we cannot guarantee the future, we can learn to deal effectively with the challenges it may throw in our paths.

REFERENCES

American Psychiatric Association. (1980). *Diagnostic and statistical manual of mental disorders* (3rd ed.). Washington, DC: Author.

Barrios, B. A., & Hartmann, D. P. (1997). Fears and anxieties. In E. J. Mash & L. G. Terdal (Eds.), *Assessment of childhood disorders* (3rd ed., pp. 230–327). New York: Guilford Press.

Bradburn, I. S. (1991). After the earth shook: Children's stress symptoms 6–8 months after a disaster. *Advances in Behavior Research and Therapy, 13,* 173–179.

Brady, K. T. (2001). Presentation and epidemiology of PTSD. *Journal of Clinical Psychiatry, 62*(11), 907–909.

Children and families need help after disasters. (1996). *Journal of the American Medical Association, 275*(22), 1714–1715.

Council on Social Work Education (CSWE). (1992a). *Curriculum policy statement for baccalaureate degree programs in social work education.* Alexandria, VA: Author.

Council on Social Work Education (CSWE). (1992b). *Curriculum policy statement for master's degree programs in social work education.* Alexandria, VA: Author.

Drake, E. B., Bush, S. E., & van Gorp, W. G. (2001). Evaluation and assessment of PTSD in children and adolescents. In S. Eth (Ed.), *PTSD in children and adolescents* (pp. 1–31). Washington, DC: American Psychiatric Press.

Dutton, M. A. (1998). Cultural issues in trauma treatment. *Centering: Newsletter of the Center. Posttraumatic Disorders Program, 3*(2), 1–3.

Everly, G. S., & Mitchell, J. T. (2001, Summer). Americans under attack: The "10 commandments" of responding to mass terrorist attacks. *International Journal of Emergency Mental Health, 3*(3), 133–135.

Federal Emergency Management Agency (FEMA). (1989). *Coping with children's reactions to hurricanes and other disasters* (Document No. 1989 0-941-901). Washington, DC: U. S. Government Printing Office.

Federal Emergency Management Agency (FEMA). (1991). *Children and trauma* [Videotape]. Washington, DC: Author.

Fong, R. (Ed.). (2004). *Culturally competent practice with immigrant and refugee children and families.* New York: Guilford Press.

Fong, R., Boyd, C., & Browne, C. (1999). The Gandhi technique: A biculturalization approach for empowering Asian and Pacific Islander families. *Journal of Multicultural Social Work, 7,* 95–110.

Fong, R., & Furuto, S. (Eds.). (2001). *Culturally competent practice: Skills, interventions, and evaluations.* Boston: Allyn & Bacon.

Gibelman, M., & Schervish, P. (1997). *Who we are: A second look.* Washington, DC: National Association of Social Workers.

Gurwitch, R. H., Sullivan, M. A., & Long, P. J. (1998). The impact of trauma and disaster on young children. *Child and Adolescent Clinics of North America, 7*(1), 19–32.

Ho, M. K. (1987). *Family therapy with ethnic minorities.* Newbury Park, CA: Sage.

Lum, D. (Ed.). (2003). *Culturally competent practice: A framework for understanding diverse groups and social justice.* Pacific Grove, CA: Brooks/Cole.

Lyons, J. A. (1987). Posttraumatic stress disorder in children and adolescents: A review of the literature. *Journal of Developmental and Behavioral Pediatrics, 8,* 349–356.

Martin, D. (1997, November 16). Bomb attack's terrifying hold. *The New York Times,* p. 43.

Mental Health Association of New York City. (2003). *PFLASH (practical front line assistance and support for healing) training seminar.* Unpublished flyer.

Mitchell, J. T., & Everly, G. S. (2001). *Critical incident stress debriefing: An operations manual for CISD, defusing and other group crisis intervention services* (3rd ed). Ellicott City, MD: Chevron.

Nader, K. (1997). Treating traumatic grief in systems. In C. R. Figley, B. E. Bride, & N. Mazza (Eds.), *Death and trauma: The traumatology of grieving* (pp. 159–192). Washington, DC: Taylor & Francis.

Nader, K., Dubrow, N., & Stamm, B. H. (Eds.). (1999). *Honoring differences: Cultural issue in the treatment of trauma and loss.* Philadelphia: Brunner/Mazel.

Nader, K., & Pynoos, R. S. (1991). Play and drawing as tools for interviewing traumatized children. In C. Schaefer, K. Gitlin, & A. Sandgrund (Eds.), *Play diagnosis and assessment* (pp. 275–389). New York: Wiley.

Nader, K. O., & Pynoos, R. S. (1993). School disaster: Planning and initial interventions. *Journal of Social Behavior and Personality, 8,* 299–320.

Ollendick, D. G., & Hoffman, S. M. (1982). Assessment of psychological reactions in disaster victims. *Journal of Community Psychology, 10,* 157–167.

Pearlman, L. A., & Saakvitne, K. (1995). *Trauma and the therapist.* New York: Norton.

Perry, B. (1997). Incubated in terror: Neurodevelopmental factors in the "cycle of violence." In J. D. Osofsky (Ed.), *Children in a violent society* (pp. 124–149). New York: Guilford Press.

Potocky-Tripodi, M. (2002). *Best social work practice with immigrants and refugees.* New York: Columbia University Press.

Pynoos, R. S., & Eth, S. (1986). Witness to violence: The child interview. *Journal of the Academy of Child Psychiatry, 25,* 306–319.

Raphael, B., & Dobson, M. (2001). Acute posttraumatic interventions. In J. P. Wilson, M. J. Friedman, & J. D. Lindy (Eds.), *Treating psychological trauma and PTSD* (pp. 139–158). New York: Guilford Press.

Ribbe, D. P., Lipovsky, J. A., & Freedy, J. R. (1995). Posttraumatic stress disorder. In A. R. Eisen, C. A. Kearney, & C. E. Schaefer (Eds.), *Clinical handbook of anxiety disorders in children and adolescents* (pp. 317–356). Northvale, NJ: Aronson.

Ryan, K. (1999). Self-help for the helpers. In N. B. Webb (Ed.), *Play therapy with children in crisis* (2nd ed.): *Individual, group, and family treatment* (pp. 471–491). New York: Guilford Press.

Saylor, C. F., Swenson, C. C., & Powell, P. (1992). Hurricane Hugo blows down the broccoli: Preschoolers' post-disaster play and adjustment. *Child Psychiatry and Human Development, 22,* 139–149.

Shalev, A. Y., & Ursano, R. J. (2003). Mapping the multidimensional picture of acute responses to traumatic stress. In R. Orner & U. Schnyder (Eds.), *Reconstructing early interventions after trauma: Innovations in the care of survivors* (pp. 118–129). New York: Oxford University Press.

Solomon, S. D. (1989). Research issues in assessing disaster's effects. In R. M. Gist & B. Lubin (Eds.), *Psychosocial aspects of disaster* (pp. 308–340). New York: Wiley.

Stoesen, L. (2003, January). Sniper stress built gradually. *NASW News,* p. 11.

Tabor, M. B. W. (1993, March 2). Blast trauma lingers, but mostly for parents. *The New York Times,* p. A1.

Titchener, J. L., & Kapp, F. T. (1976). Family and character change at Buffalo Creek. *American Journal of Psychiatry, 133,* 295–299.

Webb, N. B. (1999). School-based crisis assessment and intervention with children following urban bombings. In N. B. Webb (Ed.), *Play therapy with children in crisis* (2nd ed.): *Individual, group, and family treatment* (pp. 430–447). New York: Guilford Press.

Webb, N. B. (Ed.). (2001). *Culturally diverse parent–child and family relationships: A guide for social workers and other practitioners.* New York: Columbia University Press.

Yehuda, R. (2001). Pathophysiology of PTSD. *Journal of Clinical Psychiatry, 62*(11), 909–910.

Yehuda, R., Spertus, I. L., & Golier, J. A. (2001). Relationship between childhood traumatic experiences and PTSD in adults. In S. Eth (Ed.), *PTSD in children and adolescents* (pp. 117–158). Washington, DC: American Psychiatric Press.

Appendix

Child Abuse and Neglect
Elsevier Science, Inc.
360 Park Avenue South
New York, NY 10010-1710
Phone: 212-989-5800
Fax: 212-633-3990

Journal of Family Violence
Kluwer Academic Publishers
P.O. Box 358
Accord Station
Hingham, MA 02018-0358
Phone: 781-871-6600
Fax: 781-681-9045
http://www.kluweronline.com

Journal of Traumatic Stress
Kluwer Academic Publishers
P.O. Box 358
Accord Station
Hingham, MA 02018-0358
Phone: 781-871-6600
Fax: 781-681-9045
http://www.kluweronline.com

Trauma and Loss: Research and Interventions
National Institute for Trauma and Loss in Children
900 Cook Road

Grosse Pointe Woods, MI 48236
Phone: 313-885-0390, 877-306-5256
http://www.tlcinst.org

Trauma, Violence and Abuse
Sage Publications Ltd.
6 Bonhill Street
London, EC2A 4PU, UK
Phone: +44 (0)20 7374 0645
Fax: +44 (0)20 7374 8741
http://www.sagepub.co.uk

PROFESSIONAL ORGANIZATIONS WITH TRAUMA-RELATED TRAINING AND/OR CONFERENCES

American Academy of Experts in Traumatic Stress
368 Veterans Memorial Highway
Commack, NY 11725
Phone: 631-543-2217
Fax: 631-543-6977
http://www.aaets.org

American Academy of Pediatrics
141 Northwest Point Boulevard
Elk Grove Village, IL 60007-1098
Phone: 847-434-4000
Fax: 847-434-8000
http://www.aap.org

American Association of Suicidology
4201 Connecticut Avenue NW, Suite 408
Washington, DC 20008
Phone: 202-237-2280
http://www.suicidology.org

American Medical Association
515 North State Street
Chicago, IL 60610
Phone: 312-464-5000
http://www.ama-assn.org

American Professional Society on the Abuse of Children
940 Northeast 13th Street

CHO #B-3406
Oklahoma City, OK 73104
Phone: 405-271-8202
Fax: 405-271-2931
http://www.apsac.org

American Psychiatric Association
1000 Wilson Boulevard, Suite 1825
Arlington, VA 22209-3901
Phone: 703-907-7300
http://www.psych.org

American Psychological Association
750 First Street NE
Washington, DC 20002-4242
Phone: 800-374-2721, 202-336-5510
http://www.apa.org

American Red Cross
National Headquarters
2025 E Street NW
Washington, DC 20006
Phone: 202-303-4498
http://www.redcross.org

Annie E. Casey Foundation
701 St. Paul Street
Baltimore, MD 21202
Phone: 410-547-6600
http://www.aecf.org

Association for Death Education and Counseling
342 North Main Street
West Hartford, CT 06117-2507
Phone: 860-586-7503
Fax: 860-586-7550
http://www.adec.org

Association for Play Therapy
2050 North Winery Avenue, Suite 101
Fresno, CA 93703
Phone: 559-252-2278
Fax: 559-252-2297
http://www.iapt.org

Association of Traumatic Stress Specialists
7338 Broad River Road
Irmo, SC 29063
Phone: 803-781-0017
Fax: 803-781-3899
http://www.atss-hq.COM

EMDR International Association
P.O. Box 141925
Austin, TX 78714-1925
Phone: 512-451-5200
http://www.emdria.org

International Critical Incident Stress Foundation
3290 Pine Orchard Lane
Ellicott City, MD 21042
Phone: 410-750-9600
Fax: 410-750-9601
http://www.icisf.org

International Society for Traumatic Stress Studies
60 Revere Drive, Suite 500
Northbrook, IL 60062
Phone: 847-480-9028
Fax: 847-480-9282
http://www.istss.org

National Association of Social Workers
750 First Street NE, Suite 700
Washington, DC 20002-4241
http://www.naswdc.org

National Institute for Trauma and Loss in Children
900 Cook Road
Grosse Pointe Woods, MI 48236
Phone: 313-885-0390, 877-306-5256
http://www.tlcinst.org

ADDITIONAL TRAUMA RESOURCES

ARCH National Respite Network and Resource Center
Chapel Hill Training–Outreach Project
800 Eastowne Drive, Suite 105

Chapel Hill, NC 27514
Phone: 919-490-5577
Fax: 919-490-4905
http://www.archrespite.org

Children's Defense Fund
25 E Street NW
Washington, DC 20001
Phone: 202-628-8787
http://www.childrensdefensefund.org

Child Welfare League of America
440 First Street NW, 3rd Floor
Washington, DC 20001-2085
Phone: 202-638-2952
Fax: 202-638-4004
http://www.cwla.org

Child Witness to Violence Project
Boston Medical Center
91 East Concord Street, 5th Floor
Boston, MA 02118
Phone: 617-414-4244
http://www.bostonchildhealth.org

Federal Emergency Management Agency (FEMA)
500 C Street SW
Washington, DC 20472
Phone: 202-566-1600, 800-480-2520
http://www.fema.gov

National Adolescent Health Information Center
University of California–San Francisco
1388 Sutter Street
Suite 605-A
San Francisco, CA 94109
Phone: 415-502-4856
Fax: 415-502-4858
http://www.ucsf.edu/youth

National Center for Children Exposed to Violence
Yale Child Study Center
230 Frontage Road
P.O. Box 207900

New Haven, CT 06520-7900
Phone: 203-785-7047, 877-496-2238
Fax: 203-785-4608
http://www.nccev.org

National Clearinghouse on Child Abuse and Neglect Information
330 C Street NW
Washington, DC 20447
Phone: 800-394-3366
Fax: 703-385-7565
http://www.calib.com/nccanch

National Resource Center on Child Maltreatment
P.O. Box 441470
Aurora, CO 80044-1470
Phone: 303-369-8008
Fax: 303-369-8009
http://www.gocwi.org/nrccm

Research and Training Center on Family Support and Children's Mental Health
Portland State University
P.O. Box 751
Portland, OR 97207-0751
Phone: 503-725-4175
Fax: 503-725-4180
http://www.rtc.pdx.edu

U.S. Department of Health and Human Services
Administration for Children and Families
Administration on Children, Youth and Families, Children's Bureau
330 C Street NW
Washington, DC 20447
Phone: 877-696-6775
http://www.calib.com

Zero to Three: National Center for Infants, Toddlers and Families
2000 M Street NW, Suite 200
Washington, DC 20036
Phone: 202-638-1144
http://www.zerotothree.org

Index